Mastering
Cancer Reconstructive Surgery with Free Flaps

Mastering
Cancer Reconstructive Surgery with Free Flaps

Editors

Prabha Yadav
MBBS MS (Plastic Surgery)
Professor and Head
Department of Plastic and Reconstructive Surgery
Tata Memorial Centre
Mumbai, Maharashtra, India
drprabhatata@gmail.com

Vinay K Shankhdhar
MBBS MS (General Surgery) MCh (Plastic Surgery)
Professor
Department of Plastic and Reconstructive Surgery
ACTREC, Tata Memorial Centre
Mumbai, Maharashtra, India
vinayshankhdhar@gmail.com

Dushyant Jaiswal
MBBS MS MCh (Plastic and Reconstructive Surgery)
Fellowship in Reconstructive Oncology
Associate Professor
Department of Plastic and Reconstructive Surgery
Tata Memorial Centre
Mumbai, Maharashtra, India
drdushyantjaiswal@yahoo.co.in

Forewords

RA Badwe
AK D'Cruz
KS Sharma

JAYPEE *The Health Sciences Publisher*
New Delhi | London | Panama

Jaypee Brothers Medical Publishers (P) Ltd

Headquarters
Jaypee Brothers Medical Publishers (P) Ltd.
4838/24, Ansari Road, Daryaganj
New Delhi 110 002, India
Phone: +91-11-43574357
Fax: +91-11-43574314
E-mail: jaypee@jaypeebrothers.com

Overseas Offices
J.P. Medical Ltd.
83, Victoria Street, London
SW1H 0HW (UK)
Phone: +44-20 3170 8910
Fax: +44(0)20 3008 6180
E-mail: info@jpmedpub.com

Jaypee-Highlights Medical Publishers Inc.
City of Knowledge, Bld. 235, 2nd Floor, Clayton
Panama City, Panama
Phone: +1 507-301-0496
Fax: +1 507-301-0499
E-mail: cservice@jphmedical.com

Jaypee Brothers Medical Publishers (P) Ltd.
17/1-B, Babar Road, Block-B, Shaymali
Mohammadpur, Dhaka-1207
Bangladesh
Mobile: +08801912003485
E-mail: jaypeedhaka@gmail.com

Jaypee Brothers Medical Publishers (P) Ltd.
Bhotahity, Kathmandu, Nepal
Phone: +977-9741283608
E-mail: kathmandu@jaypeebrothers.com

Website: www.jaypeebrothers.com
Website: www.jaypeedigital.com

Inquiries for bulk sales may be solicited at: jaypee@jaypeebrothers.com

Mastering Cancer Reconstructive Surgery with Free Flaps

First Edition: **2018**

ISBN: **978-93-5270-205-3**

Printed at Sanat Printers

Dedication

To every soul who enters the doors of this institute
To treat or to get treated,
To learn or to teach,
To question and to seek

Contributors

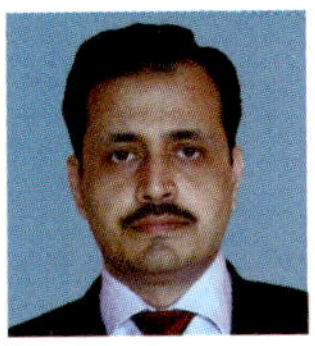

Quazi Ghazwan Ahmad
MS DNB MRCS MCh MNAMS
Consultant Plastic Surgeon
Plastic Surgery Services
Kokilaben Dhirubhai Ambani Hospital
Mumbai, Maharashtra, India
quazighazwan@gmail.com

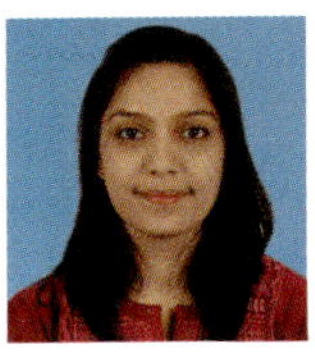

Tasneem Belgaumwala
MBBS MS (General Surgery)
MCh (Plastic and Reconstructive Surgery)
Specialist Senior Resident
Department of Plastic and
Reconstructive Surgery
Tata Memorial Centre
Mumbai, Maharashtra, India
drtasb@gmail.com

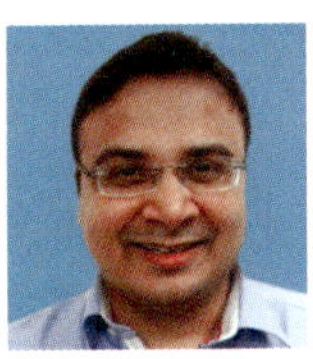

Chirag Ajay Bhansali
MS (General Surgery) MCh (Plastic Surgery)
Specialist Senior resident
Department of Plastic and
Reconstructive Surgery
Tata Memorial Centre
Mumbai, Maharashtra, India
bhansali.chirag@gmail.com

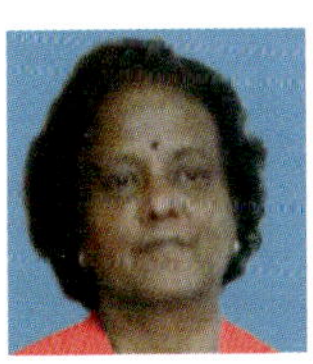

Kanchan Dholam MDS
Professor and Head
Department of Dental and
Prosthetic Surgery
Tata Memorial Hospital
Mumbai, Maharashtra, India
kdholam@hotmail.com

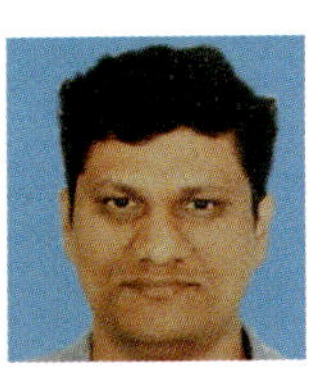

Sandeep Vivek Gurav MDS FDPO
Assistant Professor
Department of Dental and
Prosthetic Surgery
Tata Memorial Hospital
Mumbai, Maharashtra, India
drsandeepgurav@gmail.com

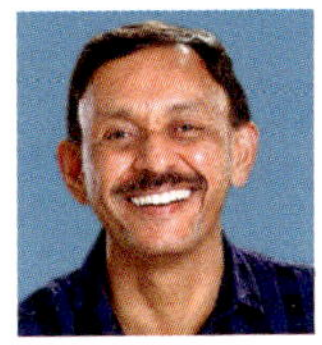

Subramania Iyer
MS MCh FRCS
Professor and Chairman
Department of Plastic and
Reconstructive surgery
Head and Neck Surgery and Oncology
Amrita Institute of Medical Sciences
Kochi, Kerala, India
subu.amrita@gmail.com

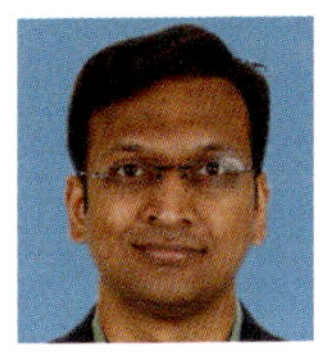

Dushyant Jaiswal
MBBS MS MCh (Plastic and Reconstructive Surgery)
Fellowship in Reconstructive Oncology
Associate Professor
Department of Plastic and
Reconstructive Surgery
Tata Memorial Centre
Mumbai, Maharashtra, India
drdushyantjaiswal@yahoo.co.in

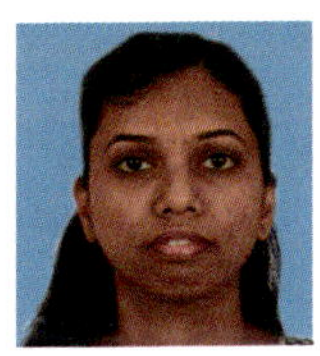

Namarata Joshi
MBBS MS (General Surgery)
Senior Resident
Department of Plastic and
Reconstructive Surgery
Tata Memorial Hospital
Mumbai, Maharashtra, India
jnamrata388@gmail.com

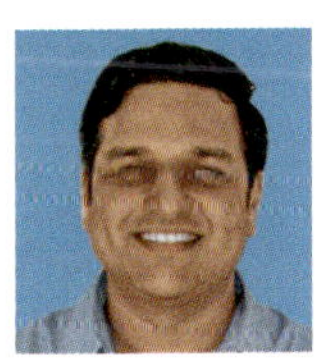

Tanmay Mohan Joshi
MBBS MS (General Surgery) MCh (Plastic and
Reconstructive Surgery) DNB
Specialist Senior Resident
Department of Plastic and
Reconstructive Surgery
Tata Memorial Hospital
tanmaymohanjoshi@gmail.com

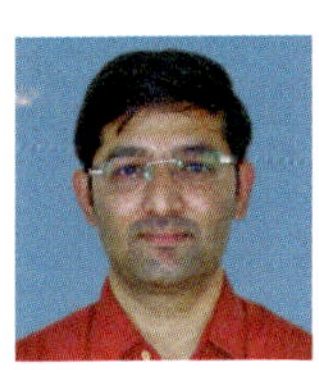

Mayur Mantri
MBBS MS (General Surgery) MCh (Plastic and
Reconstructive Surgery)
Specialist Senior Resident
Department of Plastic and
Reconstructive Surgery
Tata Memorial Hospital
Mumbai, Maharashtra, India
drmayurmantri@gmail.com

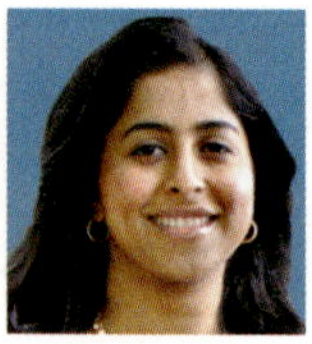

Saumya Mathews
MBBS MS (General Surgery) MCh (Plastic and Reconstructive Surgery)
Assistant Professor (Adhoc)
Department of Plastic and Reconstructive Surgery
Tata Memorial Hospital
Mumbai, Maharashtra, India
saumya_mathews@yahoo.com

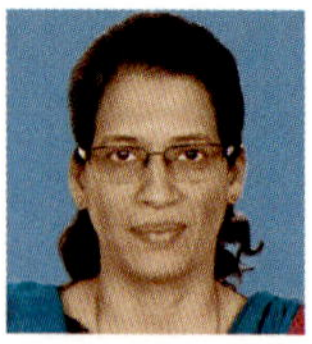

Vijaya Patil MBBS MD (Anesthesia)
Professor
Department of Anesthesiology
Critical Care and Pain Services
Tata Memorial Hospital
Mumbai, Maharashtra, India
vijayappatil@yahoo.com

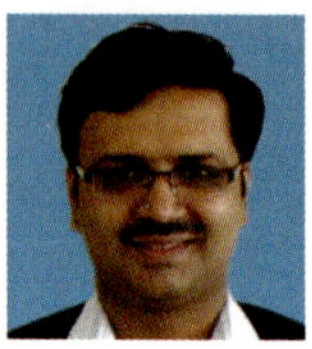

Prashant Puranik
MS MCh (Plastic Surgery) DNB (Plastic Surgery)
Fellowship in Reconstructive Oncology
Consultant
Plastic and Reconstructive Surgeon
Health Care Global Hospital
Bengaluru, Karnataka, India
prspuranik@gmail.com

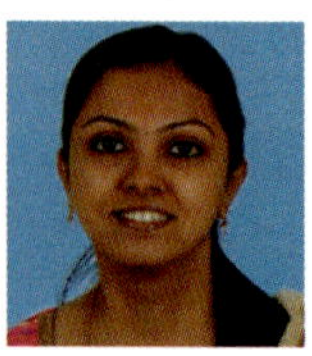

Amrita Rao
MBBS MS (General Surgery)
MCh (Plastic and Reconstructive Surgery)
Specialist Senior Resident
Department of Plastic and Reconstructive Surgery
Tata Memorial Hospital
Mumbai, Maharashtra, India
amritarao0703@gmail.com

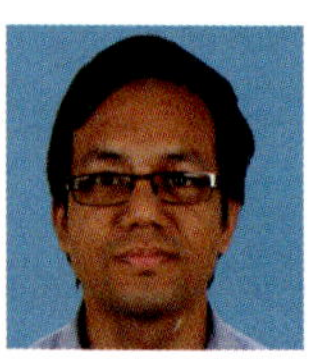

Neeraj Rao
MBBS MS (General Surgery)
Senior Resident
Department of Plastic and Reconstructive Surgery
Tata Memorial Centre
Mumbai, Maharashtra, India
Neeraj1207@gmail.com

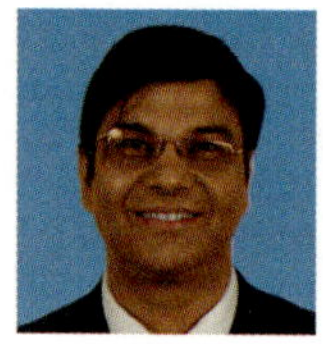

Vinay K Shankhdhar
MBBS MS (General Surgery) MCh (Plastic Surgery)
Professor
Department of Plastic and Reconstructive Surgery
ACTREC, Tata Memorial Centre
Mumbai, Maharashtra, India
vinayshankhdhar@gmail.com

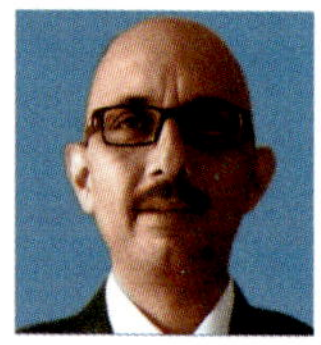

Mohit Sharma MS MCh
(Plastic and Reconstructive Surgery
St. Andrew's Fellow in Burns and Hand Surgery)
Professor
Department of Plastic and Reconstructive Surgery
Amrita Institute of Medical Sciences
Kochi, Kerala, India
ammasmohit@gmail.com

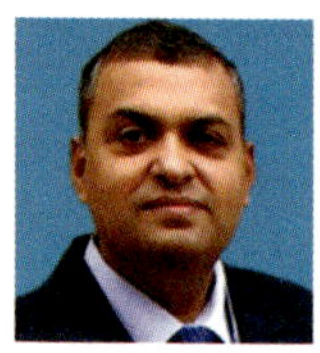

Hari Venkatramani
MS MCh DNB EDHS
Senior Consultant
Department of Plastic, Hand, Reconstructive Microsurgery and Burns
Ganga Hospital
Coimbatore, Tamil Nadu, India
drhariv@gmail.com

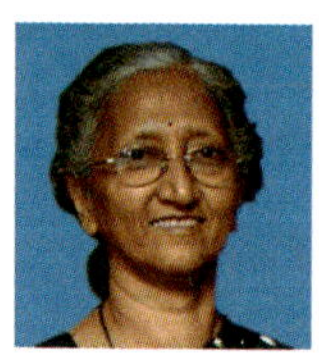

Prabha Yadav
MBBS MS (Plastic Surgery)
Professor and Head
Department of Plastic and Reconstructive Surgery
Tata Memorial Centre
Mumbai, Maharashtra, India
drprabhatata@gmail.com

Foreword

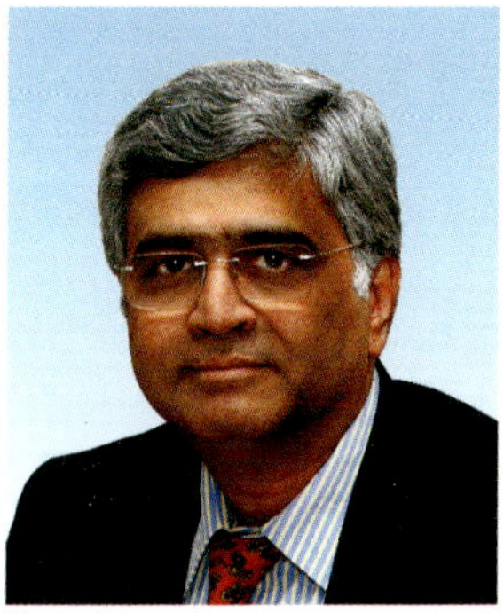

In all my years at Tata Memorial Centre, one of the most visible changes in delivery of care, is the establishment of Free Tissue Transfer as the mainstay for reconstruction. As we mastered the radicality of surgical extirpation, the Plastic and Reconstructive Surgery team, ably led by Dr Prabha Yadav, kept pace with and often beat, the 'TMH conveyer belt' of work load. This has led to establishment of free flaps as the standard of care for most reconstructions, matching the worldwide trend. Inspite of 5000 free flaps over 12 years and current state of 600 a year, the denominator is unaddressed. The dream is to ensure every resection gets the best reconstruction possible, not just at TMH but across the country. We hope to replicate this model of specialized reconstruction teaching units at our upcoming centres at Varanasi, Mohali and Vizag; and ultimately in the National Cancer Grid across the country. This book will be a great resource for all 'Eklavaya's' who wish to imbibe the philosophy and techniques of cancer reconstruction, as practiced at TMH, but do not get a chance to train here. With great pride I can say this is truly a 'Make in India' initiative. The 'Banyan tree' of cancer reconstruction is now firmly rooted at TMH, the seeds are dispersing, germinating, growing, bearing fruits and welcoming birds from far and wide to benefit from it. I wish the team all the best for this initiative

RA Badwe
Director
Tata Memorial Centre
Mumbai, Maharashtra, India

Foreword

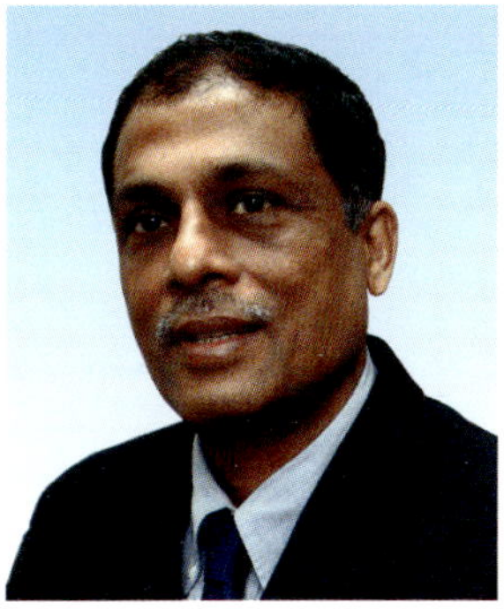

The department of Plastic and Reconstructive Surgery of Tata Memorial Hospital under the leadership of Dr Prabha Yadav has completed over 5000 microvascular free flap reconstructions in a span of 12 years. These numbers are amongst the highest for a single unit globally. I congratulate the department for now putting this vast experience into this book for the benefit of others. This book highlights the nuances and techniques as well as tips and tricks that have been garnered through the course of this journey.

There is something in this book for everybody involved in cancer free flap reconstruction from the young postgraduate to the experienced microvascular surgeon. This book differs from others in that it introduces simple cost effective practical devices that have been developed by the department which can be widely applicable in other developing countries like ours.

Emphasis in the treatment of cancer has shifted from survival to quality of life, reconstruction plays a pivotal role for the same. Free flap reconstructions are a must in the armamentarium of any reconstructive surgeon. With multiple flaps described in literature, the algorithms in the book will be useful to understand the ideal reconstruction post tumor extirpation. These have been simplified and are applicable to all regional specialties in cancer care. This book is a must read for all as,

"Only a fool learns from his own mistakes.
The wise man learns from the mistakes of others."
— Otto von Bismarck

AK D'Cruz
Director
Tata Memorial Hospital
Mumbai, Maharashtra, India

Foreword

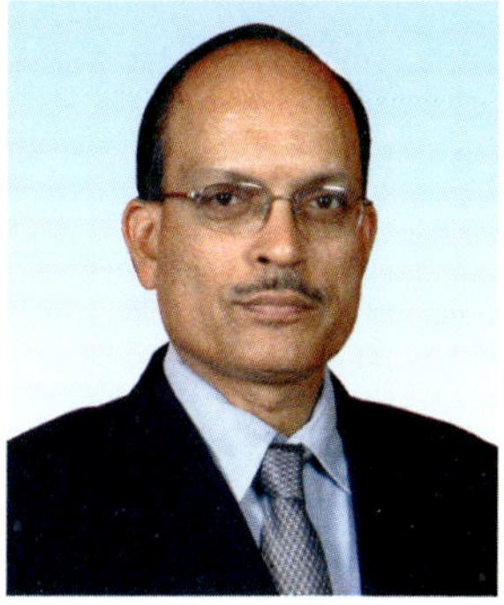

It is a great privilege and pleasure to write these words. The Plastic and Reconstructive Services at Tata Memorial Hospital are the leaders in our country for cancer reconstruction. As the Director of Academics, I am proud of their persistent efforts to train reconstructive surgeons from across the country. The MCh Plastic and Reconstructive Surgery and post super-speciality training programs are now well established at Tata Memorial Hospital Mumbai. The ONCORECON, short 5-day intensive sensitizing and training course conducted multiple times a year by the department, is a successful brand by itself. This book is the next step in the teaching initiatives of this department. The insights and wisdom imparted in it, are the nectar and ambrosia, of years of experience, thinking and tremendous hard work. The unique aspect is it is all based on 'Indian experience' with thoughtful insights into problems and solutions for Indian subcontinental populations. We wish it will further help in demystifying free tissue transfer and establish it as a routine mode of cancer reconstruction rather than a novelty. We hope that this book, inspires many youngsters to pursue cancer reconstruction with free flaps, refine those who are already doing it and instil a sense of pride in those who nurtured microsurgery in its nascent years.

KS Sharma
Director (Academics)
Tata Memorial Centre
Mumbai, Maharashtra, India

Preface

I (Prabha Yadav) joined Tata Memorial Hospital, in 2005 for my second innings in reconstructive microsurgery. Little did I realise that this opportunity would be the most fortunate professional turn in my life. Sailing in this ocean of knowledge for 12 years, with some of the best minds across fields of oncology, has been a great learning, humbling and invigorating experience.

The motto of the hospital of 'Service, Research and Education' can be felt in the very air of this August Institute.

Tata Memorial Hospital receives thousands of patients in outpatient departments daily, each waging their own battles with cancer with some help from surgery, chemotherapy and radiation. 'Evidence-based Medicine' is the core value around which most decision is taken in multidisciplinary joint clinics. The variations and experiments are restricted to research setting and exceptional circumstances. The sitewise DMG (Disease Management Group) system ensures the specialists of specialists are taking care of each patient. The Plastic and Reconstructive unit performs nine hundred plus major surgeries per year, of these around 600 are free tissue transfers. Over 12 years the number of free tissue transfers has summed up to 5000 and counting. We have mainly used three workhorses, free fibula osteocutaneous flap, free anterolateral thigh flap and free radial forearm flap to reconstruct ninety five percent of our defects. We do believe that mastering these three workhorses and riding them with maximum skill and guile can enable a reconstructive microsurgeon to ride through the obstacle of any defect.

It is a common misconception that a lot of talent, prolonged training and costly setup is required to acquire the skills to perform free flaps. Rather, microsurgery is probably the only surgical skill which can be so closely simulated for practice, outside a patient, all it takes is a microscope or loupe, some blood vessels, instruments and suture. All one needs is a little courage with lots of passion, patience and practice.

Free tissue transfer has for long been a novelty rather than the standard of care for years in this country, unlike rest of the world. The tide is now turning. Around 100 free tissue transfers are performed in India daily, a lot of which are in small towns or setups (based on a survey we conducted). We can proudly say we have done our bit in demystifying microsurgery and free flaps, by training people and propagating our philosophy.

Tata Memorial Centre is affiliated to the Home Bhabha National Institute (HBNI), a deemed university, for all its educational degrees. We are also recognized for various training courses by international agencies like WHO, IAEA and UICC. We receive numerous students for super speciality, postgraduation and fellowship courses every year. Apart from these, many join to pursue training in nursing, paramedical and non-medical fields for long and short-term courses. The Plastic surgery department plays its small role. We offer a 3-year MCh (Plastic and Reconstructive Surgery) course and post MCh specialist registrars, as long-term training programs. We also conduct multiple times in a year, a short but intensive five-day training, sensitizing and cadaver dissection program, ONCORECON. It has become a hugely successful brand by itself, receiving 16–24 trainees every year. We also get visiting observers and residents for their elective rotating postings from across the country, many of whom end up feeling inspired to pursue cancer reconstruction in their practice.

This book is a further effort to spread the seeds of microsurgery far and wide. It was long in conception and delivered in a hurry, please forgive us for the shortcomings. We have covered all basic free flaps needed for cancer reconstruction of most common sites in Indian population. We have also included concerns immediately related to surgery. A small section on refinements and what the future holds has been added.

After reading this book if a few people feel inspired, a few flaps are saved and some life is added to years of a few cancer patients, we would consider our purpose served.

Our belief—what can be resected, can be reconstructed.

Our practice—do nothing when not needed, and anything and everything when needed, every time and anytime.

Our dream—that every cancer patient receives the best of reconstruction with the least of morbidity, not just in TMH or teaching institutes but in every place across the country—where cancer is treated.

I wish to convey my heartfelt gratitude to all my teachers. Dr VN Shrikhande for initiating me into surgery. Dr NH Antia, Dr BM Daver, Dr SJ Vaidya and Dr Sudhir Karmarkar for nurturing me in my formative years in Plastic and Reconstructive Surgery. Dr AD Dias and Dr RL Thatte for providing the guiding lights of teaching and philosophy. Professor Georgio Brunelli for training me in micorsurgery. Professor Bob Acland and Professor Isao Koshima for inspiring me to achieve greater heights in reconstructive microsurgery.

Prabha Yadav
Vinay K Shankhdhar
Dushyant Jaiswal

Acknowledgments

We are grateful to Saumya Mathews for excellent editorial work.

Our colleagues and Residents in the department of Plastic and Reconstructive Surgery Neeraj Rao, Namrata Joshi, Firoz Borle, Vineet Pilania and Sumit Hadgaonkar for taking care of other work when we had to write this book.

We are thankful to Mr Jitendar P Vij (Group Chairman) and Mr Ankit Vij (Group President) of M/s Jaypee Brothers Medical Publishers for publishing this book according to our preferences. We also thank Ms Chetna Malhotra Vohra (Associate Director–Content Strategy) for her contributions while formatting this book. We also would like to thank Mr Sabrish, Mr Jaoquim, Ms Esha Saini, Mrs Kamlesh Bisht (Typesetter), Mr Himanshu Shekhar Lal and Mr Shakil (Proofreaders) for their dedication and support in getting this book published.

Dr Subash Yadav for stead fast encouragment and support for this project.

Parents, spouses and children of all involved in writing this book for supporting us through the extra hours of work and sleep deprived nights.

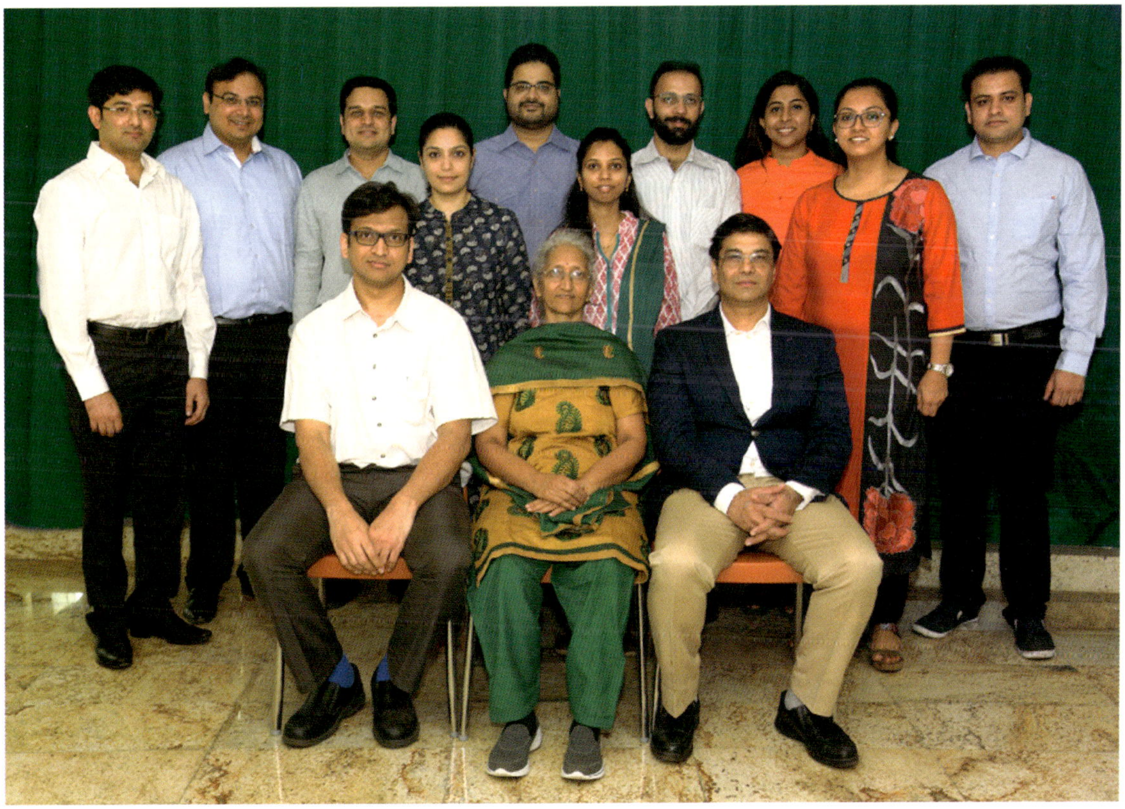

Contents

Philosophy and Current Practice of Cancer Reconstruction at Tata Memorial Hospital

Dushyant Jaiswal, Prabha Yadav, Vinay K Shankhdhar

INTRODUCTION

The current gold standard, for head neck and breast reconstruction world over, is Free tissue transfer or free flaps, as commonly called. We have performed over 5000 free flaps over the last 12 years. Currently, every year we perform around 600 free tissue transfers for reconstruction of cancer defects. Tata Memorial Centre receives 65000 patients every year. 11000 are Head Neck cancer of which 2100 undergo surgery and 500 receive a free tissue transfer. 5000 are breast cancer cases of which 1800 are operated and only 50 receive a free tissue transfer. 50 more free tissue transfers are done for limbs and trunk.

We believe that every patient should receive the best possible reconstruction.

If resection adds years to life, Reconstruction add life to those years.

Reconstructive surgeons pushing boundaries of reconstruction, to handle more and more complex and large defects, has enabled the resecting surgeons to push the limits of surgically possible resections.

We use a Reconstructive Tool Box approach for decision-making. The option which provides the best possible outcome with least donor morbidity, irrespective of difficulty level or time for surgery, is chosen over simpler options which will only heal the wound.

The option usually exercised is of microvascular free tissue transfer or free flaps.

Free tissue transfer is the 'gold standard', 'bedrock' or default option for most Head Neck reconstruction in our Plastic and Reconstructive Surgery Department.

MOST HEAD NECK DEFECTS CAN BE *MANAGED* BY THE 'THREE' FLAPS

We believe that most, up to 95%, of all defects after HN cancer excision, can be managed with the three free flaps.

Free Fibula Osteocutaneous Flap (FFOCF)

Wherever bone is needed fibula is used. The skin paddle, based on the perforators from peroneal vessels, can be used with great liberty to address the associated mucosal, skin and soft tissue defect.

Free Radial Artery Forearm Flap (FRAFF)

Provides the thin, pliable option for small defects of buccal mucosa and tongue defects.

Free Anterolateral Thigh Flap (FALT)

It is our default option whenever the flap needs more volume or surface area.

The remaining only 5% defects need a flap beyond these three. The defect might be large, complex, odd shaped or all of them needing an alternative flap. Sometimes an unfavorable donor profile, too thin or thick as compared to the defect or violated by chemotherapy might necessitate this. Very rarely an alternative choice could be made solely to reduce the donor area skin graft or muscle function loss morbidity.

The alternative flaps could be from anywhere in the body. We generally use thoracodorsal artery perforator flap (TDAP), medial sural artery perforator flap (MSAP) and deep inferior epigastric artery perforator flap (DIEP) as our options when needed.

Other few specialized free flaps needed in arsenal are:

Free DIEP Flap

For whole breast reconstruction after mastectomy

Free Jejunum Flap

For pharyngeal reconstruction after total laryngopharyngectomy

Free Latissimus Dorsi Flap

For occasional large, irregular defect on limbs with exposed implants, bone cement or vital structures.

FREE FLAPS IRRESPECTIVE

Generally, a lot of fear and timidity is associated with free flaps, especially for a beginner. This is often projected, especially in an event of thrombosis to age, comorbidities, previous surgery and radiation. Often they end up becoming a reason for not doing a free flap in a given patient, when it might be the best solution.

We routinely perform free flaps irrespective of all these factors, age, routine controlled comorbidities like diabetes mellitus/Hypertension/IHD, previous surgery and neck dissection, radiation, recurrence, size or complexity of defect, presumed short survival of the patient.

Generally, if the defect demands a free flap it gets a free flap!

Sometimes the surgery might be a little challenging technically or needs to be completed in relatively short duration. This should not be a deterrent or contraindication to free tissue transfer, all it needs an experienced surgeon as in any other case.

We would think twice before executing a free flap, only if the anesthetist expresses concern over the long duration of surgery or we are worried about the risk of exploration.

STANDARDIZATION OF SURGICAL TECHNIQUES

The surgical technique of harvest of the 'three' flaps has been almost standardized in the department. Individual harvest techniques are discussed with each chapter. This enables the beginners to scale the learning curve rapidly. It also enables easy communication about details. The deviations and tricks are also easy to understand as a basic set template exists.

EMBRACING THE PERFORATOR CONCEPT

The perforator philosophy is now firmly established in almost all flaps we do. Any flap, ALT, DIEP or the skin island with fibula is only as good as the perforator it possesses. Perforators are visualized and dissected. There is no provision for blind muscle harvest for perforator presumption or protection.

SIMULTANEOUS HARVEST

Our default option is to harvest free flaps simultaneously. Only times we harvest flaps after defect creation is, when there is uncertainty, about the size, shape and components of the final defect resulting in an altered flap choice. Sometimes it is logistically not possible to do so due to lack of space or change of position is required for flap Harvest.

VESSEL SELECTION

Choice of vessel in Head Neck and limbs should be made based on their quality, size, patency and blood flow. Name of vessel should not dictate its selection, its character should.

END-TO-END OR END-TO-SIDE

Generally, end-to-end microvascular anastomosis are done. End-to-side is considered when, tributary is unavailable or mismatch is severe. End to side anastomosis is a must in armamentarium of every microvascular surgeon doing reconstruction, especially for Head Neck. It takes away the question of vessel availability and gives a choice of doing microvascular anastomosis (MVA) on side where the flap would contour/fit better.

FLAP MONITORING

We monitor our free flaps only clinically. No mechanical monitoring real time devices are used. This is mainly due to cost constraints. With the low exploration rates, high salvage rates and overall high rates of free flap survival it might not be cost effective to use these devices.

Clinical monitoring includes visual inspection for color and turgor and needle prick/scratch for assessing the resultant bleed.

THROMBOPROPHYLAXIS

We do not use thromboprophylaxis for microvascular anastomosis (MVA) patency as a routine. Only in case of a thrombotic event is therapeutic anticoagulation started.

We do however use LMWH (Low molecular weight heparin) for deep vein thrombosis (DVT) prophylaxis at once daily dose in cases requiring immobilization.

PHOTOGRAPHY

Clinical photography is practiced for each patient. Pre, intra and post-operative and follow-up image documentation is done.

IMAGING

Currently we do not use imaging or any sort of modeling as a routine for our reconstruction planning mostly for logistic reasons. Cost if a deterrent.

Recently we have started using CT angiograms for DIEP flap planning for breast reconstruction and found them to be useful. But we intend to use imaging more liberally especially for complex, complicated defects which required customized, personalized solutions.

Very occasionally we do use stereolithography for 3D models, mostly for benign cases where primary osteointegration is done.

RAPID RECOVERY PROTOCOLS

The aim is to keep the hospital stay minimum, return to function rapid and radiation in time when needed.

Nasogastric tube feeds are started on POD 1 and oral feeds on day 4, urinary catheter removal at 24–48 hrs, tracheostomy decannulation by 5–7 days, Suture removal by 10–14 days. Speech and swallowing therapy, shoulder exercises are started before discharge. Patients are generally discharged by postoperative day 6–10.

Radiation has to be started by 4–6 weeks. Low threshold is kept for surgical intervention in marginal or partial necrosis of flaps.

THE UNADDRESSED DENOMINATOR

Tata Memorial Centre receives a huge influx of patients from the all over the country. Theatre space is limited, leading to a waiting time for surgery of 4–6 weeks.

We perform around 600 free tissue transfers a year and another 300 pedicle flaps and major surgical procedures. The number of free flaps might appear large, but it is only a third of patients who get operated at TMC and need a free flap for an ideal outcome. The denominator is yet unaddressed.

CHAPTER 2

Art and Technique of Microvascular Anastomosis

Hari Venkatramani

INTRODUCTION

Microsurgery is now a century old practice. Though the success of microsurgery depends upon various factors, basic principled technique is the key towards achieving consistent good results. The foundation of modern suturing technique relies on the concept of triangulation, first popularized by **Alexis Carrel** in 1906 and for which he received the Nobel Prize. This concept conveys that by virtue of taking three key sutures the lumen can be well-visualized and the edges are lifted adequately apart.

Julius Jacobson is credited for coining the word "**Microsurgery**" in 1960s. With advancement in skill the size of vessels anastomosed became smaller going up to 1 mm. **Isao Koshima** coined the term "**Supramicrosurgery**", to describe the anastomosis of vessel size of less than 0.8 mm. With technical expertise and improved understanding of the necessary preoperative and postoperative care, the results of microsurgery in most units risen to over 98% in free flap transfer.

The other significant advance in microsurgery was the development of microsutures and instruments pioneered by **Dr Robert D Acland** and the founders of the **S&T Company**.

MICROSURGERY INSTRUMENTS

Success in microsurgery depends a lot on the quality of instruments. Good quality instruments are expensive but can make all the difference between success and failure. Nothing is more frustrating than a jeweler's forceps not holding the adventitia well.

A basic instrument set should have the following instruments

- Two fine tip jeweler's forceps
- One piece adventitia holding forceps
- One vessel dilator
- Two curved scissors: One for dissection and one for adventitia trimming
- One straight sharp tip cutting scissors for vessel division
- One clamp applicator forceps
- One curved tip needle holder
- One small angled forceps
- Clamps: 2V, 3V, HDD and RD all two single and one double
- Two ligaclip applicator in 100 and 200 sizes and one set of clips each **(Fig. 1)**.

The instruments are manufactured in two sizes 5.5"and 11" depending on the surgeon's preference. We find the longer size instruments most useful in deeper surgical wounds that require extra reach, such as in the axilla.

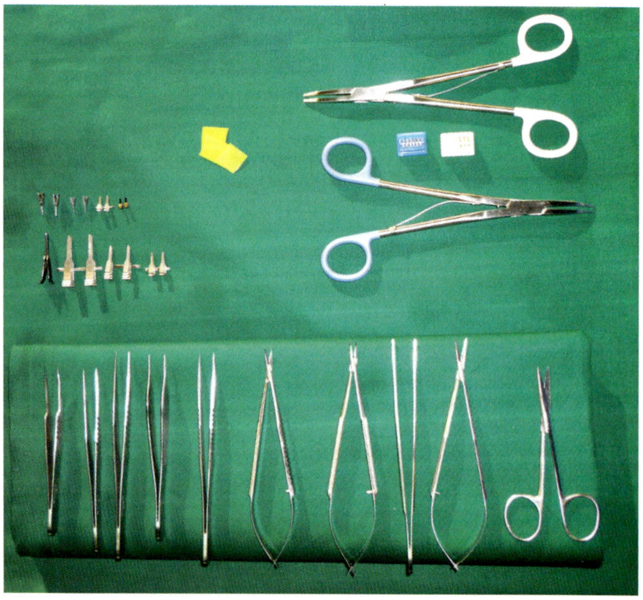

Fig. 1: Basic microvascular instrument set

SUTURE MATERIAL

Sutures for regular microvascular surgery are available through the ranges of 8.0 to 10.0. For super microsurgery in which the size of the vessels is less than 0.8 mm, finer sutures beyond in 11.0 -13.0 are also available now, but are more expensive and require special instrumentation.

The needle size of a 10.0 suture should ideally be 50–75 micron, with a tapered point with a round body that is flattened in the middle. This is ideal for 1 mm size vessels.

SUTURE SELECTION

Selection of accurate suture size is critical, smaller suture will require greater number of "bites" and larger suture will create a larger hole in the vessel wall. However, one must consider the thickness of the vessel wall to be anastomosed. Expectedly, a thicker wall will require a larger needle and suture size. The quality of needle used is determined by its ability to complete the entire repair without bending or becoming blunt. We have found in our experience that for most free flap reconstruction in which the vessel size is around 2 mm, 9.0 microsuture is ideal for use. For smaller vessels (less than 2 mm) such as in digital replantation or use in children, 10.0 is preferred. For supramicrosurgery like in lymphatico-venous anastomosis and less than 0.8 mm size vessels, 11.0 sutures are preferred.

MICROVASCULAR ANASTOMOSIS DEVICES

Microvascular anastomotic coupler device is a system, specifically designed for venous anastomosis. Thin walled veins are ideally suited. Arteries which have thicker wall and are more prone to atherosclerosis are not suitable for coupler assisted anastomosis.

For veins in the 0.8 mm to 4.3 mm size range and wall thickness of 0.5 mm or less coupler assisted intima to inti ma can be successfully achieved.

The coupler device has rings that are 1-4 mm in size and pins with shaft diameter of 0.16 mm. After determining the size of the lumen to be anastomosed, an appropriate sized coupler is used. Both venous ends are fed into the center of ring and then averted back so as to be impaled on the small pins. Once closed the device brings the two rings into opposition there by bringing the inner surfaces of the ends together. The average time taken to couple veins is under 10 minutes, with added advantage of better addressing any size discrepancy of the two ends.

The success rate is for coupling veins is very high and exceeds suture technique in many centers. The coupler can also be combined with an implantable Doppler device for postoperative monitoring.

SELECTING THE RECIPIENT VEIN

Head and Neck

When operating in neck tributaries of Internal Jugular Vein (IJV) are most frequently used. External Jugular Vein (EJV) can be used if available. End to side anastomosis with IJV is used if no tributaries are available or vessel lie is more suitable or end to end anastomosis requires dealing with severe luminal discrepancy. When operating in the vessel depleted neck, harvesting the cephalic vein from mid arm region and reversing it to the neck is an option.

Limbs

Large size veins are usually preferred. Lower limb free flap success largely depends on recipient veins. The quality of venous walls also need to be closely evaluated, as more muscular walled veins such as saphenous vein are more prone to spasm and hence need to be well dilated. Lower extremity veins are under high pressure and will therefore have some back flow. Large tributaries entering close to the site of anastomosis need to be ligated or clipped as they add to pressure in the recipient veins. We prefer use of the venae comitantes over the saphenous veins. The exception to this is when the deeper veins are very small as compared to size of flap veins, in this case the larger saphenous vein is also used along with one deeper vein.

SELECTION OF RECIPIENT ARTERY

After the defect is created, the recipient artery is dissected proximal to the defect. The ease of dissection along the vascular pedicle is an important guide for the assessing the quality of artery. Arterial flow should be brisk and expansile pulsation should be palpated. A significant length of vessel should be dissected as flap dimensions may vary. We generally prepare approximately one-inch segment and small surrounding branches are clipped. It is important for the site of anastomosis to be distant from clipped branches. Approximate length of artery dissection should allow easy flipping of the Acland clamp during back wall suturing. If the vessel size is small as in case of pediatric patients, we find it best to carry out the final dissection under microscope. Time spent at this stage of preparation and dissection reduces the overall ischemia time of flap.

We do not routinely divide the artery to check the flow and only do so if it has been previously ligated along the edge of the defect during initial debridement. If the artery needs to be divided, blood flow is assessed and lumen is flushed with heparinized saline and clipping with a ligaclip. The vessels are kept moist throughout the dissection with gauze soaked in 2% Lignocaine.

The vessels should be covered and should not be frequently disturbed to avoid spasm.

When operating in head and neck, any branch of carotid artery which is of matching lumen and good flow can be used. Facial artery is usually the first choice, as it is often ligated in neck dissection; followed by superior thyroid artery and transverse cervical artery. End to side anastomosis to external carotid can be done in vessel depleted neck.

PREPARATION OF VESSELS

Gentle but sharp dissection under good magnification is very important while preparing the vessels for anastomosis. The adventitia is both thrombogenic and carries the sympathetic nerves which are responsible for creating spasm. At least 2 mm from the edge should be trimmed. The best technique is to pull the adventitia beyond the cut edge and sharply divide it with straight adventitia cutting scissors. The technique is also called "circumcision of adventitia".

END-TO-END ANASTOMOSIS

When there is size match between the donor and recipient vessel and other vessels supplying the limb are intact end-to-end anastomosis can be safely performed.

The site of anastomosis should be placed in the center of double clamp. There should be enough space to allow flipping the clamp over **(Fig. 2)**. The repair can be performed in two ways: in the first technique we start from the extreme far corner opposite to the side of operating surgeon and then follow with a corner suture towards the surgeon and then midline along posterior side. The other technique is to start from the extreme corner and keep suturing the anterior side and then flip the clamp and then do the back wall **(Fig. 3)**.

Open-loop suturing may be used in last few sutures to maintain the visibility. Continuous sutures are taken without tightening, keeping small loops. The first loop is then tied and suture cut. Next loop is then pulled through and tied in similar manner until all the sutures have been tied.

One Way Up Technique

Here we start the anastomosis on the back wall first and then keep suturing from both sides until finally placing the center suture on the anterior wall. This technique is very useful in tight spaces where flipping the clamp is not possible. The other main advantage is avoidance of back wall suturing.

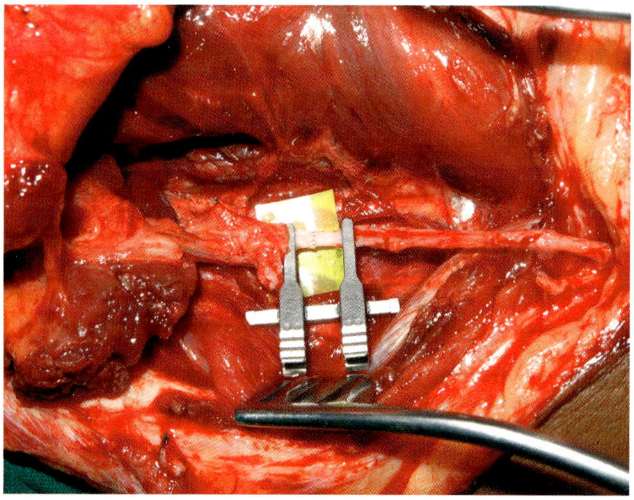

Fig. 2: Ensure that sufficient space is available for flipping the clamp

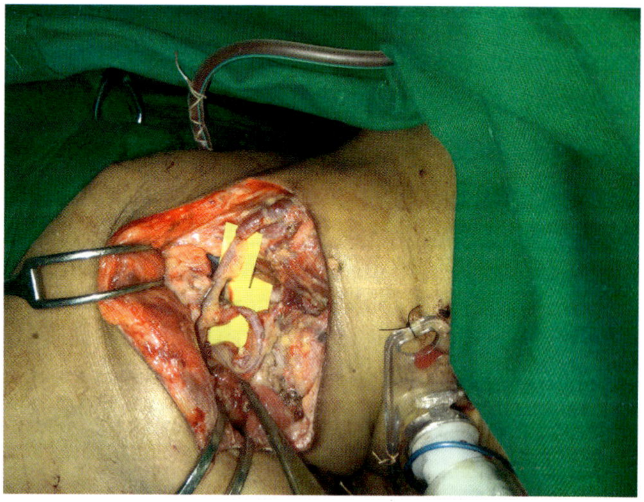

Fig. 3: Completed end-to-end anastomosis

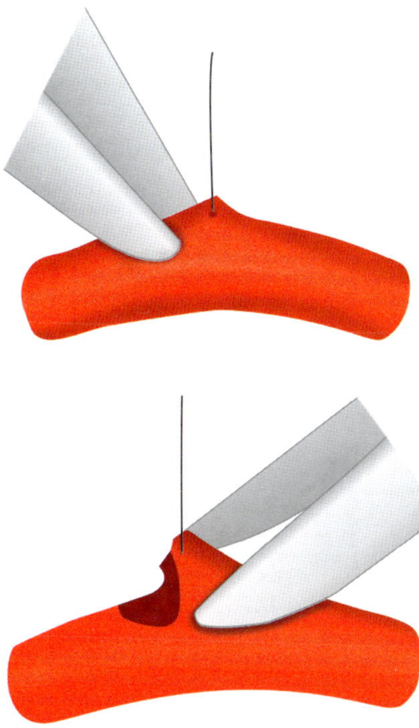

Fig. 4: Creating a venotomy for end-to-side anastomosis

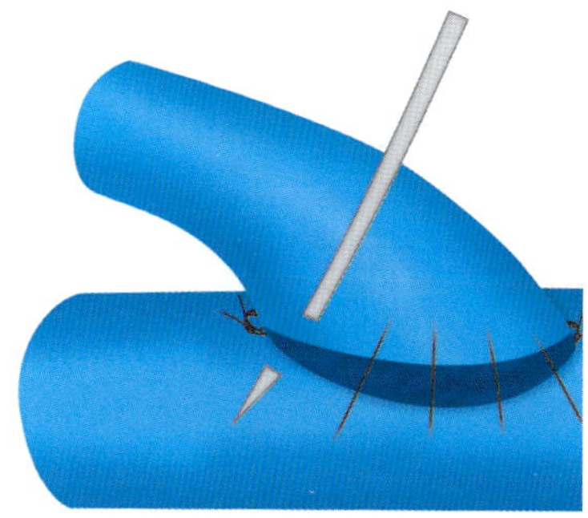

Fig. 5: End-to-side suturing technique

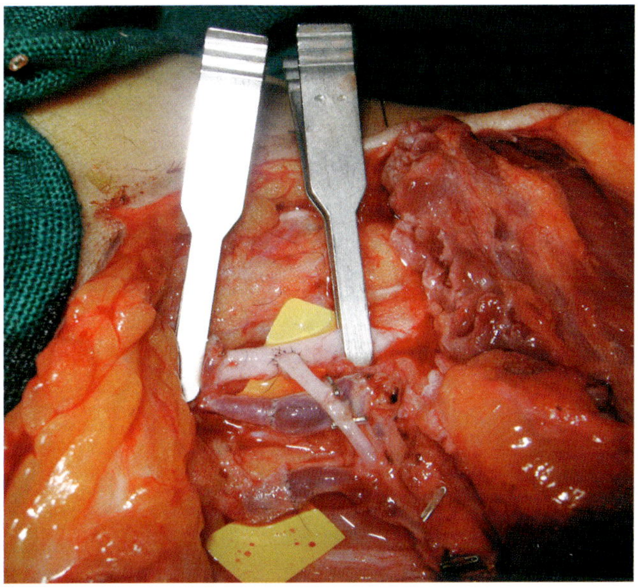

Fig. 6: Avoid kinking or stretching of the vessel

END-TO-SIDE SUTURING TECHNIQUE

End-to-side is technically more challenging. It is ideally suitable for circumstances where there is gross size discrepancy, or when there is only a single flowing vessel in the limb. The main requirement is to have a wide segment of recipient artery prepared. The flap vessels also should be of adequate length and well dissected off the accompanying veins. This is important to be able to retract the artery well for safely suturing the back wall, which is the most challenging part. We follow Dr Acland's technique in which first a 9.0 suture is taken at the site of proposed repair. The suture is held up under mild tension with a jeweler's forceps and two sharp cuts are made at 45-degree angle to achieve an oval hole which is dilated well with vessel dilator **(Fig. 4)**.

Dr Marko Godina advocated that the presence of the created side-hole in the larger vessel allows for it to be stretched without collapse and therefore increases the rates of anastomotic success.

We prefer to use two single clamps on either side during repair. A single vascular clamp like the Satinsky can be applied in head and neck to carry end to side anastomosis with jugular vein.

In the end-to-side technique, the corner sutures are placed first, the difficult back wall is then sutured keeping the flap artery retracted away towards opposite side. The front side sutures are then placed. The distal clamp is released first to visualize back flow in the vessel, followed by the proximal clamp. Once the blood flows through the anastomotic site it functions to lift the vessel with a gentle curvature, it is important to avoid kinking or stretching of the vessel **(Figs. 5 and 6)**.

SUTURING TECHNIQUES IN SPECIAL SITUATIONS

Vessel Size Mismatch

- Minimal mismatch can be managed by dilating the smaller vessel wall.

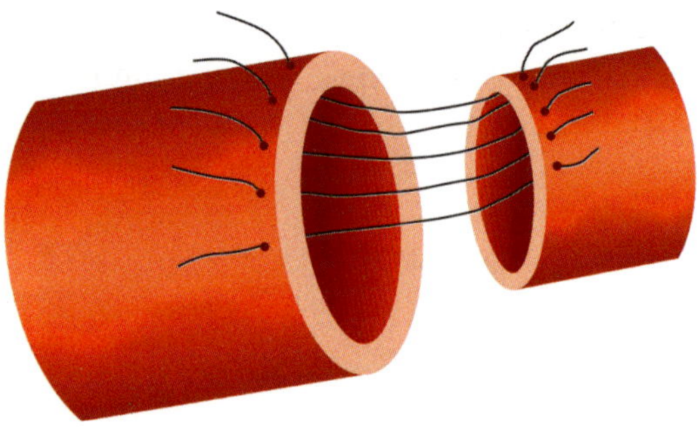

Fig. 7: Managing luminal discrepancy with unequal bites

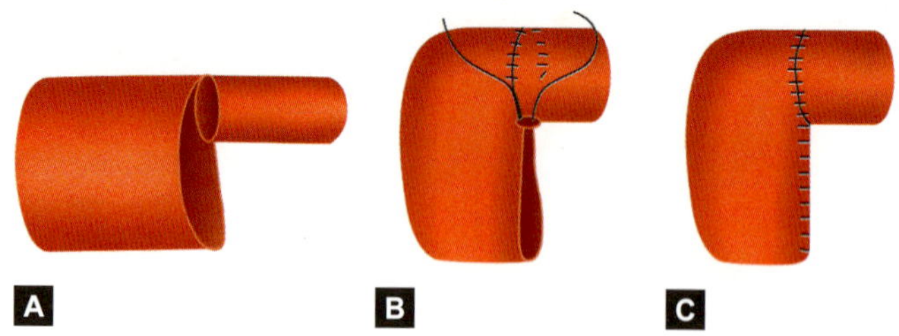

Figs. 8A to C: Managing large luminal discrepancy

- When the mismatch is 2:1, then bites in the smaller vessel should be kept closer relative to the opposite larger lumen vessel. This ratio should be maintained throughout the circumference of repair **(Fig. 7)**.
- Spatulation technique is an alternative option and involves cutting the smaller vessel obliquely and then pulling the edge into the clamp to effectively increase the lumen size.
- If the mismatch in the vein is greater than 2:1 then two vessels are sutured at one corner and then the larger vessel closed along the open margin by suturing or use of liga clip **(Figs. 8A to C)**.
- Horizontal mattress sutures can be used to adjust luminal mismatch. It has added advantage of causing good eversion of vessel wall.

Continuous suture technique: Although interrupted sutures are gold standard, continuous sutures may be used in certain situations and may give good result in experienced hands. Care must be taken to avoid purse stringing and entrapment of adventitia.

VASCULAR LOOP TECHNIQUE

When no good recipient vessels are available near the site of anastomosis, a vascular loop is very useful. A long saphenous vein graft is harvested and anastomosed between the proximal large artery and adjacent vein. This AV loop is allowed to mature and used after few days. Use of the AV loop acutely has demonstrated better success rate. The loop is divided in the center depending on the flap artery and vein length **(Fig. 9)**.

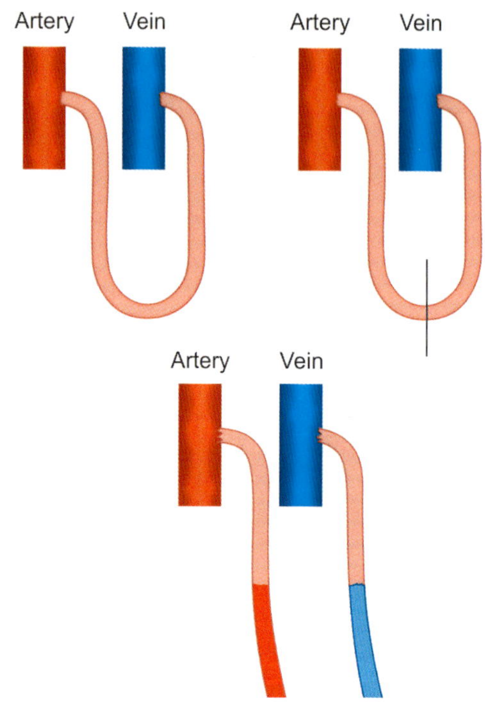

Fig. 9: Vascular loop technique

THE ANASTOMOTIC SET-UP AND TECHNIQUE

Following dissection, the vessels are brought together in the center of field, and accurately sized clamps are applied ensuring both side vessel ends are not under tension. The rough gouge for appropriate tension is observing that the diameter of the vessel matches the width of the clamp. A contrast background which is pliable and sturdy is placed under the vessel ends to cover the area between the clamps. The vessel ends within the double clamp are then trimmed of all adventitia. The lumen is flushed to remove any existing clots. The clamp on the proximal artery is opened to visualize adequate flow and then immediately re-clamped. The vessels end should be symmetrically aligned and closely approximated to "kiss". If the ends are overlapping a small scissor can be placed between the

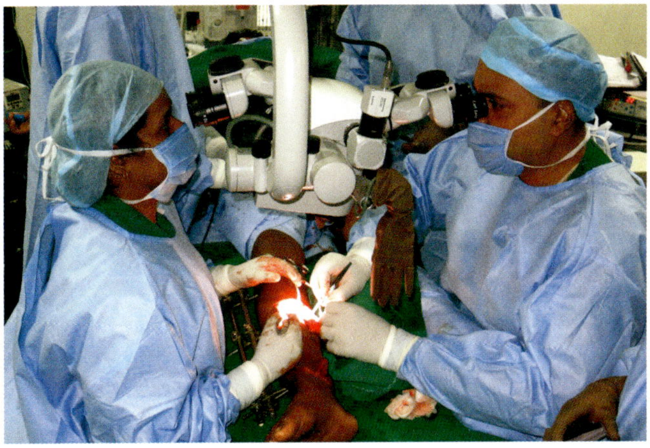

Fig. 10: Anastomotic set-up and positioning

double clamp to spread, it apart and ensure appropriate close approximation of the vessels. Small gauze is then used around to absorb any remaining irrigation fluid in the field and to provide a contrast for the suture. Constant irrigation is carried out with heparinized saline. The surgeon and assistant's elbows should be well supported and eye piece of microscope should be parallel to the eye of the surgeon **(Fig. 10)**.

CONCLUSION

Successful microvascular surgery depends on great attention to detail and technique. Clean dissection, adequate trimming of adventitia, atraumatic handling of vessel walls and finally good proximal flow in the artery are key element of success. Investing in good instruments, operating loupes and microscopes makes a significant difference in the ability to achieve success.

CHAPTER 3

Preoperative Issues

Prashant Puranik, Chirag Ajay Bhansali

Microvascular flaps are at the highest rung of reconstructive ladder and technically complex. Good preoperative planning is often more important than the actual harvest of the flap. A good preoperative plan can often be the difference between success and failure.

DEFECT ASSESSMENT

On the OPD visit of the patient the likely defect, its size (length, breadth and thickness), shape and components (Buccal mucosa, skin, muscle) should be imagined and the reconstructive plan should be made. In cases requiring complex reconstructions, plan should be made after consultation with the oncosurgeon.

FLAP/DONOR SITE ASSESSMENT

Ideal flap should be replacement of like with like tissues. Flap chosen should match defect in its structure, geometry and tissue character. Objective assessment, inspection and palpation, of the donor site should be done rather than judgment by the general appearance of the patient. Donor sites should be evaluated for skin thickness and pliability, thickness of subcutaneous tissue, color match and hair growth. Consideration to anatomical variables, like vascular pedicle length and caliber and donor site morbidity should be taken into account for decision making. Major injury or scars at any flap territory precludes use of flap.

FLAP-WISE CONSIDERATIONS

Free Radial Artery Forearm Flap

- Nondominant hand is preferred for the harvest.
- History of intravenous cannula insertion for chemotherapy taken. Chemotherapeutic injection can cause vasculitis and thrombosis of vessel. Cephalic vein is common site for venous cannulation. This makes radial forearm flap harvest a relative contraindication.
- Allen's test should be done at wrist level. Any cannulation on planned side should be avoided and instructed.

Free Fibula Flap

- Skin changes in patient suffering from varicose veins and peripheral vascular disease should be evaluated.
- Peripheral pulses of the dorsalis pedis and posterior tibial artery should be evaluated. If any pulse not palpable Doppler evaluation is done. CT angiogram is rarely needed.
- Range of movement of ankle, knee and hip joint should be noted. Any restriction of flexion, will limit achieving optimal position for flap harvest.

Free Flaps from Abdomen

- Volume of abdominal pannus is evaluated with pinch test.
- Tone of the abdominal muscles must be evaluated with head raising test.
- Umbilical or abdominal wall hernias are ruled out.
- Previous longitudinal incisions are noted; flap may need augmentation of vascularity if full pannus is used.
- Pfannenstiel incision may limit the height of flap but does not interfere with venous drainage.
- It is advisable to perform CT angiography of deep inferior epigastric arterial system which provides valuable information about perforator location, patterns of venous drainage, vascular anatomy and dominance of superficial epigastric system.

Anterolateral Thigh Flap

- Thickness, pliability and likely primary closure of the thigh are evaluated by the pinch test.
- Hand held Doppler is used to locate the perforators preoperatively.

SPECIAL INVESTIGATIONS

In previously operated patients or irradiated patient of head and neck cancers status of neck vessels can be concern. Preoperative color Doppler of the neck or CT angiography can provide information about the status of blood vessels.

ANESTHESIA CONSIDERATIONS

Pre-anesthetic preparation of these patients is like any other patient. Counseling and consent for anesthesia should be taken. Details in Chapter on Anesthesia Concerns.

COUNSELING AND CONSENT

- Patients concerns, expectations should be understood.
- Flap counseling should focus on various donor sites, various flap components and a mention about microvascular anastomosis.
- Common surgical complications like infection, bleeding, flap complications like vascular thrombosis should be explained as also donor site scarring and aesthetic result.
- Postoperative pressure garments, drain tubes, Ryles tube and Foleys catheters should be counseled.
- Informed consent should be taken preferably in vernacular language.
- Head neck resection can be unpredictable at times. To account for this unpredictability all possible flaps that might be used in the reconstruction should be counseled about.
- Coverage of the donor site with skin grafts and also the sites of skin graft harvest should be explained.

Implant/Mesh Issues

Patients are counseled that the surgery will involve implantation of foreign objects like titanium mesh/plates, screws, prolene mesh and liga clips.

Cost Counseling of Surgery and Exploration

Information regarding the cost of surgery, cost of implants and disposables, should be provided to the patients. Sensitization regarding additional cost in case of exploration for thrombosis or any other complication and their sequelae, should be done.

Explanation of Risk/Exploration

Possibility of arterial and venous thrombosis which may require re-exploration of the flap should be explained to the patient in detail. Consent regarding vein grafts and a new flap pedicle or free should be taken prior to re-exploration.

CHAPTER 4

Anesthesia and Free Flaps

Vijaya Patil

INTRODUCTION

We the surgeons at Tata Memorial Centre are fortunate to have an excellent department of **Anesthesia, Critical Care and Pain**. The integrated services provides excellent peroperative care to our patients. Needless to say, the long hours of anesthesia and prompt response to a need for thrombotic exploration are a prerequisite for a microvascular unit. We can not thank enough our Anesthesia, Critical Care and Pain colleagues for providing relentless services and intellectual support to us.

Microvascular free flap for complex and extensive defects has revolutionized many surgeries, involving massive cancer resections.

The technique of free tissue transfer is complex. Initial flap failure rates reported in early '60s may have ranged as high as 40% to 50% but the overall failure rate quoted in recent literature is around 1-5 %. Despite improvement in surgical skills, loss of free flap represents major problems.

Anesthesia plays a major role in improving the success rate of this type of surgery by controlling the global hemodynamics and the regional blood flow. Many factors that an anaesthetist controls influence free flap microcirculation such as blood volume, vasoactive drugs usage, use of regional blocks, maintaining perioperative body temperature etc.

Free flap surgeries are different from other surgeries due to certain peculiarities of the flap.

- Usually only a single feeder artery and vein.
- Subject to warm ischemia during transfer making it susceptible to ischemia reperfusion injury on revascularization
- Denervated but responds to physical and chemical stimuli
- There is significant reduction in original blood flow in first 24-48 hours due to reperfusion injury
- No intact lymphatic drainage leading to increased risk of interstitial edema.

PHYSIOLOGIC CONSIDERATION

The guiding principle of anesthesia for free flap surgery is the maintenance of optimum blood flow to free revascularized tissue. The determinants of flow are summarized by the Hagen-Poiseuille equation

$$\text{Blood flow} = \Delta P \pi r^4 / 8 \eta l$$

Where ΔP = pressure difference between two ends of a tube, r = radius of the tube, η = viscosity and l = length of the tube.

From this we may deduce that the goals of anesthesia for free flap surgery are maintaining vasodilatation, good perfusion pressure and low viscosity.

ANESTHESIA MANAGEMENT

Preoperative Assessment

Principles of preoperative assessment and management remain same as for any other surgery. This includes proper history taking to assess functional status of patient, underlying pre-existing medical condition and eliciting relevant drug history followed by ordering for relevant investigations and finally optimizing for surgery.

In addition, different subsets of patients will have different set of problems peculiar to that patient population. Patients with head and neck malignancies are often elderly, poorly nourished, heavy smokers and drinkers and may have significant underlying cardiac and respiratory dysfunction. They are likely to have difficult airway due to primary malignancy or secondary to radiotherapy.

Postoperatively these patients are likely to have urinary catheters, nasogastric tubes and many a times endotracheal tube or tracheostomy. Preoperative counseling should include explanation of all these devices otherwise inability to talk or void urine can lead to agitation and irritation, excess movements and uncooperative state.

Conduct of Anesthesia

Balanced general anesthesia with adequate analgesia to reduce the stress response and catecholamine release is technique of choice. Since most of these surgeries are prolonged duration surgeries many anesthetists choose to avoid N_2O and use oxygen air mixture.

Volatile anesthetic agents remain preferred agents for maintenance of anesthesia. Almost all inhalational agents lead to decrease in blood pressure due to their effect on peripheral vascular resistance and myocardial contractility.

Studies using laser Doppler flowmetry to measure total flap flow in Guinea pigs have showed that during normovolemic conditions flap flow remains well maintained in both with halothane and isoflurane anesthesia; however, during mild to moderate hypovolemia flap flow decreases markedly with halothane anesthesia while it remains unchanged with isoflurane suggesting superiority of isoflurane.[1] Sevoflurane and Desflurane are probably the volatile agents of choice due to a combination of relatively stable cardiovascular conditions and rapid offset after prolonged surgery. In addition, the preconditioning effects of sevoflurane can protect endothelial cells against ischemia-reperfusion injury and become agent of choice in free vascular tissue transfers.[2] Also it has been demonstrated that sevoflurane, when compared with intravenous anesthetics such as Propofol, could have beneficial effects on the microcirculation by decreasing extravasation of plasma into the interstitial space, and thus limiting flap edema.[3]

Opioids constitute major part of anesthetic management as they are potent analgesic, minimize stress response to intubation, reduce requirement of volatile anaesthetic agents and have minimal effect on myocardial contractility or peripheral vascular resistance. Fentanyl, remifentanyl or alfentanyl are preferred drugs of choice due to their shorter half-lives allowing better titration and rapid recovery.

One can also use nonsteroidal anti-inflammatory agents that would maintain postoperative analgesia as well as will have opioid sparing effects.

The majority of patients can be extubated at the end of surgery. Emergence and extubation can be very challenging. At the time of extubation one should aim to have awake cooperative patient but at the same time care should be taken to minimise haemodyanamic responses and avoid movements at operative site. This is especially true in head and neck surgery and it is vital to ensure optimal analgesia before discontinuing the anesthetic.

Fluid Management

Traditional teaching has been to use hypervolemic hemodilution during anesthesia for free tissue transfer to maintain good flap flow by decreasing viscosity, increasing cardiac output and avoiding vasoconstriction.

However, studies do not support this assumption, rather almost all studies looking at fluid therapy in free flap surgeries have shown increased complication rates associated with more fluids. As free flaps have no lymphatic drainage they are prone to interstitial edema and so excessive fluid administration may in fact be detrimental.[4,5]

Achieving a balance between flap perfusion and prevention of hypervolemia is a major task of anesthetist. Maintenance of an adequate mean arterial blood pressure (MAP) and cardiac output is crucial. Combination of crystalloids and colloids to maintain good blood pressure and urine output of 0.5 mL/kg/hr can be used as a goal for fluid therapy. Retrospective analysis of 241 head and neck reconstruction has shown that more than 7 liters fluid infusion in entire intraoperative period was associated with increased flap complications.[6]

Crystalloid volume greater than 130 mL/kg/24 hrs was an independent predictor for medical complications in retrospective evaluation of 185 patients undergoing free flap reconstruction following ablation of head and neck cancer.[7] Another study showed increased complications of flap when patients received >6 mL/kg/hrs fluids.[8] All these findings suggest excess fluid is harmful and caution should be exerted while infusing fluids for these surgeries.

Role of Regional Anesthesia

Most of the studies in this field are done using epidural analgesia. Epidural analgesia provides good analgesia and by blocking sympathetic system induces vasodilatation, both of which should be beneficial in flap surgery. However, one has to take precautions so as to maintain normal blood pressure otherwise hypotension associated with sympathetic blockade will produce MAP dependent fall in flap blood flow.

A 'steal phenomenon' has also been proposed with blood flow diverted away from the denervated free flap to vasodilated vessels. Study done in human patients have shown that epidural block did not cause any change in microcirculatory flow in the intact skin and muscle, however, it resulted in a 20–30% decrease in microcirculatory blood flow in all the free flaps studied along with significant decrease in MAP.[9] However a recent case series has reported successful use of epidural anesthesia for gracilis free flap suggesting epidural anesthesia can be used in carefully selected patient.[10] Use of upper extremity blocks have been found to be effective over plain GA both regarding postoperative pain relief and microvascular flow in flap for microvascular surgeries in upper limb.[11,12]

Achieving Specific Goals of Microvascular Surgery

Maintaining Vasodilatation

1. **Avoid hypothermia**: Temperature control is very important for microvascular surgeries both during and after surgery. Hypothermia causes vasoconstriction and increases blood viscosity, both detrimental to flap perfusion. Minimize heat loss by keeping patient well-covered, using forced air warming blankets, warming mattresses and blood and fluid warmers. Many times preventing hypothermia is difficult task as multiple sites of surgeries or large operative fields increase heat loss and prevent application of effective warming measures. In such cases one can raise OT ambient temperature after discussion with surgeons.
2. **Maintain euvolemia**: Hypovolemia leads to vasoconstriction. In microvascular free flap surgeries there are more than one operating site that can increase insensible fluid loss. Also patients with faciomaxillary or intraoral malignancies tend to have difficulty in swallowing resulting in hypovolemic state preoperatively. Assessment of intravascular volume status and avoidance of hypovolemia is very important for good flap perfusion
3. **Good analgesia**: Pain is powerful stimulant for sympathetic stimulation leading to vasoconstriction. These patients need good analgesia in view of multiple incision sites, drains and sometimes awkward positions. Good analgesia reduces the level of circulating catecholamines and avoids the vasoconstrictor response to pain.
4. **Maintain normocapnea**: CO_2 is most potent systemic vasodilator. Hypocapnia commonly seen under anesthesia is not a benign clinical entity and leads to vasoconstriction and decrease in blood flow across various vascular beds including flap blood flow. There is increasing evidence that hypocapnia induces substantial adverse physiological and medical effects and should be avoided.

Maintaining Perfusion Pressure

The preservation of a good perfusion pressure is essential to flap survival. Appropriate anesthetic depth and proper fluid management are usually all that is needed.

During the dissection stages of surgery, especially for major tumor resection, surgeons might request for controlled hypotension to improve the surgical field and reduce blood loss which can be accomplished by increasing depth of anesthesia, infiltration of local anesthetic and vasoconstrictor, and optimum position to achieve unobstructed venous drainage.

After resection of primary site, during harvesting and anastomosis of the flap, mean arterial blood pressure should be maintained at a normal or slightly elevated level to ensure an adequate perfusion pressure through the graft tissue bed.

There is very little evidence to show that systemically administered catecholamines adversely affect flap blood flow. Almost all studies done are animal studies and have shown that blood flow to flap is directly proportional to MAP irrespective of the agent used.

In a study conducted on porcine model by Banic et al.[13] it was shown that systemic phenylephrine in a dose that increased the systemic vascular resistance and arterial pressure by 30% showed no adverse effects on blood flow in free musculocutaneous flaps.

Sodium nitroprusside, however, in a dose causing a 30% decrease in systemic vascular resistance and arterial pressure, caused a severe reduction in free flap blood flow despite maintaining cardiac output suggesting importance of perfusion pressure.

Suominen et al. compared dobutamine, dopamine and placebo on effect on blood flow in recipient and donor blood vessels in TRAM flap for breast reconstruction and concluded that if vasoactive agents are needed during microvascular surgery, dobutamine seems to be more advantageous than dopamine.[14] The recent study by Messy et al. in porcine model compared phenylephrine and epinephrine on their effect on blood flow across pedicled artery and microvasculature in flap. Results showed that epinephrine consistently increased both flows across the entire dose range whereas phenylephrine consistently decreased the pedicle artery blood flow and the microvascular perfusion. Furthermore, epinephrine-induced increases in cardiac output correlated well with the observed increases in pedicle artery blood flow and microvascular perfusion.[15]

Thus, the general recommendation is to use inotropes like dobutamine or adrenaline after ensuring that patient is not hypovolemic.

Prevention of Deep Vein Thrombosis (DVT)

Significant number of patients undergoing major surgery under general anesthesia develop DVT.[16] Though incidence of clinically relevant DVT is low, nonetheless if it happens it results in significant morbidity and mortality.

The eighth ACCP conference on antithrombotic and thrombolytic therapy make a strong recommendation for use of thromboprophylaxis to all major surgical procedures (procedures lasting for >1 hour) and prolong immobilization.[17]

One can use either unfractionated heparin 5000U SC bid or low molecular weight heparin once a day.

For patients at high bleeding risk one may consider using mechanical thromboprophylaxis. In surgeries, where bleeding can be a major problem, the surgeon should use Intermittent Pneumatic Compression devices both before and during the operation and in the early postoperative period. When it is deemed appropriate, anticoagulation should then be commenced.[18]

Maintaining Low Viscosity

The ideal hematocrit for patients undergoing free tissue transfer procedures are unknown.

For years physicians used the "10/30" rule (Hb of 10 and hematocrit of 30), but various[19] studies have shown that this is no longer a clinically useful value. There is a non-linear relationship between blood viscosity and hematocrit; viscosity rises steeply when the hematocrit exceeds 40%.

Studies have shown that most critically ill and surgical patients can tolerate much lower hemoglobin levels without adverse effects, but a safe threshold above which red cell transfusion is clearly unnecessary has not been established. Many observational studies have shown an association between red cell transfusions and infection[20,21] multiple organ failure,[22] increased ICU and hospital length of stay,[23,24] and mortality. In a pig model comparing partially well-perfused and partially ischemic flap, normovolemic hemodilution increased flap blood flow and increased oxygen tension in ischemic flap, with the optimum Hb being around 9 mg% and Hct just less than 30.[25] Recent observational cohort study done by Rossmiller and colleagues did not show increased flap failures by lowering transfusion threshold to hematocrit 25.[26]

Postoperative Care

Principles of postoperative care are same as for any other surgery which include keeping patients warm, pain free and hemodyanamically stable.

Coughing or vomiting can reduce flap flow by increasing venous pressure and should be avoided.

One can use intravenous patient controlled analgesia or continuous nerve blocks for analgesia.

In addition care has to be taken to maintain unobstructed venous flow by giving proper position and keep patient relatively immobile to avoid stress on vascular anastomosis. Since most of these patients remain immobilized or minimally mobilized for prolonged postoperative duration, thromboprophylaxis should be integral part of postoperative care in these patients. Patients requiring postoperative ventilation are generally admitted to ICU.

Glycemic Control

Perioperative period is a highly diabetogenic state due to hypermetabolic stress response which increases glucose production and causes insulin resistance.

In surgical patients, perioperative hyperglycemia has been shown to increase risk of postoperative mortality, and cardiovascular, respiratory, neurologic, and infectious morbidity.[27]

American Diabetes Association and the American Association of Clinical Endocrinologists currently recommend targeting blood sugar between 140–180 mg% with use of insulin infusion.[28]

Monitoring of Flap

Since microvascular flap depends on feeding artery and vein for its survival till development of collateral capillary circulation, flap needs continuous monitoring to identify problems of perfusion. The frequency with which flap observations should take place depends on individual practitioner and varies from as frequent as every 30 minutes to every 4–6 hours. The traditional methods of monitoring include mainly clinical observation of skin colour, capillary return and temperature of free skin flaps. However, the best of the currently available methods is laser Doppler flowmetry which allows more reliable and objective method of assessment of microcirculation of free flap. As the level of care required by patients of free flap surgery is, most centers prefer to admit them to high dependency unit (HDU).

CONCLUSION

Along with good surgical technique, good anesthesia technique and proper postoperative management are important contributors to outcome in free flap surgeries. Application of good physiological principles helps to attain these goals.

REFERENCES

1. Sigurdsson GH, Banic A, Wheatley AM, et al. Effects of halothane and isoflurane anesthesia on microcirculatory blood flow in musculocutaneous flaps. Br. J. Anaesth. 1994; 73:826-32.
2. Lucchinetti E, Aguirre J, Feng J, et al. Molecular evidence of late preconditioning after sevoflurane inhalation in healthy volunteers. Anesth Analg. 2007;105:629-40.
3. Bruegger D, Bauer A, Finsterer U, et al. Microvascular changes during anesthesia: Sevoflurane compared with propofol. Acta Anaesthesiol Scand. 2002;46:481-87.
4. Booi DI. Perioperative fluid overload increases anastomosis thrombosis in the free TRAM flap used for breast reconstruction. Eur J Plast Surg. 2011;34:81-6.
5. Neinstein, R; Hofer S OP, Zhong T, et al. Fluid considerations to minimize early postoperative complications in free flap breast cancer reconstruction. Plastic & Reconstructive Surgery. 2010; 126:90.
6. Haughey BH, Wilson E, Kluwe L, et al. Free flap reconstruction of the head and neck: analysis of 241 cases. Otolaryngol Head Neck Surg. 2001;125:10-7.
7. Clark JR, McCluskey SA, Hall F, et al. Predictors of morbidity following free flap reconstruction for cancer of the head and neck. Head Neck. 2007;29:1090-1101.
8. Franklin J, Yoo J, Matthews TW, et al. Morbidity associated with perioperative fluid management in free-flap reconstruction of the head and neck. Laryngoscope. 2002;112:765-6.
9. Erni D, Banic A, Signer C, et al. Effects of epidural anesthesia on microcirculatory blood flow in free flaps in patients under general Anesthesia. European Journal of Anesthesiology. 1999;16:692-8.
10. Alam NH. Haeney JA. Platt AJ. Three episodes of gracilis free muscle transfer under epidural anesthesia. Journal of Reconstructive Aesthet Surgery. 2006;59:1463-6.
11. Kurt E, Ozturk S, Isik S, et al. Continuous brachial plexus blockade for digital replantations and toe-to-hand transfers. Ann Plast Surg. 2005;54:24–7.
12. Inberg P, Kassila M, Vilkki S, et al. Anesthesia for microvascular surgery in children. A combination of general anesthesia and axillary plexus block. Acta Anaesthesiol Scand. 1995;39:518-22.
13. Banic A, Krejci V, Erni D, et al. Effects of sodium nitroprusside and phenylephrine on blood flow in free musculocutaneous flaps during general anesthesia. Anesthesiology. 1999;90:147-55.
14. Suominen S, Svartling N, Silvasti M, et al. The effect of intravenous dopamine and dobutamine on blood circulation during a microvascular TRAM flap operations. Annals of Plastic Surgery. 2004;53: 425-31.
15. Massey MF, Gupta DK. The effects of systemic phenylephrine and epinephrine on pedicle artery and microvascular perfusion in a pig model of myoadipocutaneous rotational flaps. Plast Reconstr Surg. 2007;120:1289-99.
16. Sakon M, Maehara Y, Yoshikawa H, et al. Incidence of venous thromboembolism following major abdominal surgery: A multi-center, prospective epidemiological study in Japan. J Thromb Haemost. 2006;4:581.
17. American College of Chest Physicians Antithrombotic and thrombolytic therapy, 8th ed. Chest. 2008;1336 suppl: 1293-533.
18. Venturi ML, Davison SP, Caprini JS. Prevention of venous thromboembolism in the plastic surgery patient: Current guidelines and recommendations. Aesthetic Surgery Journal. 2009;29:421-8.
19. Antal G Hudetz, James D Wood, Bharat B Biswal, et al. Effect of hemodilution on RBC velocity, supply rate, and hematocrit in the cerebral capillary network Kampine. Journal of Applied Physiology. 1999;87: 505-9.
20. Landers Df, Hill Ge, Wong KC, et al. Blood transfusion-induced immunomodulation. Anesth Analg. 1996;82: 187–204.
21. Carson J, Altman D, Duff A, et al. Risk of bacterial infection associated with allogeneic blood transfusion among patients undergoing hip fracture repair. Transfusion. 1999;39:694–700.
22. Zallen G, Offner P, Moore E, et al. Age of transfused blood is an independent risk factor for postinjury multiple organ failure. Am J Surg. 1999;178:570–2.
23. Keller M, Jean R, LaMorte W, et al. Effects of age of transfused blood on length of stay in trauma patients: a preliminary report. J Trauma. 2002;53:1023-5.
24. Malone D, Dunne J, Tracy K, et al. Blood transfusion, independent of shock severity, is associated with worse outcome in trauma. J Trauma. 2003;54:898-907.
25. Schramm S, Wettstein R, Wessendorf R, et al. Acute normovolemic haemodilution improves oxygenation in ischemic flap tissue. Anesthesiology. 2002; 96:1478-84.
26. Rossmiller SR, Cannady SB, Ghanem TA, et al. Transfusion criteria in free flap surgery. Otolaryngology-Head and Neck Surgery. 2010;142:359-64.
27. Duncan AE, Abd-Elsayed A, Maheshwari A, et al. Role of intraoperative and postoperative blood glucose concentrations in predicting outcomes after cardiac surgery. Anesthesiology. 2010;112(4):860-71.
28. Moghissi ES, Korytkowski MT, DiNardo M, et al. American Association of Clinical Endocrinologists and American Diabetes Association consensus statement on inpatient glycemic control. Endocr Pract. 2009;15(4):353-69.

CHAPTER 5

Thromboprophylaxis for Free Flaps

Quazi Ghazwan Ahmad, Amrita Rao

INTRODUCTION

The advent of microsurgery has opened up a new era in plastic surgery. Microsurgical procedures to be not free from complications and failure rate vary between 5 and 10% across institutes. Antithrombotic pharmacological prophylaxis has been proposed in an attempt to improve free tissue transfer success rates. The three commonly used drugs used are Heparin, Dextran and Aspirin. Although numerous animal and few prospective clinical studies were conducted with these three drugs no consensus on treatment guidelines has been reached. No studies were able to conclusively demonstrate a statistically significant improvement in free tissue transfer success rates with the usage of these drugs.

A randomized clinical control trial to evaluate the use of anticoagulant for prophylaxis of thrombosis was conducted at Tata Memorial Centre between 2005 and 2008 enrolling almost 600 patients. It was a multiphase trial. We are summarizing the yet unpublished data.

Our Study: Role of anticoagulants in Head and Neck microvascular reconstruction. A Randomized Controlled Trial to evaluate its use for prophylaxis of thrombosis

Authors of this study: Dr Quazi Ghazwan Ahmed, Dr Prabha Yadav, Dr Vinay Kant Shankhdhar , Dr Kanti Shetty

This study at our centre was conceptualized by (late) Dr Rajendra Prasad.

Patients included in the study were all patients undergoing free flap reconstruction in head and neck region and were classified as ASA I and II by anesthesiologists.

Aims of the Study

- The primary objective of the study was to find whether there is need for pharmacological thromboprophylaxis in free flap microvascular reconstruction done for head and neck region and if yes, is there an ideal drug
- Secondary objectives were to evaluate the benefit and risk of anticoagulants.

Postoperative flap monitoring was mainly based on clinical findings which included warmth, color and pin prick examination at 3 hourly intervals for the first 48 hours followed by 6 to 8 hourly for the next 3 days in all free flap cases.

In **Phase I**, 148 patients were randomized into two groups. The first group of patients received dextran infusion for 72 hours post-surgery and the second group received low molecular weight heparin at induction of surgery followed by once daily for 72 hours post-surgery. Each group was further randomized into two subgroups. The control subgroup which received no further treatment after 72 hours the Aspirin subgroup which received 150 milligrams of Aspirin daily for the next 5 days. So in effect we had a total of 4 subgroups.

Result of this phase of the study:

- ***The difference in distribution of cases of thrombosis in the different groups was not statistically significant***
- Low molecular weight heparin led to increased incidence of wound hematoma.
- Prepondcrance for chest complications in the dextran group
- 1 case of renal complication in the low molecular weight heparin group
- When data was analyzed for effect of other comorbid conditions like hypertension, diabetes smoking, previous chemotherapy or previous radiotherapy, none of these were found to have any significant effect on the success rate of microvascular surgery.

Phase I of this study led to the conclusion that there was no statistically significant difference in thrombotic events in the multiple arms of the study.

To the answer the question whether any thromboprophylaxis is needed in the first place and whether these drugs lead to any additional risk and cost the **Phase II** of the study was started. In this Phase 200 patients were randomized into two groups. Group 1 received Dextran infusion for 72 hours post-surgery. Group 2 was control group in which no thromboprophylaxis was used.

Phase II concluded that:

- There was no statistically significant difference in the rate of microvascular thrombosis between the 2 groups
- There is a statistically significant increase in chest complication in the dextran group and one case of Renal complication

To consolidate data, the study was continued for another year (Phase III) in which 200 patients for accrued and as a protocol no thromboprophylaxis drug was used in these patients.

Conclusions after 3 Phases of the randomized control trial showed that:

- *The difference in the incidence of thrombosis is not significant in different groups of thrombus prophylactic drugs vis-a-vis no use of these drugs.*
- There was no statistically significant difference in the success rate over the three phases of the study
- Use of low molecular weight heparin is associated with higher incidence of wound Hematoma.
- Use of dextran is associated with higher incidence of chest complication.
- Both dextran and heparin have a minimal risk of renal complication
- The morbidity with the use of thromboprophylactic drugs was significantly higher.

Summarization of the study			
	I	II	III
Success rate	95.81%	96.85%	95.82%
Thrombosis	11.18% (16/143)	5.79% (11/191)	7.85% (15/191)
Chest complications	4.19% (6/143)	4.18% (8/191)	1.04% (2/191)
Hematoma	10.48% (15/143)	5.23% (10/191)	1.04% (2/191)

Comparison of the thromboprophylactic drugs currently used:

Drug/Side effect	Ease of dosage	Respiratory complications	Renal complications	Hematoma	Cost	Risk of allergy
Heparin	2 or 3 divided doses intravenously (best if given by continuous infusion)-cumbersome	None	None but its route of excretion is renal and hence must be used with care in those with renal insufficiency	Risk high especially if high dose infusion is given. Also risk of heparin induced thrombocytopenia	Low cost	High and can develop during treatment
Low molecular weight heparin	Twice daily subcutaneous injection	None	Similar to heparin	Lower as half-life is longer and hence stable bioavailability	High cost	Lower than heparin
Aspirin	Oral tablet once daily	None	Can occur especially in those with hyperuricemia and gout as it impairs the kidneys ability to eliminate uric acid	Present	Low cost	Present with small risk of Angioedema
Dextran	Continuous intravenous infusion-cumbersome	High. Occurs secondary to pulmonary edema	High	Present	High cost	Present

Current Protocol at Tata Memorial Centre

Based on this study the current Protocol in our unit is; no antithrombotic prophylaxis for microvascular anastomotic patency is used as a routine, irrespective of age and comorbidities.

We do begin single dose low molecular weight heparin for Deep Vein Thrombosis prophylaxis in all patients receiving free flap surgery which is continued until they are adequately mobilized.

In those patients who have either vascular thrombotic event during primary surgery or undergo exploration for the same within 5 days of surgery we begin therapeutic prophylaxis with twice daily low molecular weight heparin administered subcutaneously. In these patients, pharmacological therapy is continued for 3 weeks by either continuing subcutaneous low molecular weight heparin or changing it to oral warfarin (titrated with PT-INR monitoring).

A drug which can guarantee patency and no thrombosis would be a dream for all of microvascular surgeons. In the past, we have searched for one such elusive drug and many still continue to do so. Many others continue to use one of the drugs mentioned in this chapter despite lack of adequate evidence of benefit. But as our knowledge and experience has grown we now have the wisdom that there is no replacement to a meticulous surgical technique.

CHAPTER 6

Anterolateral Thigh Flap

Dushyant Jaiswal, Tasneem Belgaumwala

INTRODUCTION

The Anterolateral Thigh Flap (ALT) was first described by Song et al. The earliest largest series were published by Fu Chen Wei et al., this led to immense popularity of the flap.

It has become the 'workhorse' for defects in cases where soft tissue bulk is needed in addition to skin.

ALT has been used widely across the globe, from head to toe and in numerous shapes, sizes and forms. It is now an indispensable, often first line, element in the armamentarium of any reconstructive microvascular surgeon.

The size of the thigh also allows large amounts of flap to be harvested with primary closure of the donor site. Even larger flaps are possible if a skin graft is accepted at the donor site.

At TMH it is the most common free flap performed, even more than fibula. We now use it for a lot of indications where we earlier used Free Radial Artery Forum flap (FRAFF).

HARVESTING THE ALT FLAP

Right or Left Thigh

We generally harvest from the left thigh as a matter convenience with regards to the operating room setup. But if there is a significant difference in the hand held Doppler signal the better side could be chosen. Occasionaly, when chimeric flap is planned, side choice could be guided by the Doppler. We do not routinely image (CT or Duplex) the thigh for perforators as a routine.

Hand-held Audio Doppler

We use 8 Mhz probe low sensitivity, high specificity Doppler machine (avoids false positives). A good Doppler signal helps in choosing left or right thigh and the location of initial incision. Doppler only tells us the presence of a perforator reaching the dermis, little else. It cannot tell us the size, course (septocutaneous or musculocutaneous), pedicle of origin or the size of flap it can sustain.

Preparation

Anterior Superior Iliac Spine (ASIS) to Patella should be exposed in the surgical field. The Doppler signal points can be marked with ink or a superficial scratch **(Fig. 1)**.

Marking

The surface marking of the septum (between Rectus Femoris and Vastus Lateralis) is between ASIS and Superolateral border of the patella. The midpoint of this line with a circle around it of 3 cm diameter is supposed to have high perforator yield. The flap can be centered around this midpoint or around the best Doppler signal marking. Generally, an ellipse is planned permitting

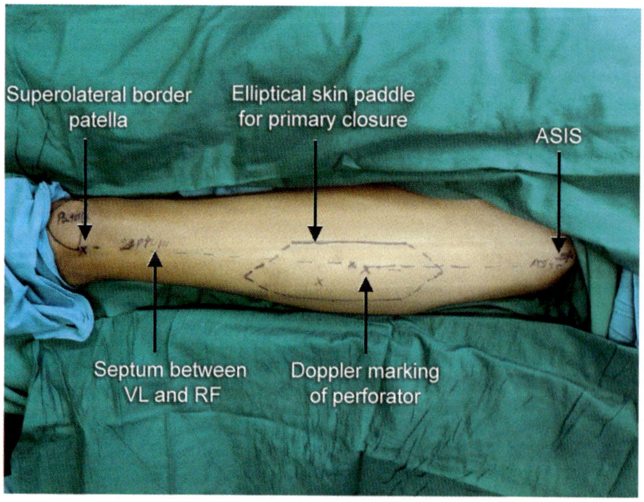

Fig. 1: Preparation of the thigh and marking of the ALT flap VL: Vastus lateralis; RF: Rectus femoris; ASIS: Anterior superior iliac spine

primary closure of the donor. If larger flap is needed and precludes primary closure of donor, flap can be planned in reverse as per the defect and centered around the best perforator.

Anterior Incision and Subfascial Approach

We prefer the anterior incision first and Subfascial approach. It enables the visualization of septocutaneous and some musculocutaneous perforators early in course of surgery. Conversion to Anteromedial thigh (AMT) or Tensor fascia lata (TFL) flap is easy. Relocating the flap superiorly or inferiorly is also more convenient **(Fig. 2)**.

Once the incision is made on the deep fascia, the Rectus Femoris is identified by its bipinnate arrangement of fibers around a central raphe **(Fig. 3)**.

RF is then retracted medial to visualize the space/septum between RF and VL **(Fig. 4)**.

Any Septocutaneous perforator should be visualized now **(Fig. 5)**.

If no perforator is visualized the deep fascia should be dissected off the VL muscle to search for a perforator. If still no perforator is visualized incision can be extended superiorly or inferiorly and perforator searched for. Dissection can also proceed medial to search a medial perforator for AMT flap, or way proximal for a TFL perforator flap **(Fig. 6)**.

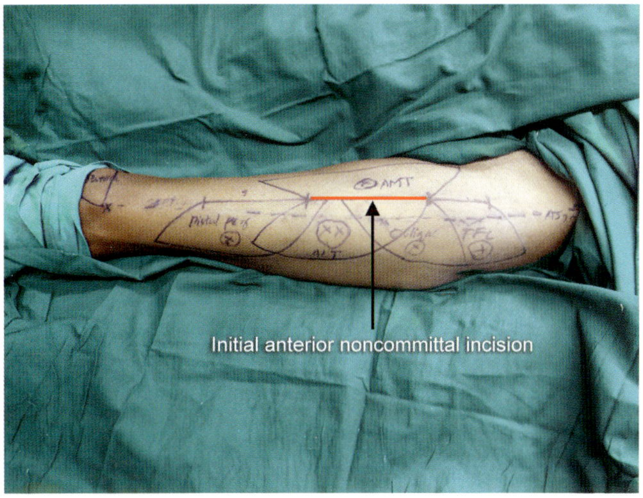

Fig. 2: Anterior noncommittal incision permitting flexibility in flap design

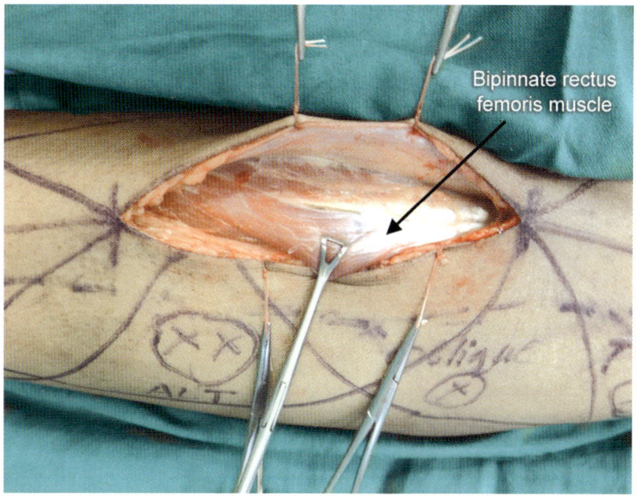

Fig. 3: Rectus muscle identification

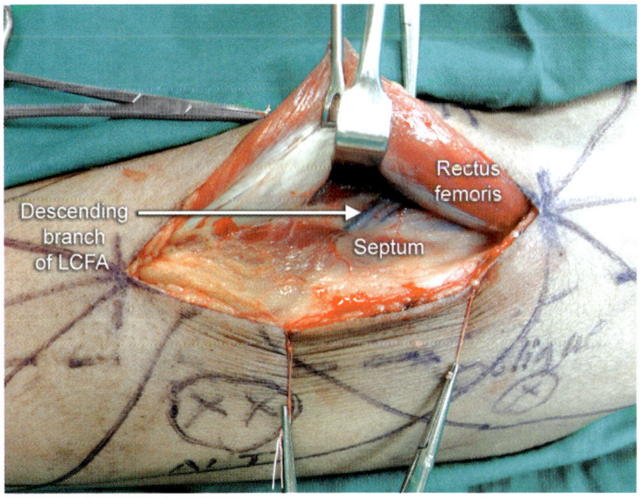

Fig. 4: Septum between RF and VL
LCFA: Lateral circumflex femoral artery

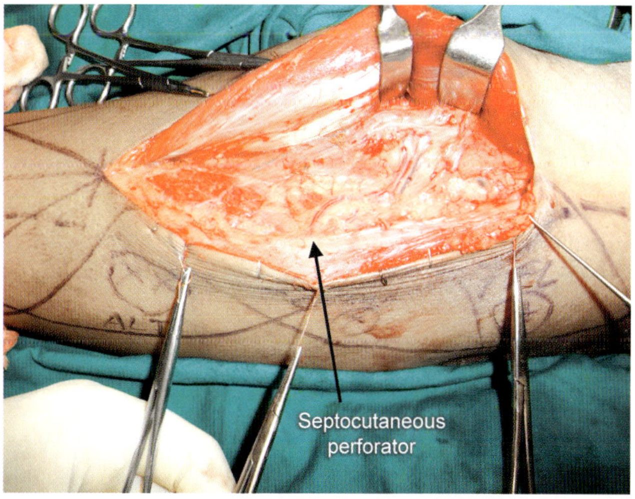

Fig. 5: Septocutaneous perforator

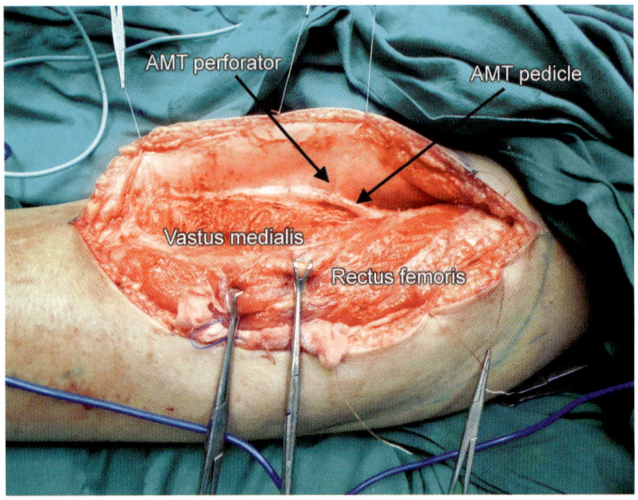

Fig. 6: AMT perforator medial to the rectus muscle
AMT: Anteromedial thigh

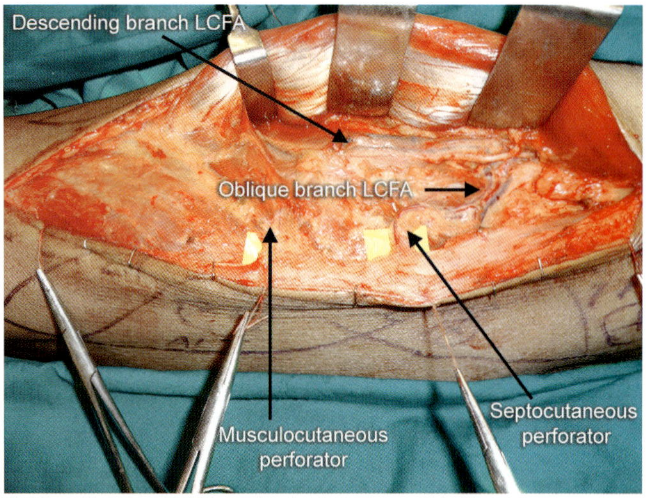

Fig. 7: Musculocutaneous and septocutaneous perforators
LCFA: Lateral circumflex femoral artery

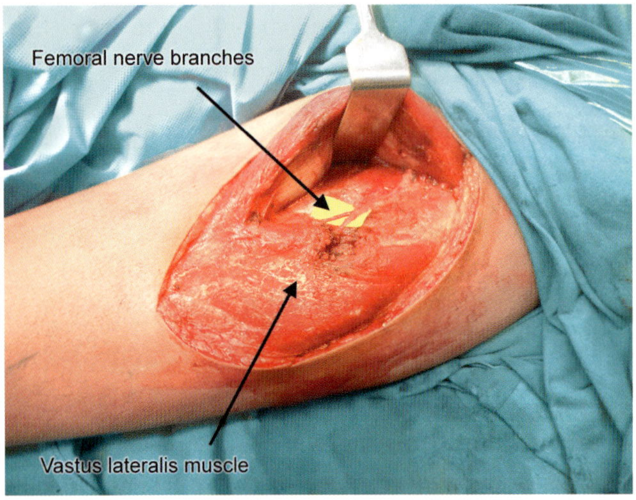

Fig. 8: Preserved nerve and muscle after septocutaneous perforator dissection

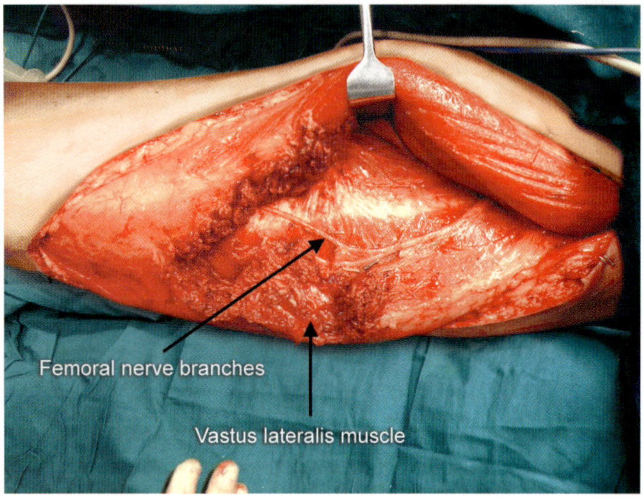

Fig. 9: Preserved nerves and muscle split for deroofing and dissecting musculocutaneous perforator

Perforator to Pedicle Dissection

The perforator is searched for, found, then only the dissection proceeds.

The perforator/s is dissected to its source pedicle, irrespective of its course septocutaneous or musculocutaneous **(Fig. 7)**.

Muscle and Nerve Preservation

All possible nerves to vastus lateralis and the muscle itself should be preserved. This is only possible when the perforators are dissected without any muscle harvest **(Figs. 8 and 9)**.

Should you Harvest VL Muscle with ALT?

Unless muscle is needed for functional muscle transfer or for bulk/filler in an extremely thin thigh, there is no indication for harvesting VL with ALT.

Vastus lateralis (VL) harvest, does not assure perforator harvest or protection. Any amount of muscle cannot guarantee safe harvest of a perforator, unless it is seen clearly and harvested cleanly. The variable course in muscle of perforators and tricky paths to reach their source pedicle, make any harvest without visualization of the perforator dangerous. This is often responsible for situations where the anastomosis is patent, VL surviving but the skin paddle is lost. There is also an incidence of partial necrosis as the best perforator is injured and only minor perforator sustaining the skin paddle.

We do concede that we were recommending VL harvest with ALT for presumption of perforator capture and protection, but time and experience have made us change to the above said perforator based approach **(Figs. 10A to D)**.

Perforator based approach ensures inclusion of the vascular soul in the body of the flap. There is also revealed assurance of perforator integrity or injury, thus leaving no ambiguity.

How Large a Flap can you Harvest without Muscle?

Any size if the best/most/needed perforators in the flap are harvested and reperfused. Muscle is incidental, ultimately perforators are the only thing which matter.

If 2 perforators are widely separated and in the flap with different pedicle of origin, supercharging or turbocharging is needed, muscle will not help at al. **(Figs. 11A to D)**.

When to do AMT or TFL Flap?

Sometimes the predominant axis/pedicle of perforator origin in the chosen thigh is medial (AMT pedicle) or proximal (TFL pedicle). In them perforators from the ALT will be absent or few and insignificant. They would not sustain a flap of large or even small size, leading to partial or total flap necrosis in postoperative period. The logical thing to do here is to harvest the flap based on perforators from the vascular axis nature has bestowed the patient's thigh with, AMT or TFL **(Figs. 12 and 13)**.

AMT and TFL can also be used in case of an ALT perforator injury, as a part of chimeric flap or as a matter of choice for a thicker flap.

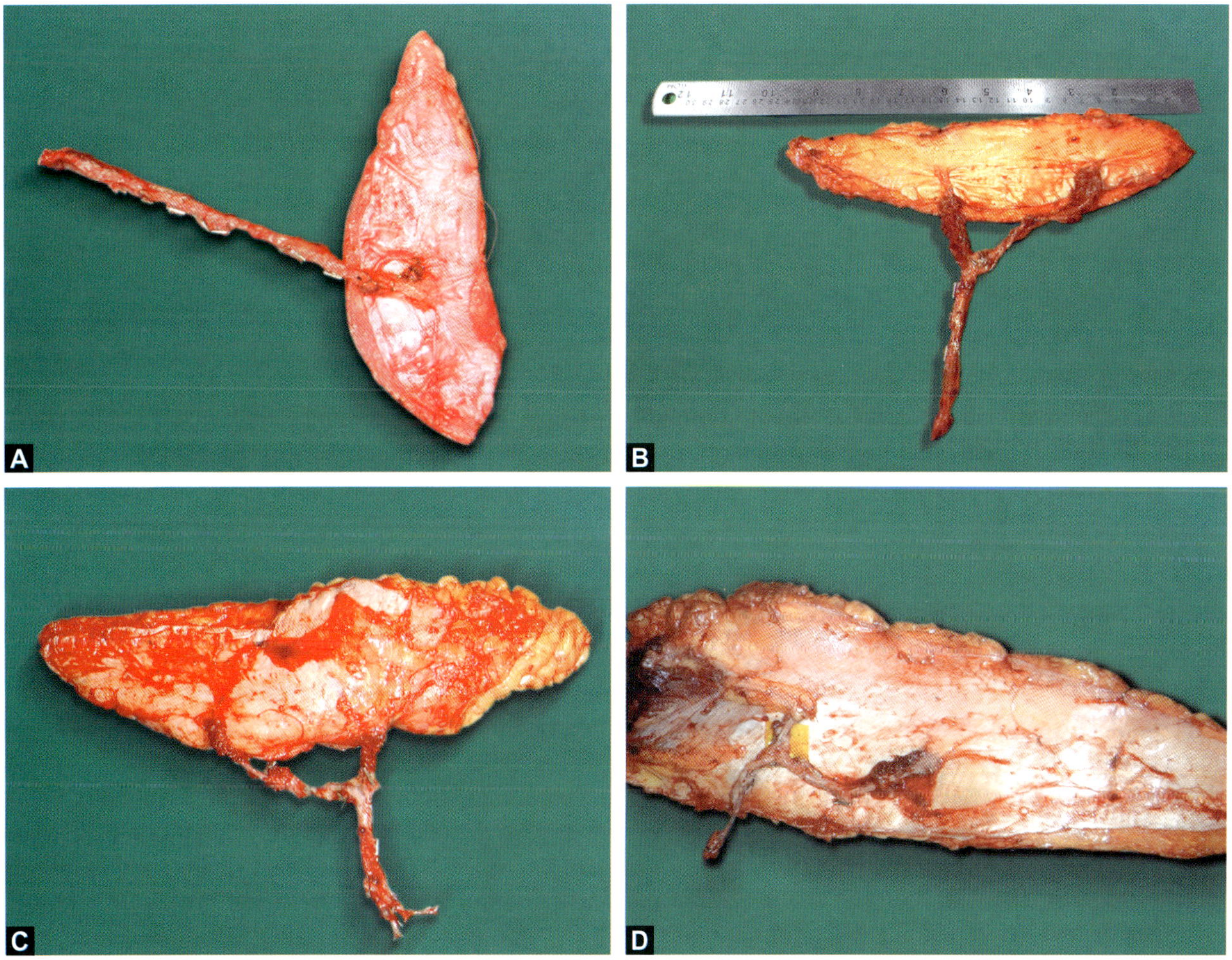

Figs. 10A to D: ALT perforator flap, no vastus lateralis harvest. (A) Septocutaneous perforator; (B) musculocutaneous perforators; (C) musculocutaneous perforator and (D) septocutaneous and 1 musculocutaneous perforator

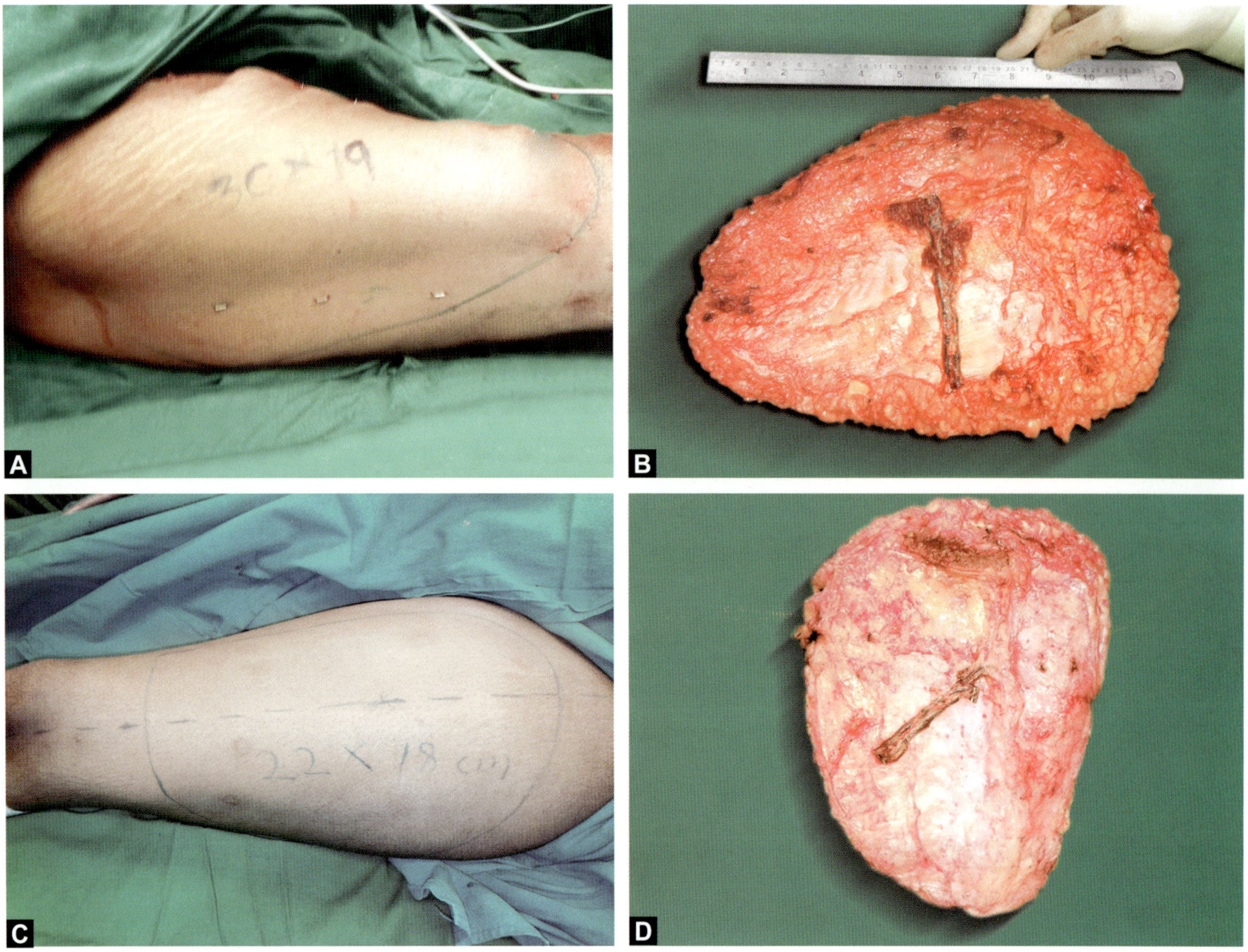

Figs. 11A to D: Large ALT flaps on few perforators, no muscle harvest. (A) 30 × 19 cms flap; (B) single perforator; (C) 22 × 18 cms flap; (D) single perforator

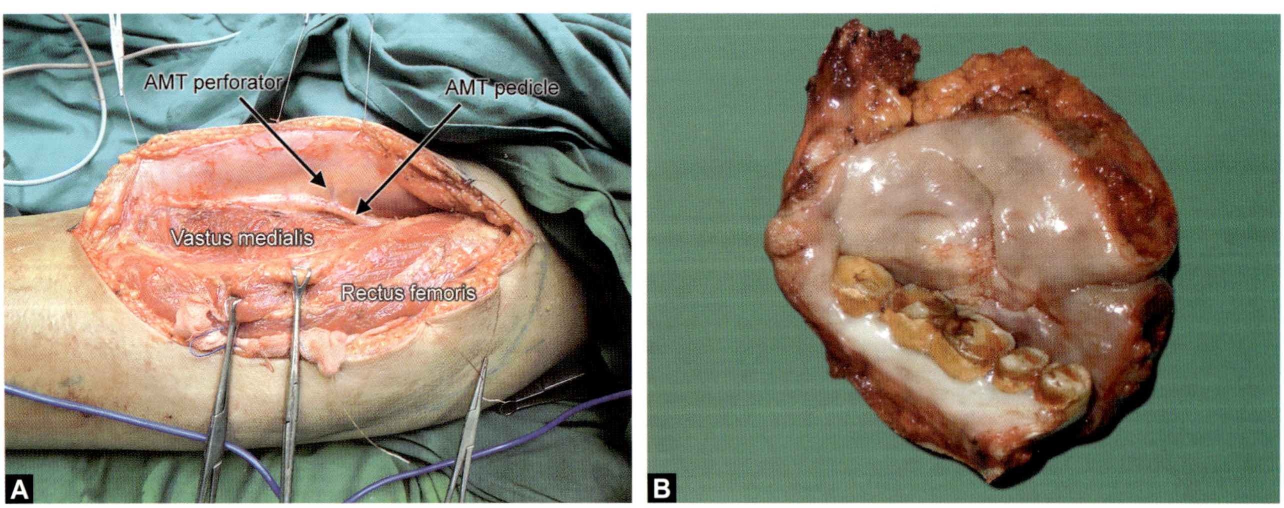

Figs. 12A and B: AMT flap in absence of ALT perforators. (A) Septocutaneous AMT perforartors in absence of ALT perforators; (B) buccal mucosa and skin defect

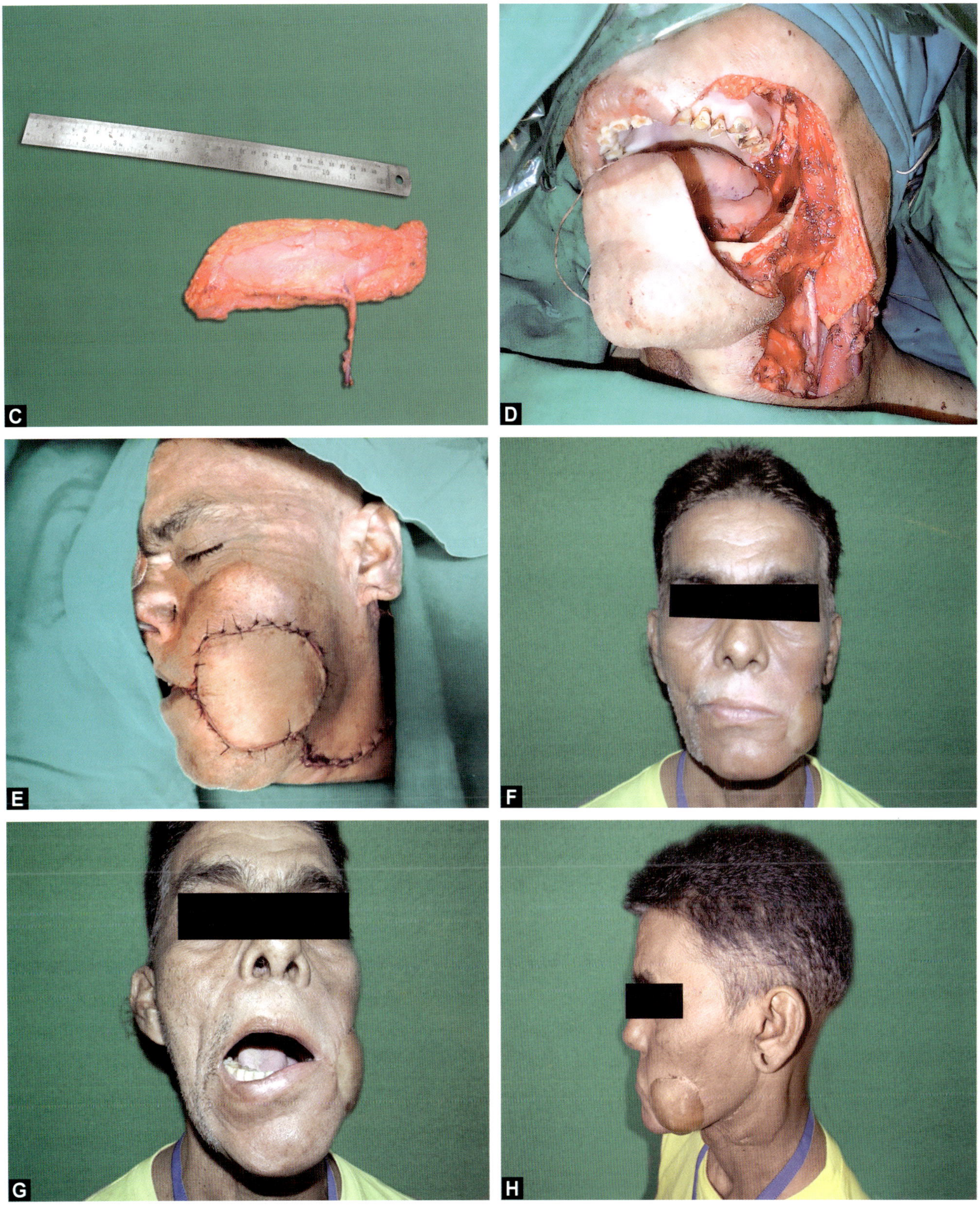

Figs. 12C to H: AMT flap in absence of ALT perforators. (C) AMT flap harvested; (D) defect with marginal mandiblectomy; (E) flap at completion; (F) 1 year postoperative front view; (G) mouth opening after RT; (H) Lateral view

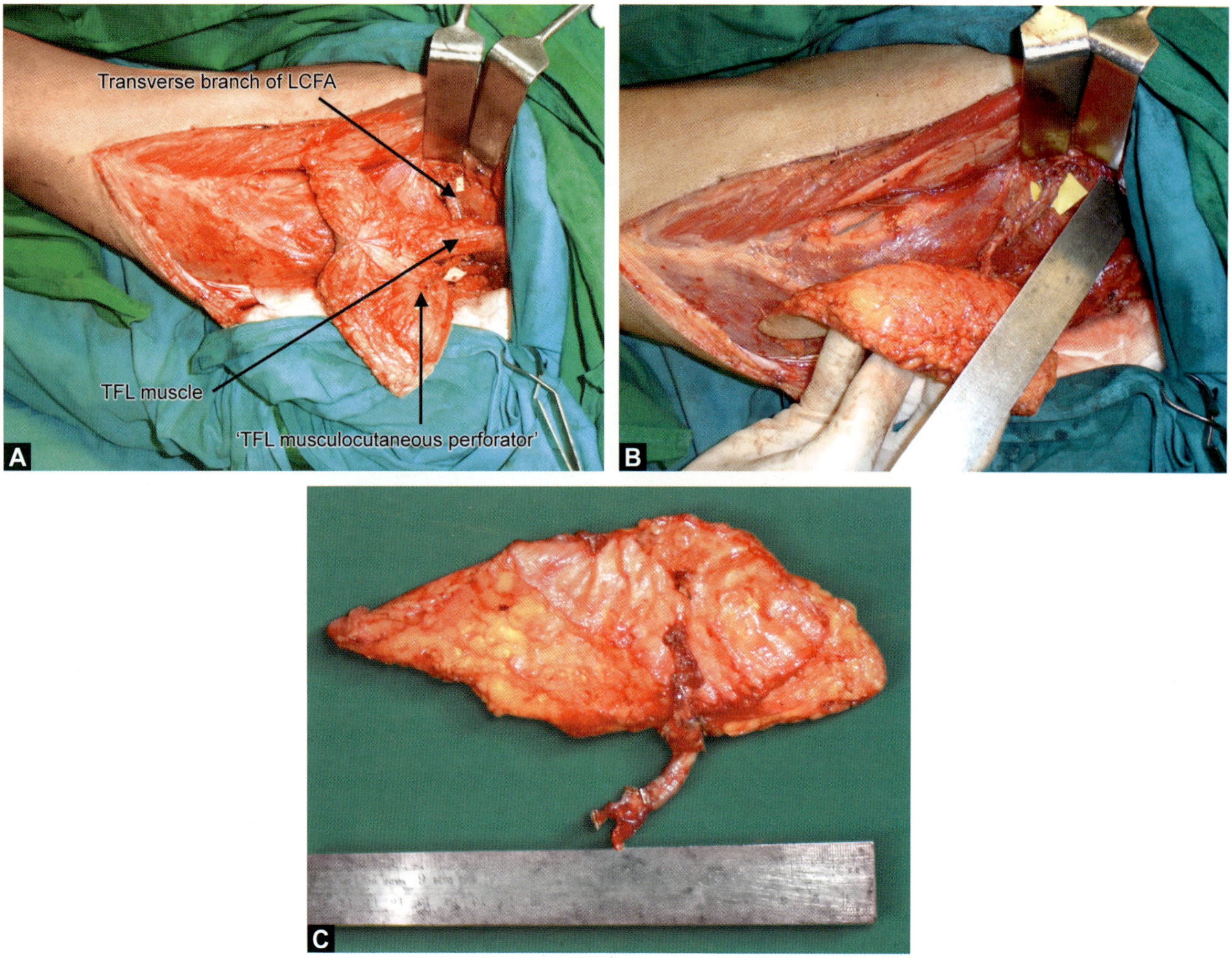

Figs. 13A to C: TFL flap in absence of both ALT and AMT perforators. (A) TFL perforator flap; (B) sufficient pedicle length; (C) TFL intramuscular perforator dissected

The common argument against these two is flap thickness. In Indian patient's thigh is often not as thick and head neck defects often need bulky flaps for fill. Surgical thinning can also be employed to control the thickness.

Chimeric Flaps

Multiple perforators can be harvested with physically separated skin paddles based on them, the perforators joining the same source pedicle.

Chimeric flaps find great utility in complex or composite defects needing multiple skin islands with ability to move differentially for a more assured inset or better cosmetic result.

Chimerism could be on multiple perforators of ALT or ALT + AMT or ALT + TFL **(Figs. 14 and 15)**. For details see chapter on Refinements.

In case the perforators do not meet a single source pedicle, 2 sets of anastomosis can be employed to achieve the same result.

DONOR SITE MANAGEMENT

Most flaps are designed as an ellipse to permit primary closure of the donor site. When relatively large flaps are needed donor, site may need to be covered with a split thickness skin graft. A small STSG is preferable to an excessively tight closure which is certain to dehisce in the postoperative period. A suction drain is placed with primary closure for 48 hrs. The knee is immobilized in extension to relax the closure and stabilize the STSG. Early weight-bearing is started with the splint in place by 4th day. Knee can be flexed in a graduated manner, starting at 2 weeks or earlier, depending on the tension in the primary closure.

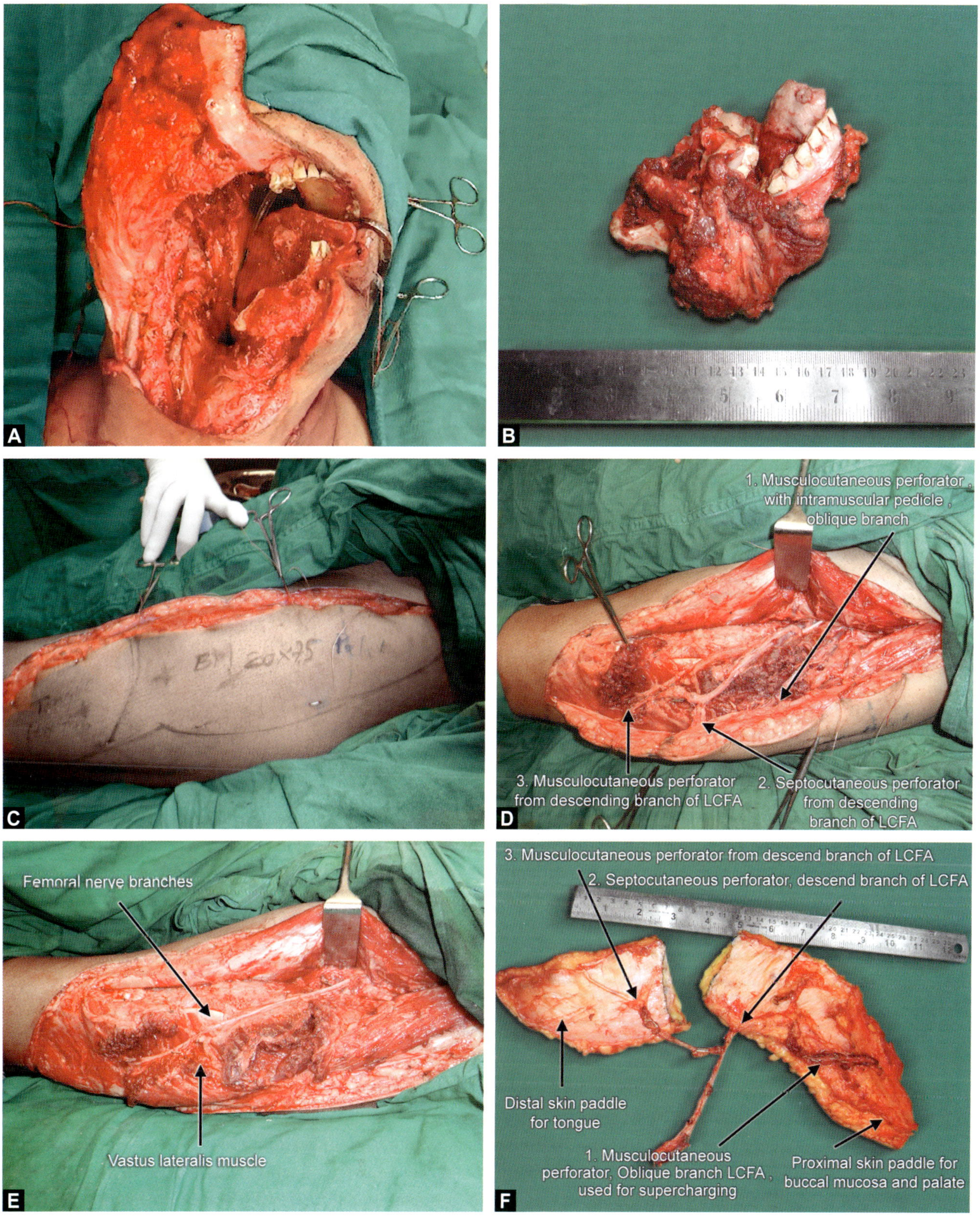

Figs. 14A to F: ALT 2 perforators. (A) Defect hemimandiblectomy, right buccal mucosa, hemiglossectomy, soft palate, left retromolar trigone; (B) specimen; (C) ALT flap planning; (D) resources available, 3 perforators on 2 pedicles; (E) preserved nerves and deroofed but preserved muscle; (F) chimeric flap, 2 skin paddles

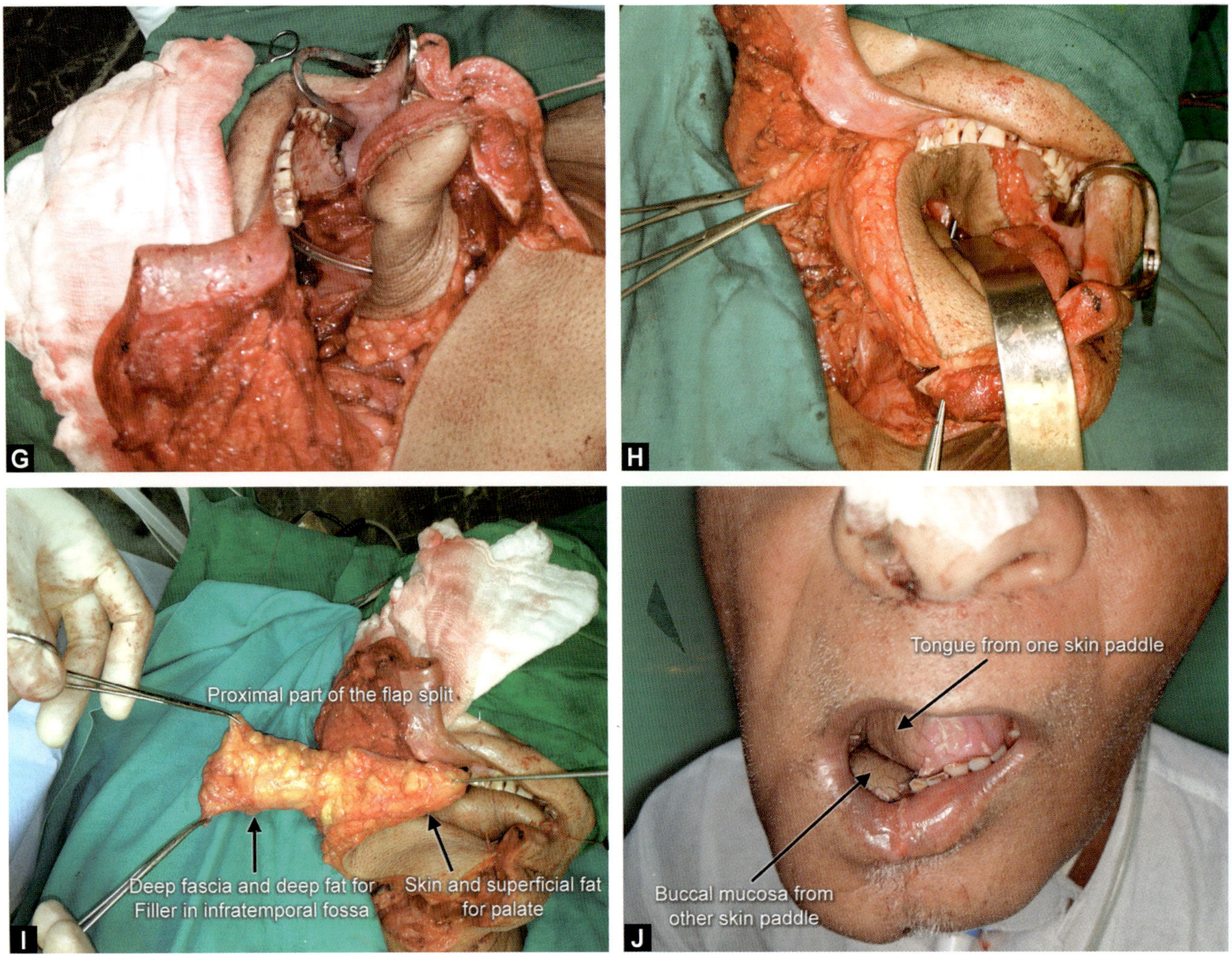

Figs. 14G to J: ALT 2 perforators. (G) Distal skin paddle used for tongue defect; (H) Proximal skin paddle used for buccal mucosa and palate; (I) Proximal most part of the flap split , skin part used for palate and deep fat used for ITF filler; (J) Postoperative

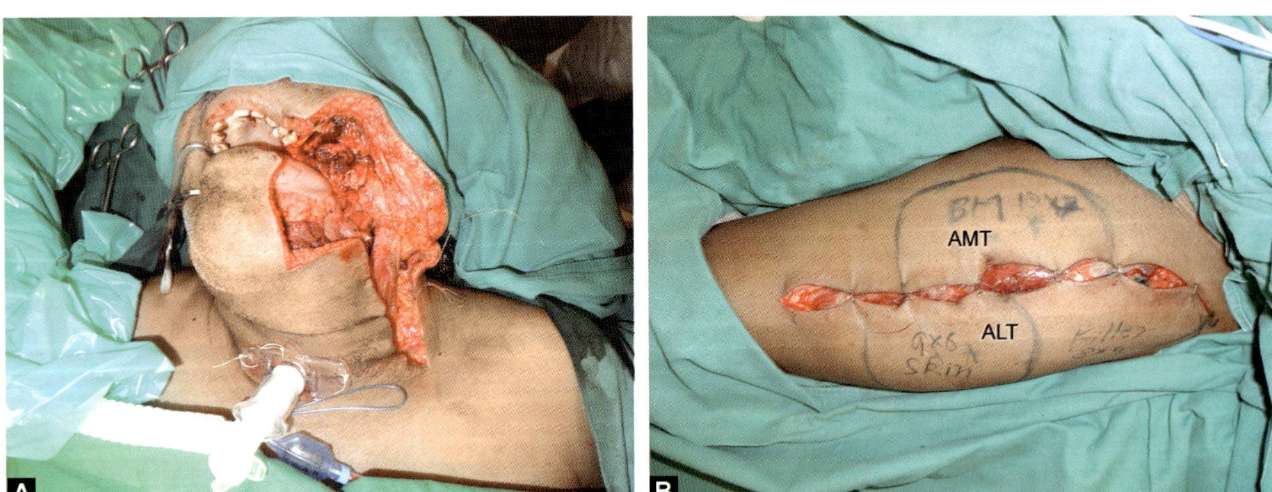

Figs. 15A and B: ALT + AMT. (A) Hemimandiblectomy with large skin and ITF defect; (B) planning of ALT plus AMT flap

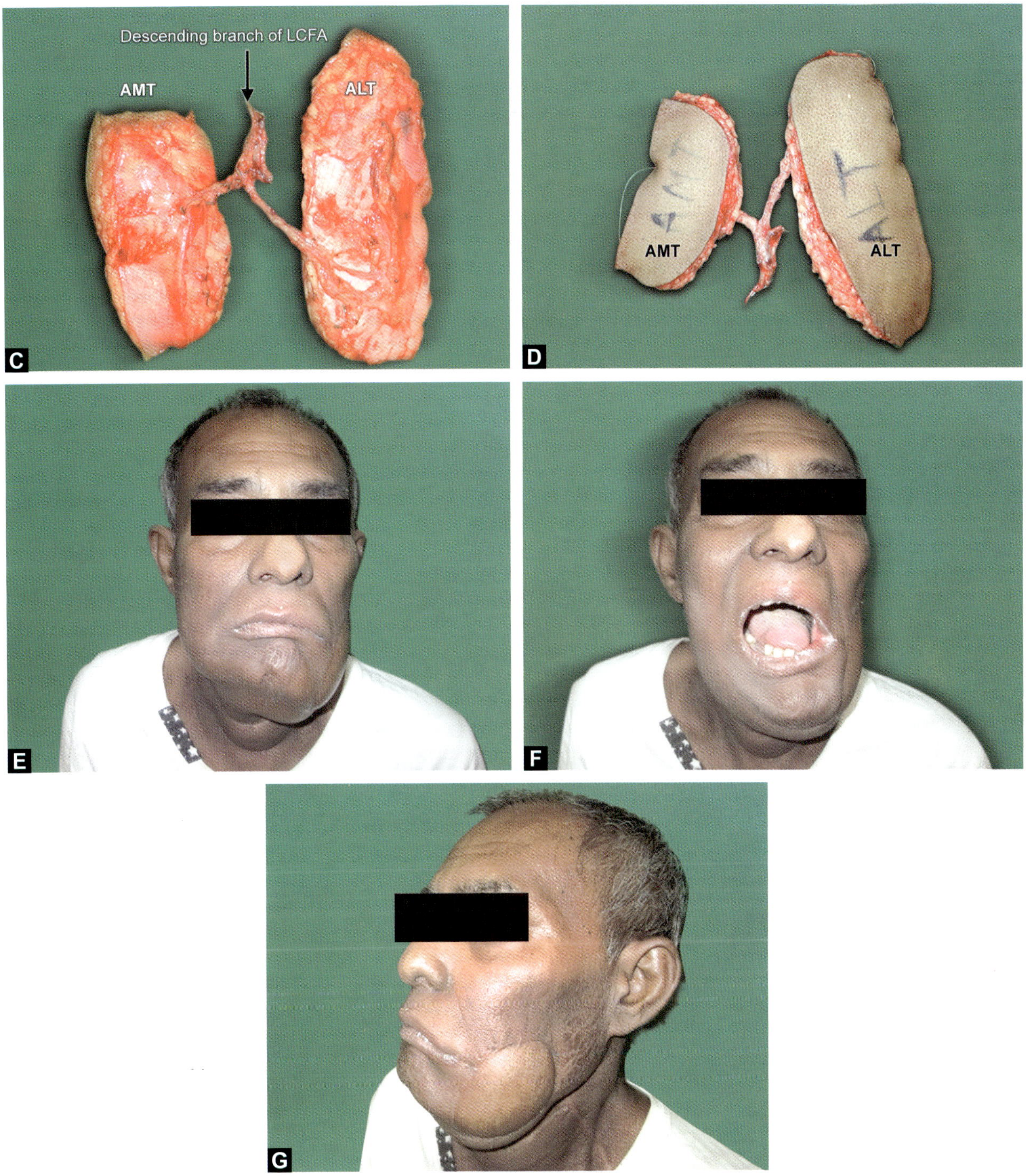

Figs. 15C to G: ALT + AMT. (C) Flap perforators and pedicles joining each other; (D) chimeric skin islands; (E) postoperative; (F) mouth opening; (G) lateral view

INDICATIONS FOR THE ALT FLAP

In our department ALT is the most commonly done free flap. It is the default choice unless otherwise stated for any skin and soft tissue defect, barring a few exceptions. Listed below are our most common uses of ALT in our department, in order of descending frequency.

1. Buccal mucosa defect lining—whenever there is a thickness associated with the defect as in with marginal mandiblectomy, posterior segmental mandiblectomy,

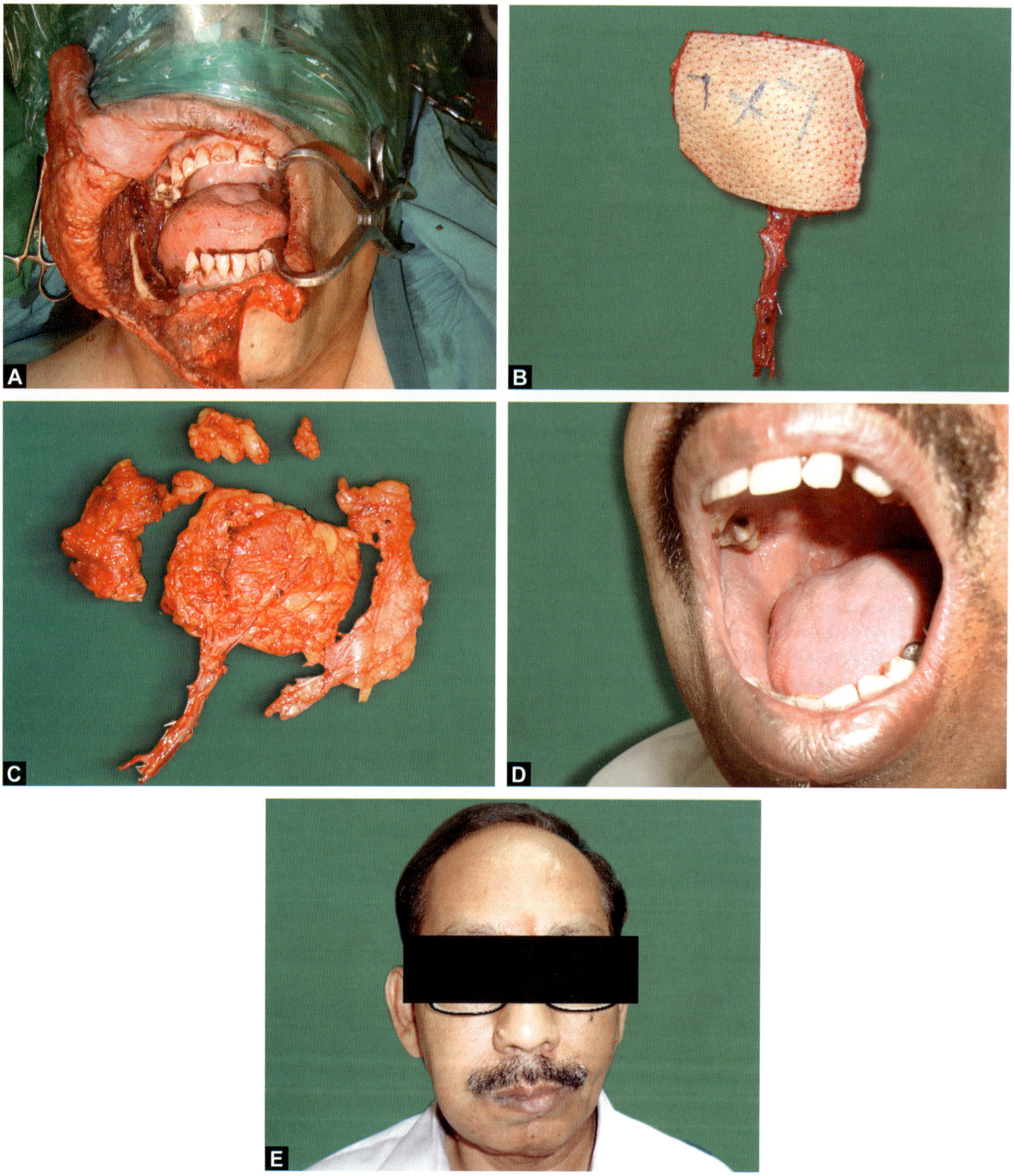

Figs. 16A to E: Buccal mucosa. (A) Buccal mucosa , RMT and marginal mandiblectomy defect; (B) ALT flap 7 × 7cms; (C) Surgical thinning for countouring; (D) Late postoperative with mucosalized flap; (E) Good contour preservation unlike a thin pliable flap

ITF clearance, upper alveolectomy to maxillectomy **(Figs. 16A to E)**.

2. Composite Buccal mucosa and skin defect **(Figs. 17A to D)**, Lip defect **(Figs. 17E to G)**.
3. Skin and soft tissue defect of Head Neck—any surface defect parotid, scalp, orbital Exentration **(Figs. 18 to 20)**.
4. Pharyngeal reconstruction—rarely as a patch or tube for restoring oesophageal continuity **(Figs. 21A to D)**.

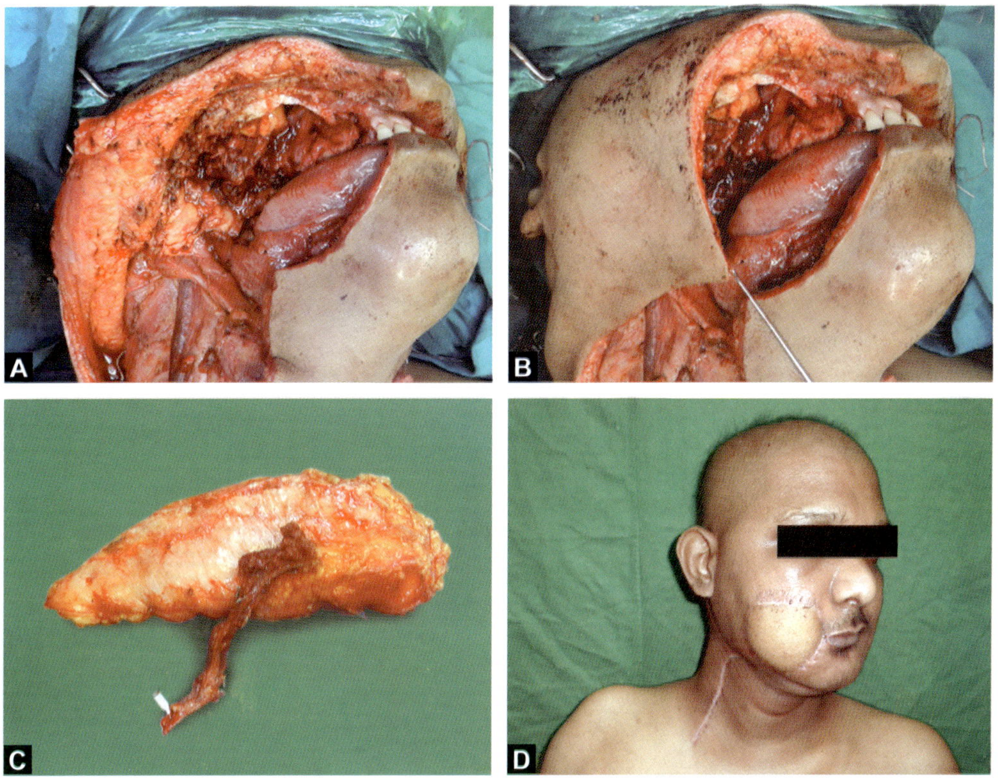

Figs. 17A to D: Buccal mucosa + skin. (A) Hemimandiblectomy and upper alveolectomy; (B) associated skin excision; (C) ALT flap on 1 musculocutaneous perforator; (D) postoperative

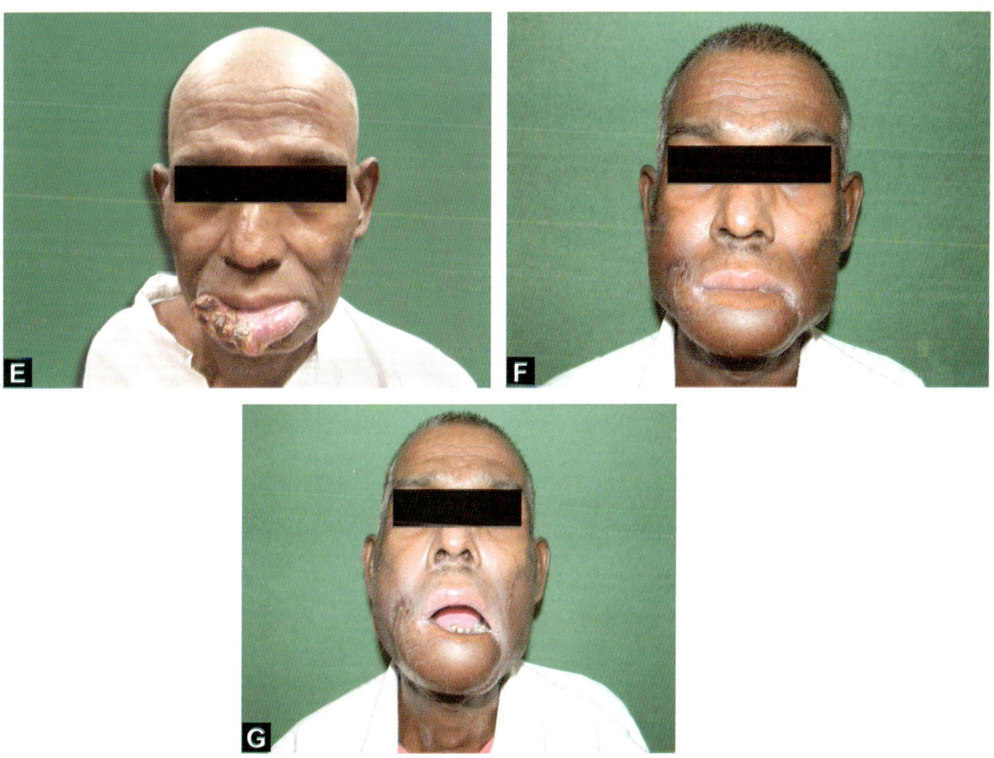

Figs. 17E to G: ALT for lip defect. (E) Fungating lip lesion; (F) ALT flap for Lower Lip with good competence; (G) good mouth opening

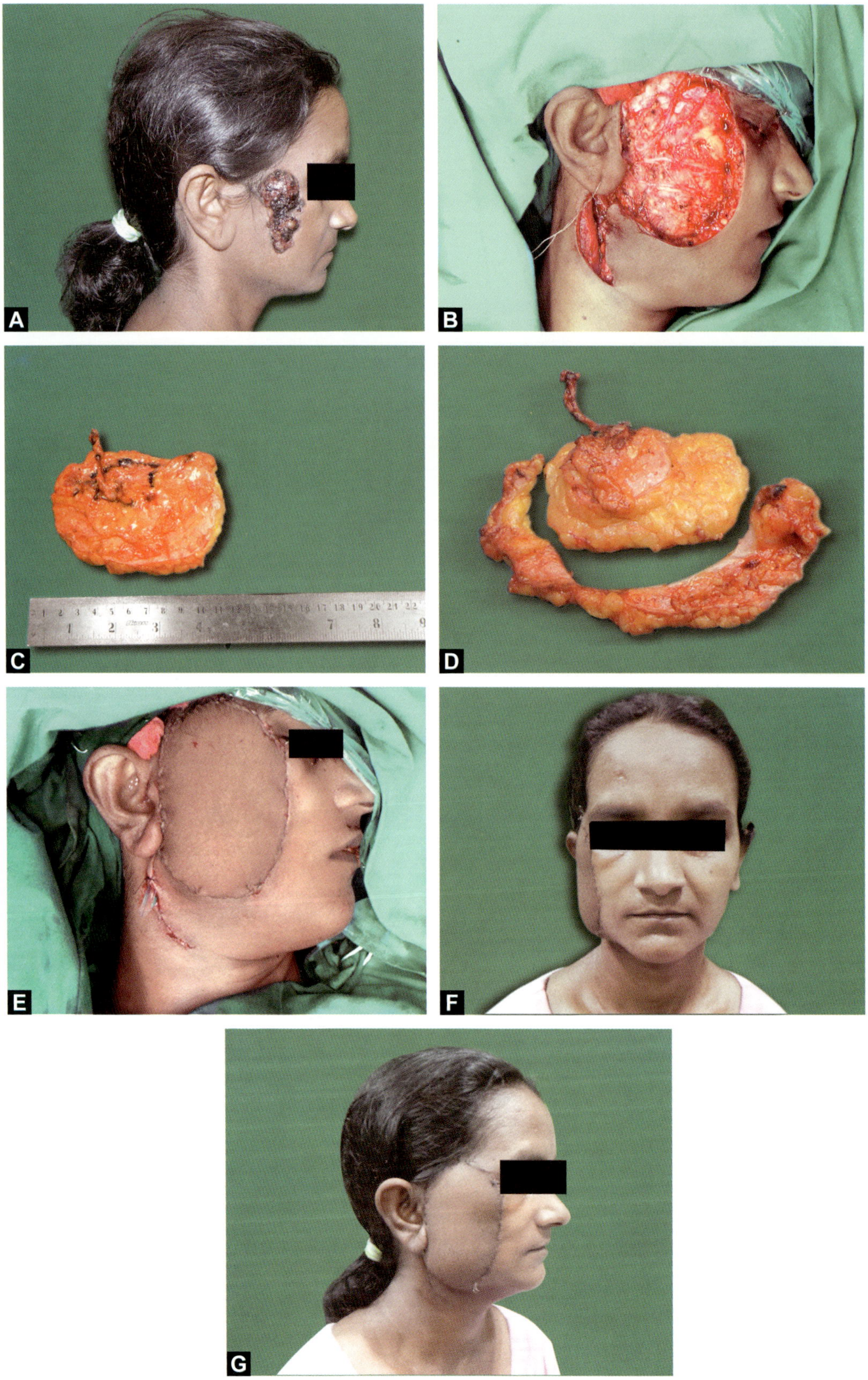

Figs. 18A to G: ALT for parotid. (A) Skin malignancy, parotidectomy with skin excision; (B) defect with facial nerve intact; (C) harvested ALT flap; (D) surgically thinned flap; (E) at completion of surgery; (F and G) late follow-up

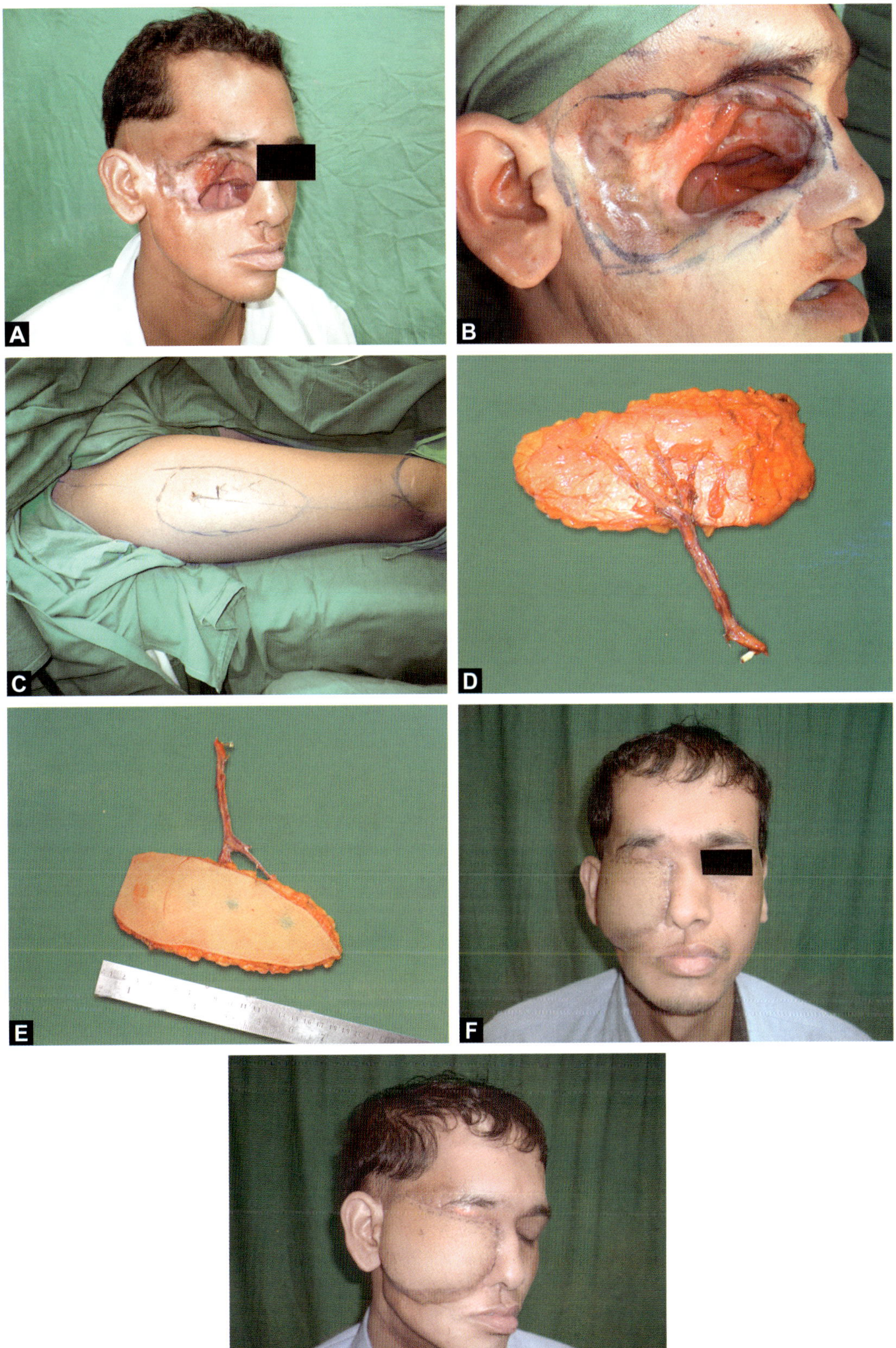

Figs. 19A to G: ALT for orbital exentration. (A) orbital exentration, breakdown after RT; (B) defect creation; (C) ALT flap planned; (D) 3 musculocutaneous perforator in ALT; (E) harvested ALT flap; (F and G) late follow-up

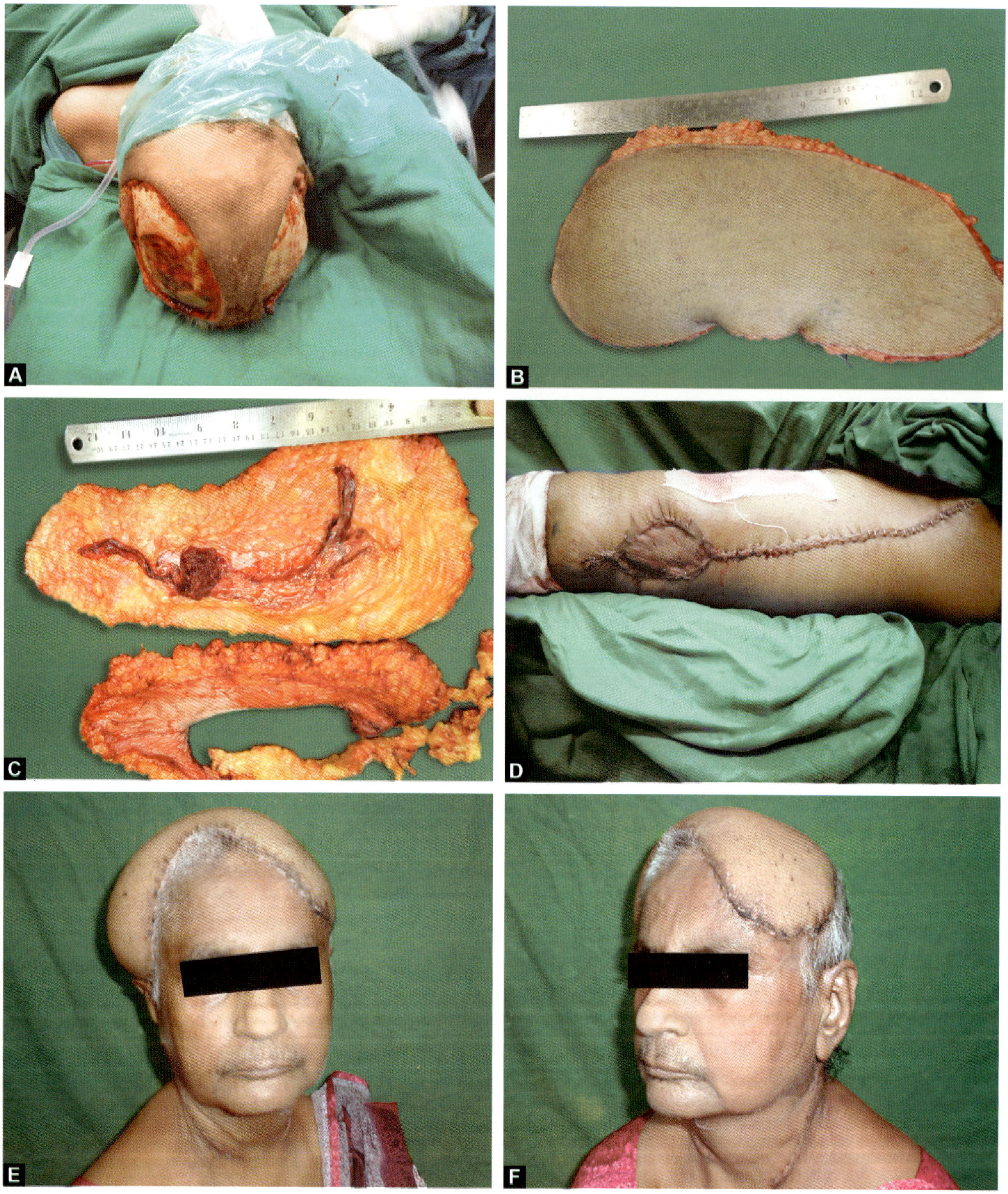

Figs. 20A to F: ALT for scalp. (A) Bilateral scalp defect following excision of angiosarcoma; (B) Harvested ALT flap 30 x 13 cm, with 2 perforators from different pedicles; (C) ALT flap thinned surgically from 900 gm to 600 gm; (D) Donor site 30 × 13 cm almost closed primarily, only 7 × 5 cm skin graft; (E and F) Follow-up

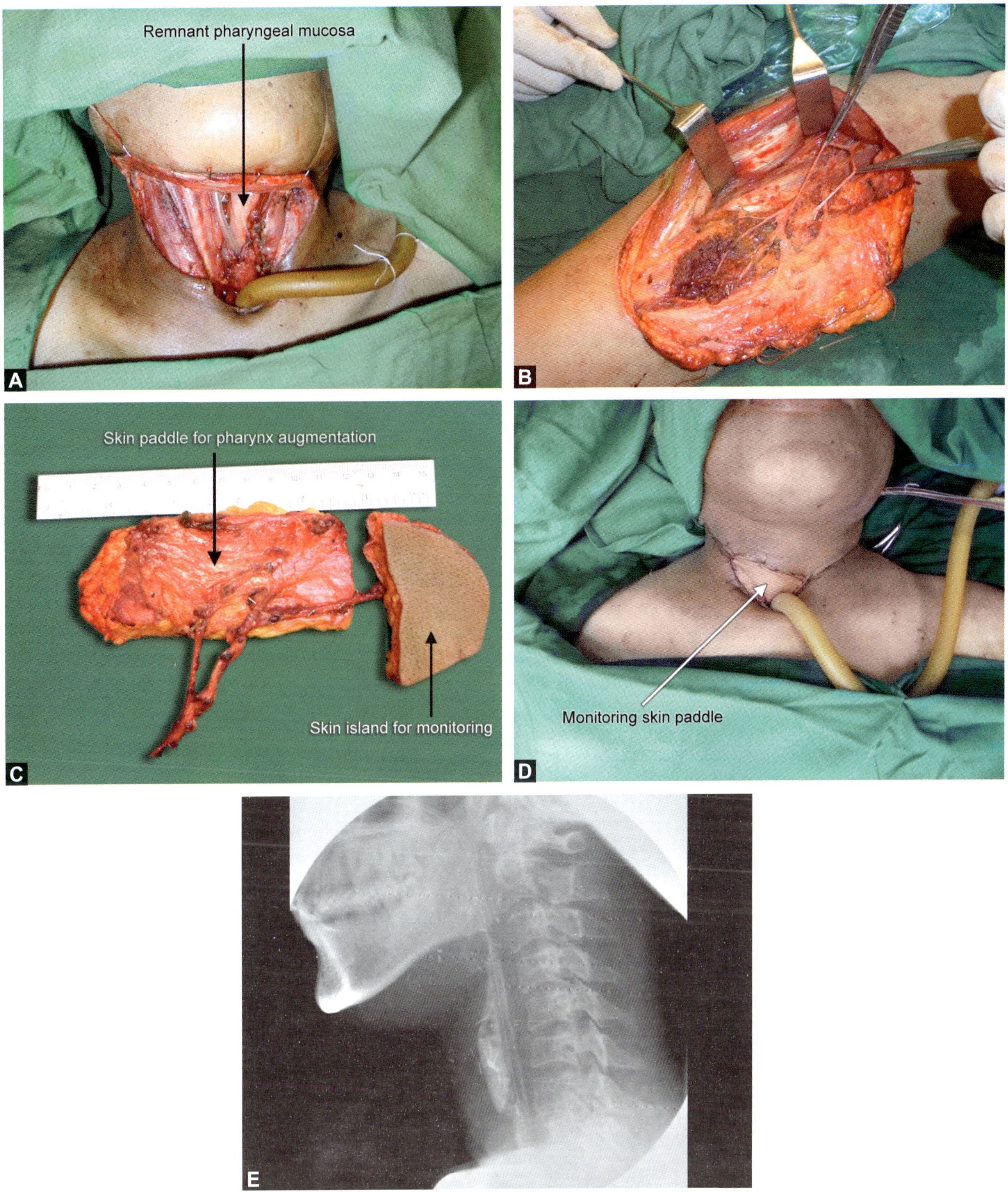

Figs. 21A to E: ALT for patch pharynx. (A) Total laryngectomy with partial pharyngectomy; (B) chimeric flap planned, one skin paddle for Pharynx, other for skin defect and monitoring; (C) Harvested chimeric ALT; (D) immediate postoperative; (E) conray image at 2 weeks showing no leak

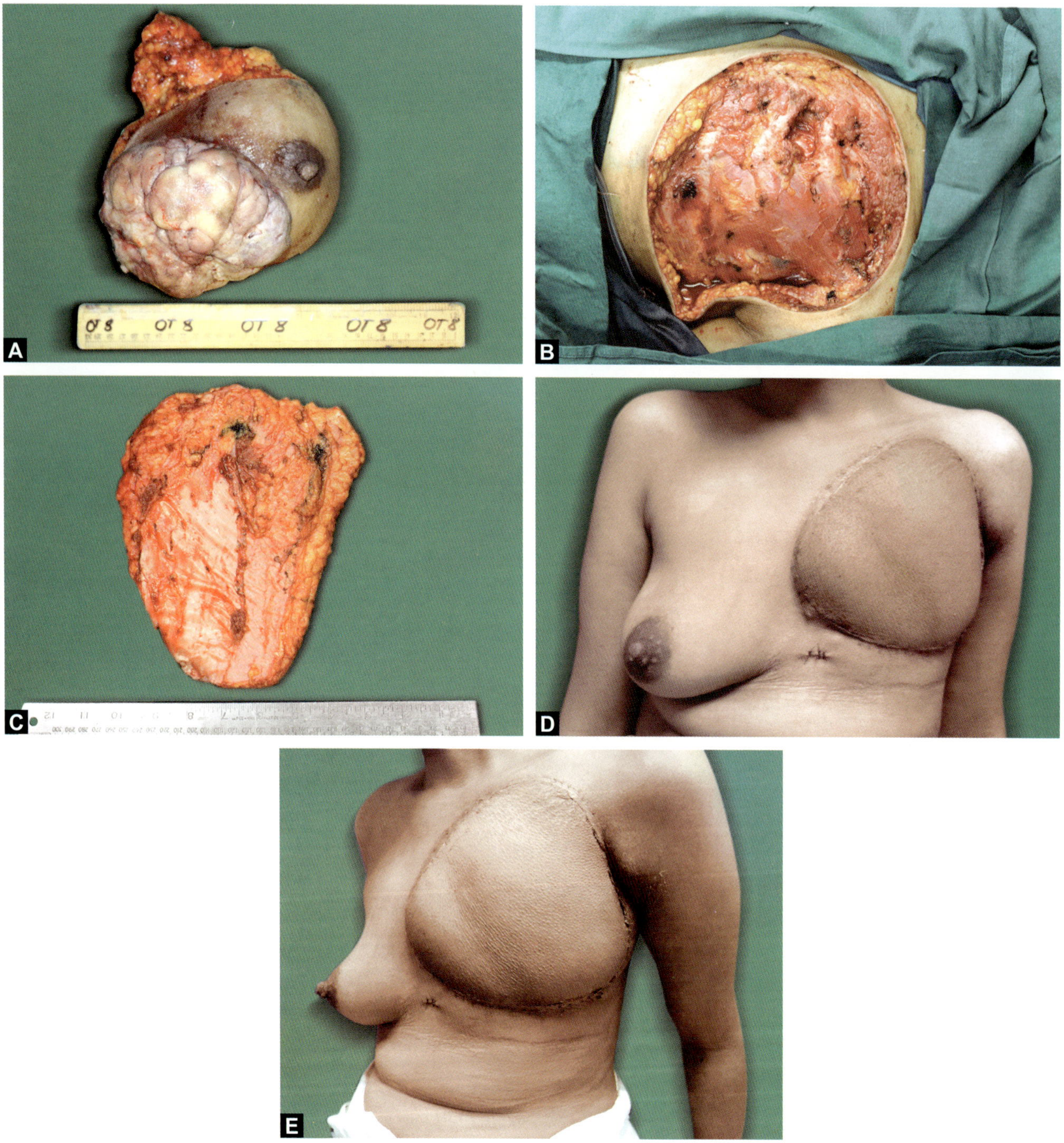

Figs. 22A to E: ALT for chest wall. (A) Radical mastectomy specimen; (B) large surface defect; (C) 25 Ú 18 cm ALT, no muscle harvest; (D and E) postoperative

5. Chest wall cover—generally after a recurrent carcinoma breast or a very large primary tumour, sometimes with a rigid chest wall reconstruction **(Figs. 22A to E)**.
6. Upper limb, lower limb—cover exposed orthopaedic implants or after soft tissue sarcoma excision **(Figs. 23 and 24)**.
7. Pedicle flap for groin defects after groin node dissection with skin excision. It can also be used for pelvis and perineal defects

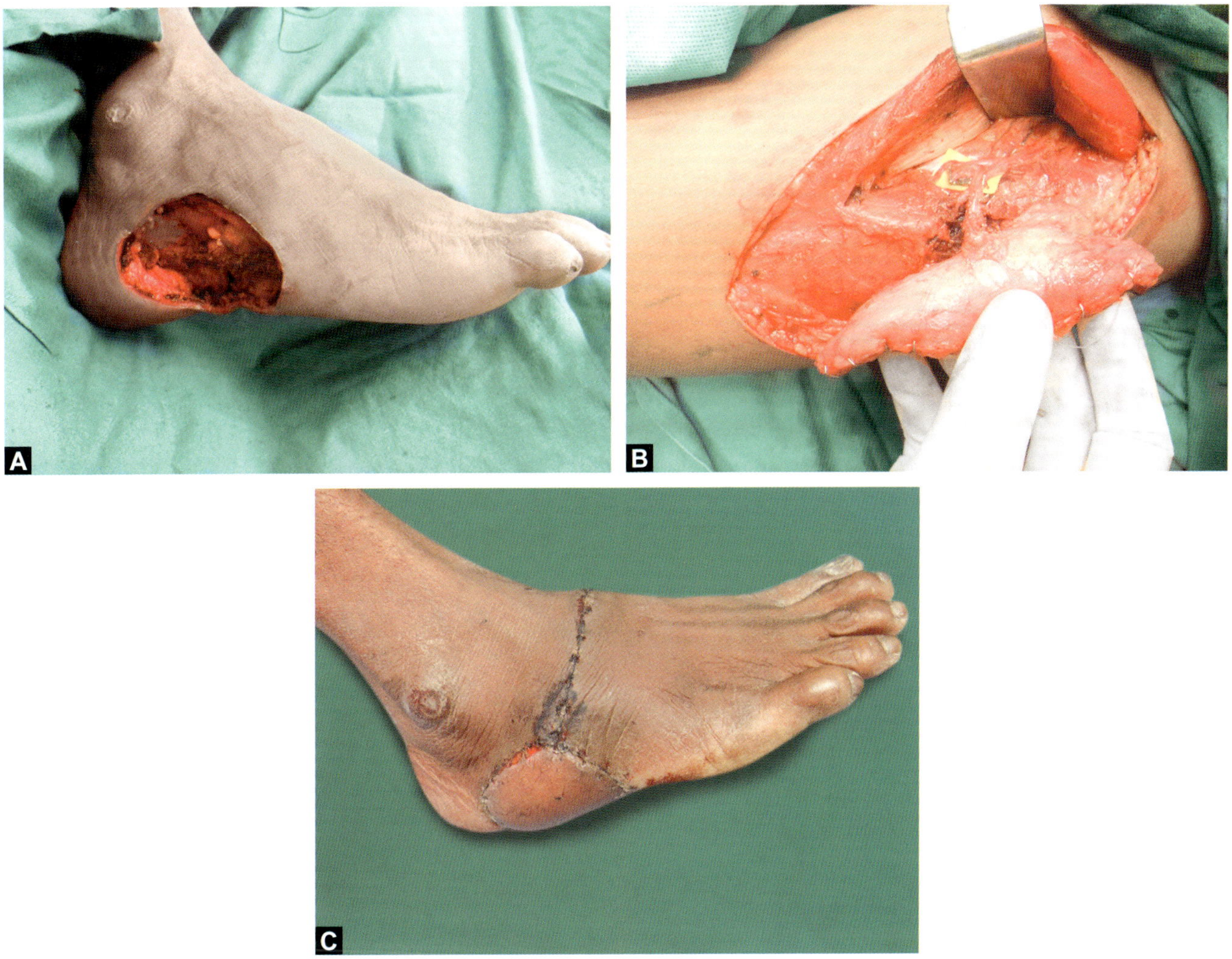

Figs. 23A to C: ALT for LL. (A) Foot defect around 7 × 5 cm; (B) septocutaneous perforator in ALT; (C) postoperative

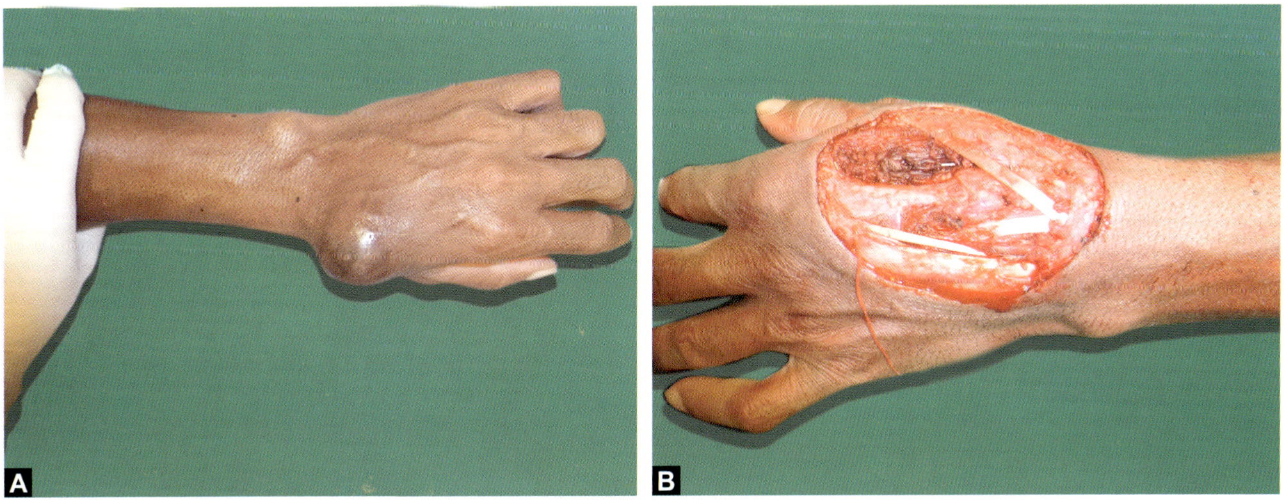

Figs. 24A and B: ALT for UL. (A) Hand sarcoma; (B) defect after excision

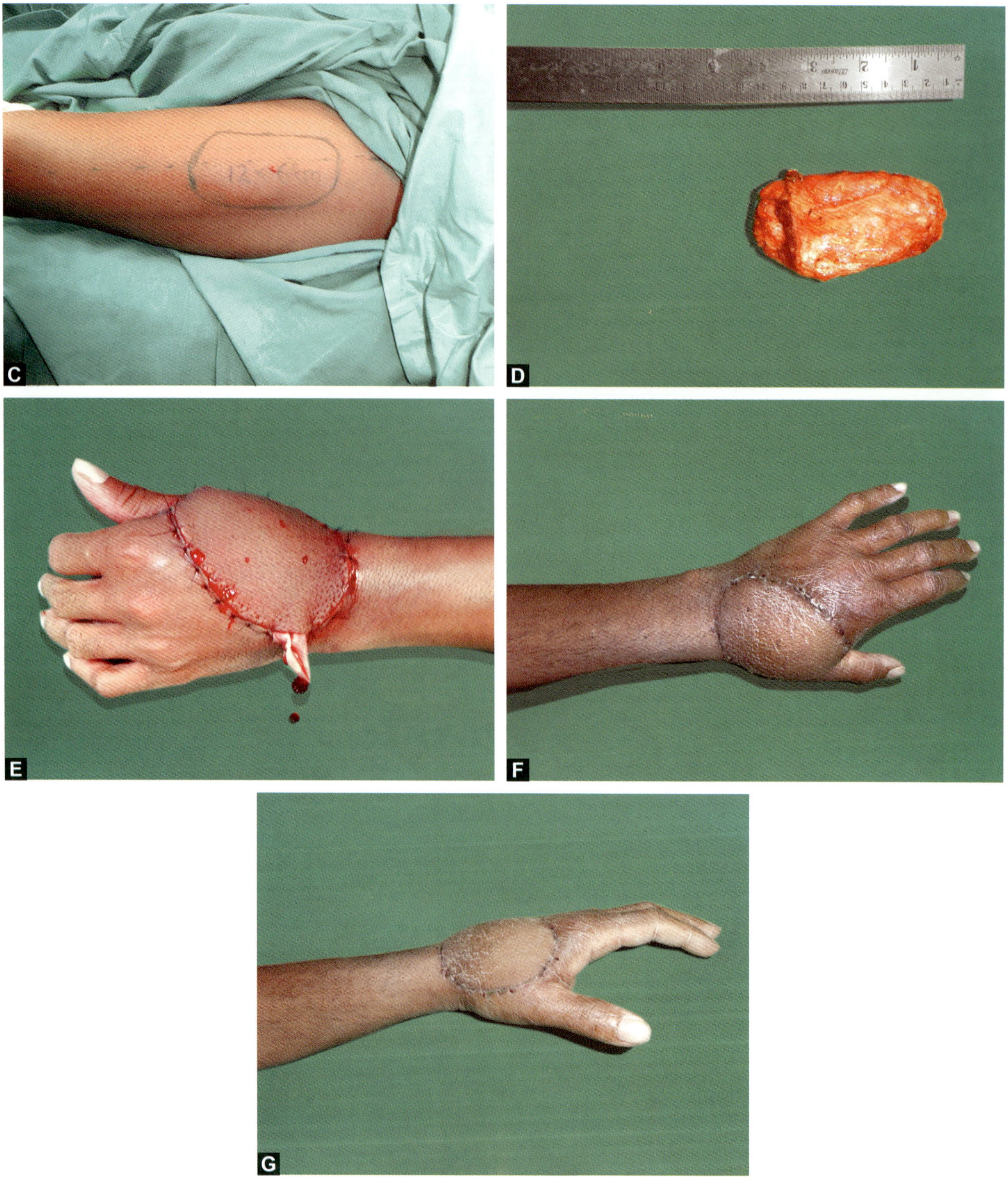

Figs. 24C to G: ALT for UL. (C) ALT flap planned, 12 × 6 cm; (D) harvested flap; (E) immediate postoperative; (F) late follow-up; (G) late follow-up

CHAPTER 7

Free Fibula Flap

Prabha Yadav, Tasneem Belgaumwala

INTRODUCTION

Free Fibula Osteocutaneous flap (FFOCF) is our flap of choice when bony reconstruction is needed. It is used as such for long bone reconstruction or contoured for mandible and maxilla. Fibula is an expendable bone as it has no direct role in weight-bearing. It provides adequate length of cortical bone with sizeable pedicle length and vessel caliber for microvascular anastomosis. Associated skin paddle can be harvested for addressing the skin defect. Soleus or flexor hallucis muscle is harvested in case additional soft tissue needs to be reconstructed. Dual blood supply of the fibula bone enables multiple osteotomies. Donor area morbidity is minimal if only bone is harvested.

ANATOMY

The fibula is a long cortical bone not directly involved in weight-bearing. It is quadrangular at the lower end but may be triangular, grooved or quadrangular at the upper end. Proximal articulation is with the tibia alone. The distal articulation with the tibia and the talus is responsible for ankle stability. The shafts of tibia and fibula are connected by an interosseous membrane.

The peroneal artery arises from the tibioperoneal trunk in the distal part of popliteal fossa.

Peroneal vessels come close to the fibula at about 7 to 8 cm from the upper end. It then supplies the fibula at around the midpoint of the bone by an endosteal nutrient artery and multiple segmental, periosteal and septal branches. Peroneal vessels run between the tibialis posterior and flexor hallucis longus muscle in the deep posterior compartment and it travels away from fibula at about 7 to 8 cm from its lower end. It then reaches the inferior tibiofibular syndesmosis, where it divides into calcaneal branches. Peroneal artery gives off some muscular branches that supply the soleus, tibialis posterior, flexor hallucis longus and peroneal muscles. The fibular head receives its blood supply from anterior tibial artery **(Fig. 1)**.

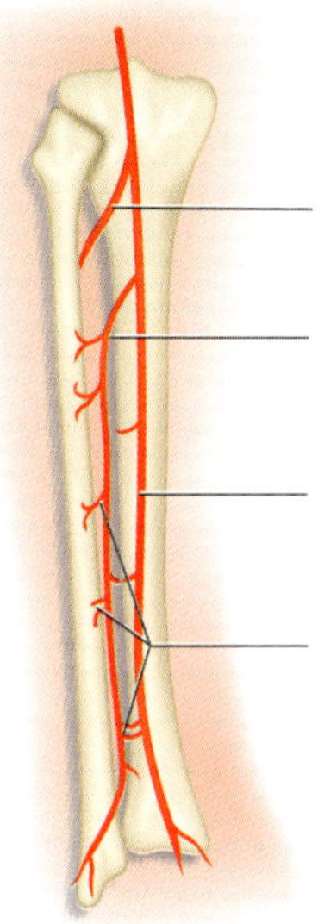

Fig. 1: Blood supply of fibula

The peroneal artery is about 1.5 to 2.5 mm in diameter.

Septocutaneous perforators supplying the overlying skin run along the posterolateral septum attached to the posterior border of fibula. They may have a variable course, running through the flexor hallucis longus or the soleus. Therefore careful dissection of the perforators is required, when muscle sparing harvest is intended. Both the anterior tibial neurovascular bundle (anterior to the interosseous septum) and the posterior tibial neurovascular bundle (deep to the soleus and medial to the flexor hallucis longus muscle) are encountered during the dissection, and a thorough knowledge of the anatomy and careful dissection are important to prevent injury to these structures **(Fig. 2)**.

Perforators supplying skin reach via the posterolateral septum. Almost all skin on lateral side of the leg can be harvested along with the bone flap.

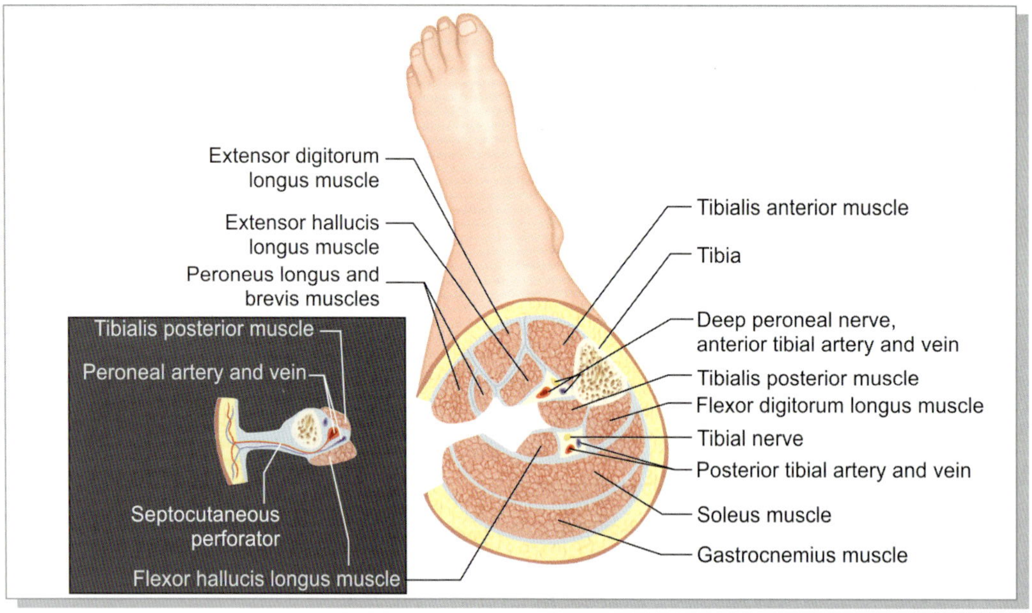

Fig. 2: Cross section of fibula

Advantages of Fibula Flap

- 20 to 30 cm of thick cortical bone
- Long pedicle with adequate vessel diameter for microvascular anastomosis
- Reliable skin paddle
- Ease of harvest
- Good hemostasis with minimal blood loss since harvested under tourniquet control
- Simultaneous harvest is possible
- Expendable bone with relatively less donor site morbidity, especially if only bone is harvested
- Bone unites well with native bone even in compromised situations like post radiotherapy.
- Implant-based dental rehabilitation is possible

Preoperative Evaluation

- Clinical history to rule out peripheral vascular and deep vein thrombosis.
- Palpate dorsalis pedis and posterior tibial artery pulsations.
- In case of doubt color Doppler is advised to check and confirm triphasic flow in anterior tibial, posterior tibial and peroneal artery. CT angiography is not done as a routine. It is advised in case of previous trauma.
- Quality and adequacy of skin and soft tissue is noted as per anticipated defect to assess for requirement of second free flap

Contraindications

- Severe peripheral vascular disease
- Prior trauma precluding flap harvest
- Peronea magna.

FLAP HARVEST

The fibula may be harvested as bone only or along with skin paddle. Some muscle in the form of flexor hallucis longus or part of soleus is harvested along with flap.

- Harvest is done in supine position with flexion at the hip and knee joint
- Placing a pillow beneath the ipsilateral hip prevents straightening of leg during flap harvest
- Stabilize the leg by tying the ipsilateral knee across the OT table to prevent it from falling over
- Tourniquet is applied at mid-thigh level **(Figs. 3A and B)**.

Marking

- Mark outline of the fibula and the posterolateral septum
- Mark osteotomy sites, leaving 6 cm from upper end to protect the lateral peroneal nerve, and 6 cm from the lower end to retain ankle stability.
- Use Doppler to localize the perforators. Mark anterior extent of the skin paddle with approximate width as per defect requirement **(Fig. 4)**.

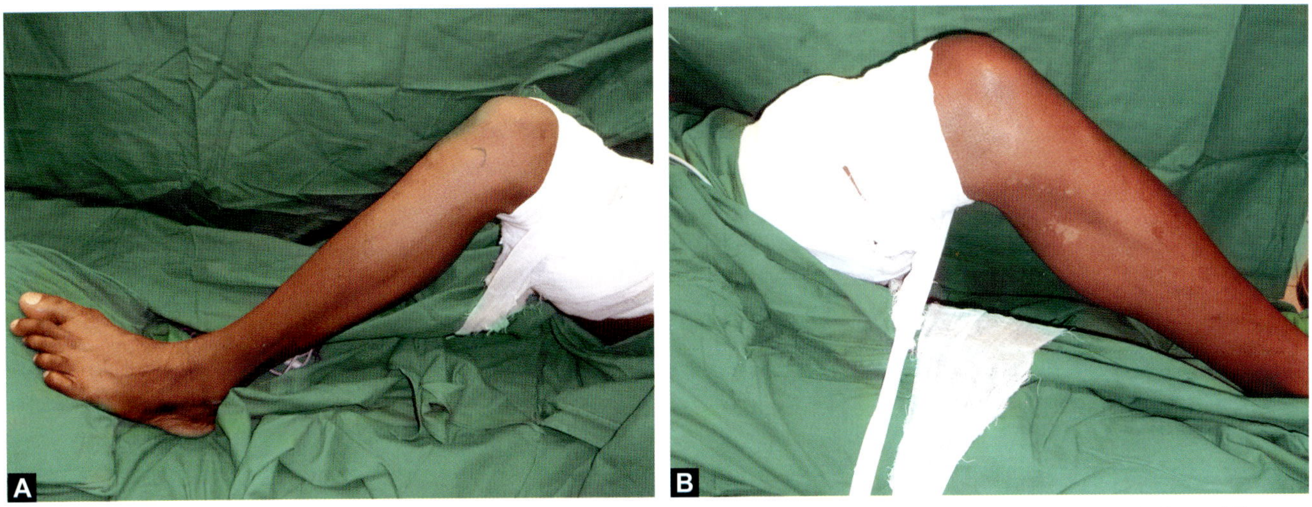

Figs. 3A and B: (A) Tourniquet application and leg position for fibula harvest; (B) leg tied to opposite side of table for stability

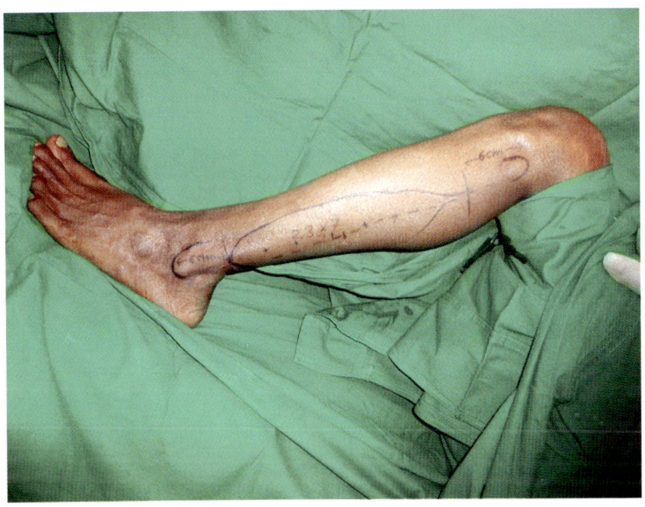

Fig. 4: Marking of skin paddle

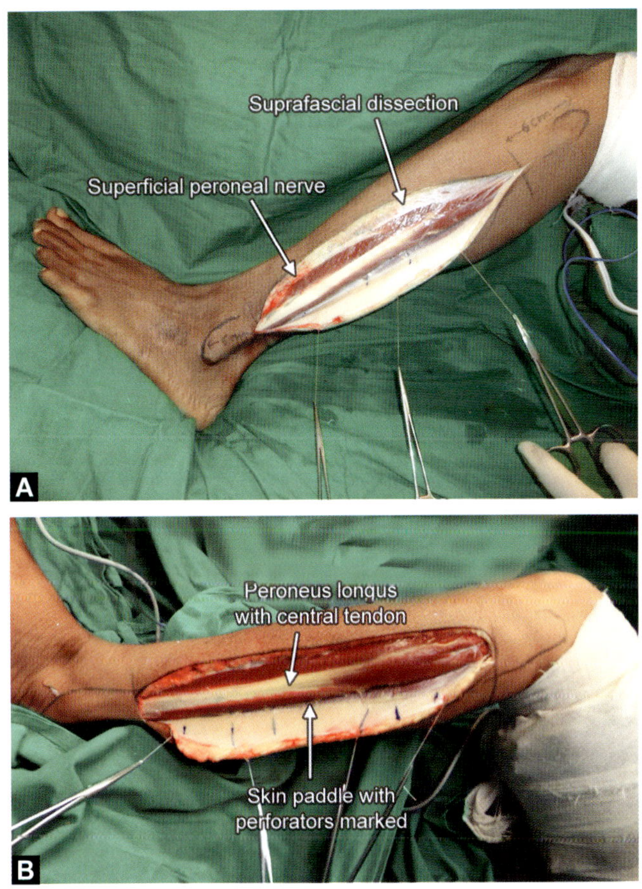

Figs. 5A and B: Suprafascial harvest; (B) infrafascial dissection up to septum to reveal perforators

Steps of Harvest

- Incise anterior skin up to the deep fascia. Continue with suprafascial dissection of the skin paddle till the superficial peroneal nerve is identified and preserved to avoid sensory loss over dorsum of foot.
- Cut deep fascia and tag it to the skin paddle to prevent shearing between skin paddle and fascia. This exposes the peroneal muscles in the lateral compartment of leg
- Infrafascial dissection is done till the posterolateral septum is identified. Note the septocutaneous perforators in septum **(Figs. 5A and B)**.
- Feel the lateral surface of the fibula and dissect the peroneal muscles off the bone in an extraperiosteal plane leaving 2–3 mm cuff of muscle behind to protect the underlying periosteum, till the anterolateral septum is reached.
- Cut this septum parallel to the bone to enter the anterior compartment.

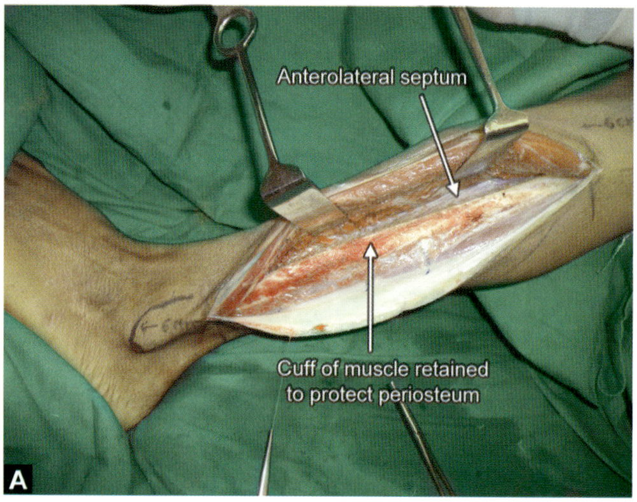

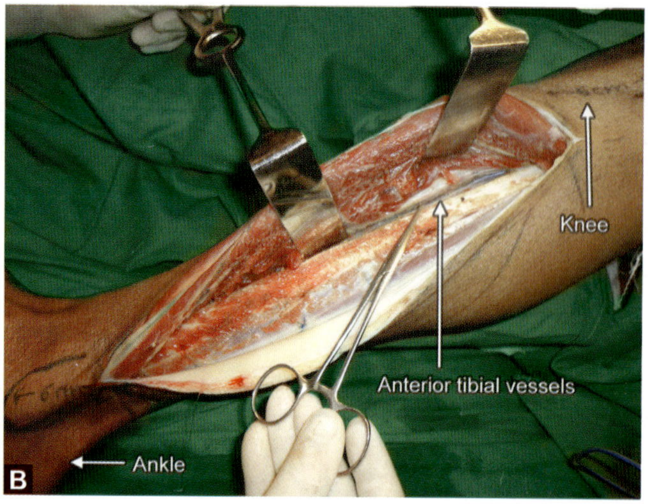

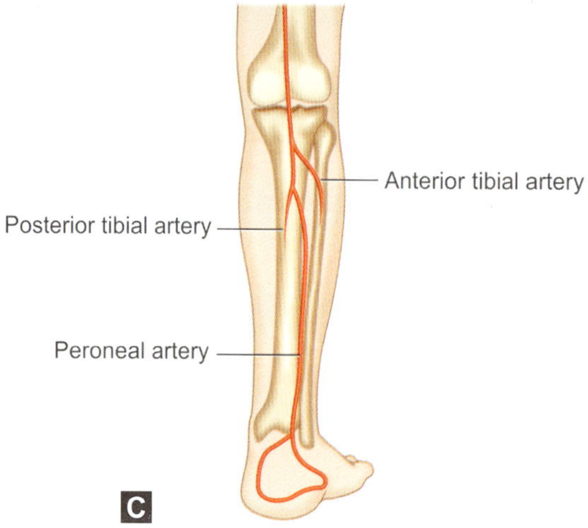

Figs. 6A to C: (A) Dissection to reveal the interosseous membrane; (B) visualization of anterior tibial vessels; (C) peronea magna

- Intraoperative inspection of the entire course of the anterior tibial artery is necessary. If the vessel is getting narrow toward ankle joint, chance of peronea magna is high. Sometimes the division of peroneal trunk may be halfway down the length of fibula, in such cases, one may need to ligate the posterior tibial vessels. If the patency of the anterior tibial vessels is doubtful, harvest may be abandoned **(Figs. 6A to C)**.
- Separate the extensor compartment muscles from the medial surface of fibula till the interosseous membrane is visualized.
- Cut the interosseous membrane close to the fibula while protecting the anterior tibial vascular bundle to enter the posterior compartment **(Fig. 7A)**.
- Osteotomies are done at the previously marked sites, subperiosteally, with the help of a Gigli saw wire to facilitate further dissection **(Fig. 7B)**.
- Retract the fibula laterally using a fibula holder **(Fig. 8)**.
- The bipennate muscle that comes into view is the tibialis posterior, peroneal vessels will be seen behind this

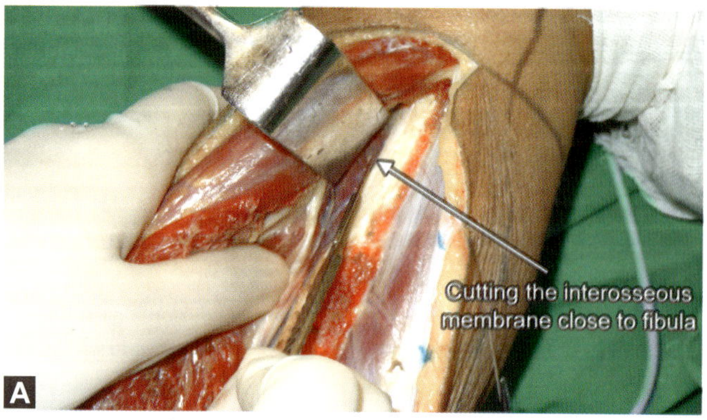

Fig. 7A: Cutting the interosseous membrane to reach posterior compartment

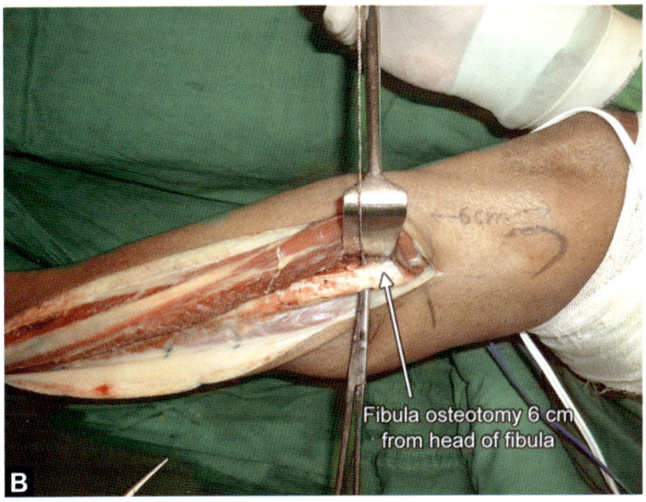

Fig. 7B: Fibula osteotomy

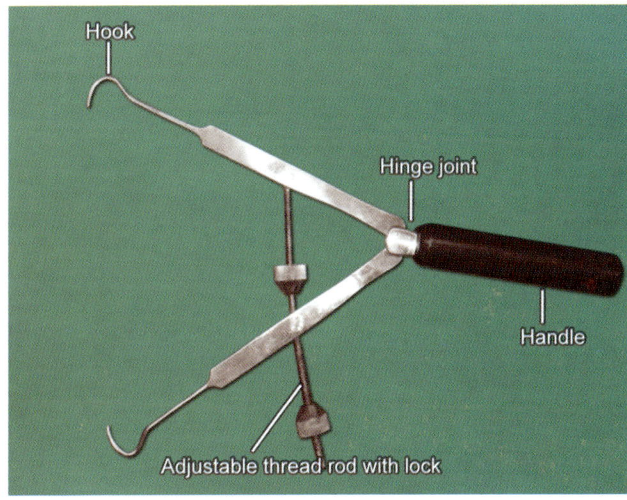

Fig. 8: Fibula holder

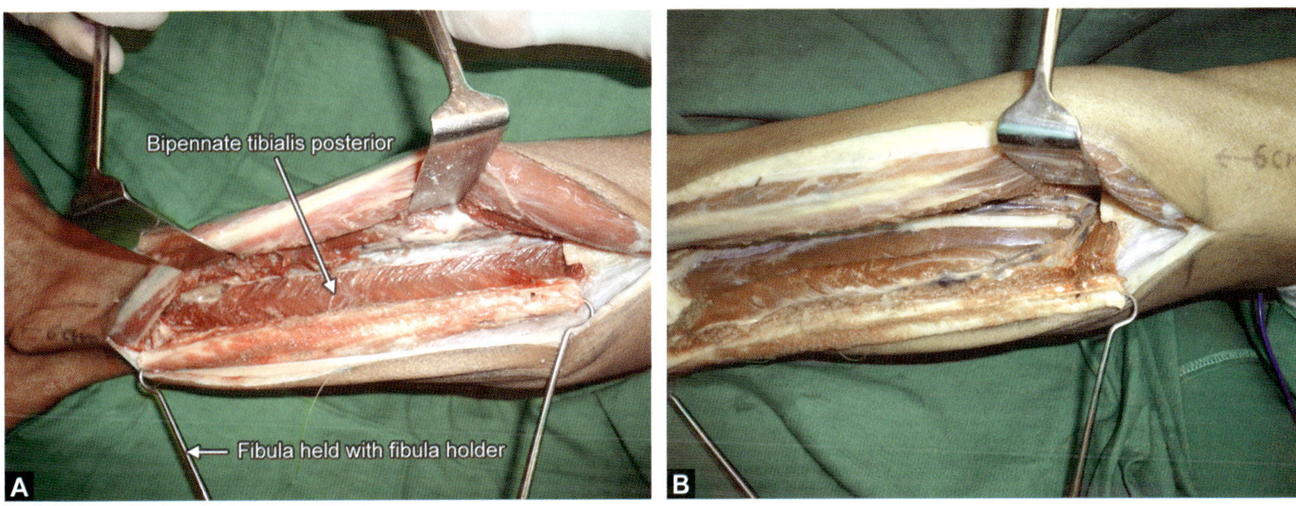

Figs. 9A and B: (A)Tibialis posterior; (B) division of tibioperoneal trunk into peroneal and posterior tibial

at the lower osteotomy site. The muscle behind the personal vessels is the flexor hallucis longus.

- Dissect the tibialis posterior muscle off the fibula taking care to ligate the branches passing through it. The peroneal vessels will be seen running along the bone with the flexor hallucis longus. Dissect the peroneal vessels up to its division from the tibioperoneal trunk **(Figs. 9A and B)**.
- Dissect the peroneal vessels at the lower end of the fibula, ligate and divide them at this level.
- Dissect the communicating branches between the peroneal and the posterior tibial vessels, clip and then divide. Divide the flexor hallucis longus (FHL) at the lower end of the fibula.
- We harvest the fibula flap with the flexor hallucis longus, as it makes dissection easy, protects the perforators and it can be used as a filler if required. The remanant FHL generally undergoes ischemic contracture resulting in flexion deformity of the great toe as the peroneal artery is usually its sole blood supply.
- Once the anterior dissection is completed, the defect is assessed for skin requirement. The skin paddle size is curtailed accordingly. The posterior incision decided, marked and incised **(Fig. 10)**.
- Infrafascial dissection is done up to the posterolateral septum.
- Take care of the perforators as they may have a short course through the soleus before turning toward the peroneal side. Observe the branching pattern, to determine if the perforator is arising from the peroneal vessel. If the proximal perforator is not arising from

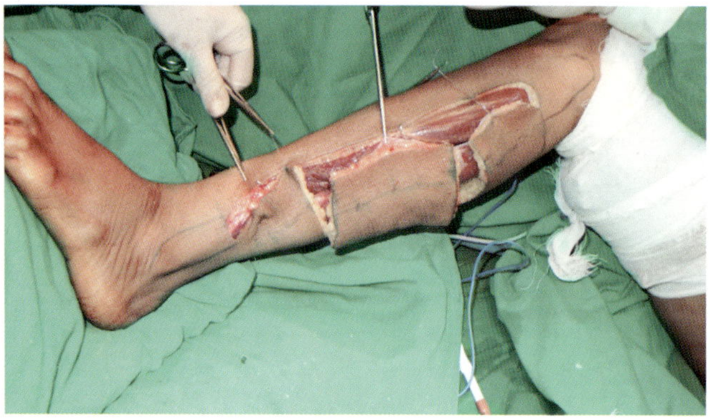

Fig. 10: Sizing of skin paddle

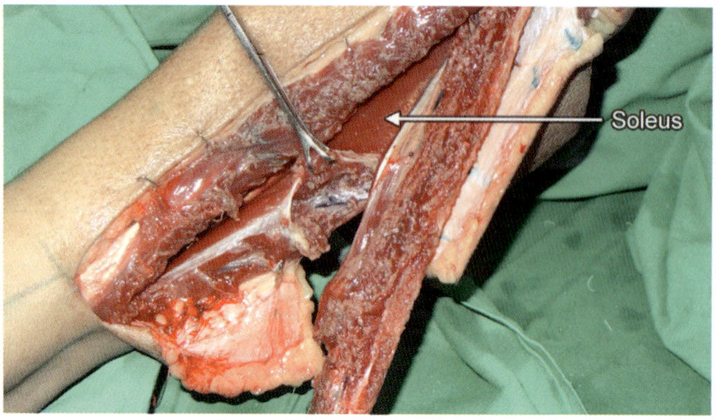

Fig. 11: Perforator dissection

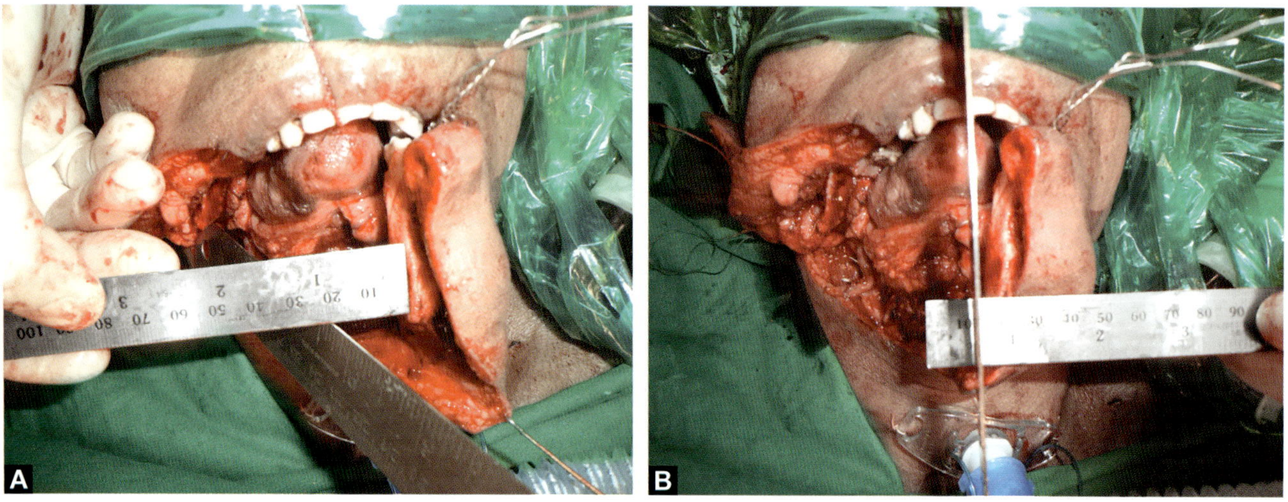

Figs. 12A and B: (A) Defect assessment; (B) checking for midline

the peroneal vessels its dissection is continued till a sizeable vessel caliber is encountered. This is done to harvest a second free flap from the same donor area if it is required for the external skin defect **(Fig. 11)**.

- Flap is freed from distal to proximal and prepare vessels for division.
- Release the tourniquet, check bleeding, achieve hemostasis and then clip and detach the flap.
- Close donor area primarily if only bone is harvested with the help of a split thickness skin graft to prevent compartment syndrome.
- Give below knee plaster of Paris slab.

Postoperative Care

- Bed rest with leg elevation.
- First check dressing of STSG is done on 5th postoperative day.
- Partial weight-bearing with the aid of walker is allowed after 5th postoperative day.
- Full weight-bearing is allowed with elastocrepe bandage support once graft is well healed.

Defect Assessment and Osteotomy Planning

Defect assessment should be done by examination of excised specimen, as well as examination of the created defect. Assessment with regards to what part or segment of bone is lost, soft tissue deficit, skin loss, need for inner lining, or tongue or palatal defect is done **(Figs. 12A and B)**.

Recipient vessels availability must be assessed.

CONTOURING FOR MANDIBLE RECONSTRUCTION

- Peroneal surface of fibula is used for plate fixation. Mark required segment from distal end to proximal end taking care of the perforators to be used **(Fig. 13).**
- Bone discarded proximally gives additional pedicle length.
- Osteotomy is planned using the excised specimen, prefabricated plate or stereolithographic models. K wire template is more convenient, yielding results which are functionally and esthetically good **(Figs. 14A and B)**.

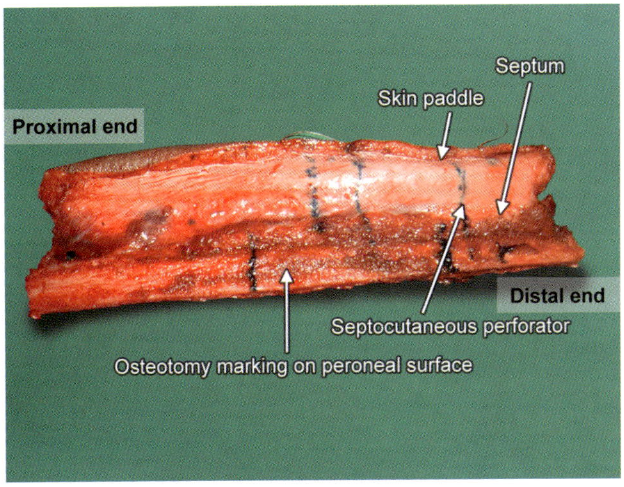

Fig. 13: Osteotomy planning

- Mandible is about 7 cm from angle to canine-premolar junction and intercanine distance is about 2.5 cm. It forms an angle of 120 degrees at canine-premolar junction. This template measures 7 cm - 2.5 cm - 7 cm from angle to angle with 120 degree angle at canine premolar level. It resembles the central part of the mandible **(Fig. 15)**.
- To bend the straight fibular bone at 120 degree, closing wedge osteotomy of 60 degree is done. Base of the triangle is always on the opposite side of the peroneal surface.
- In case of contouring for the ramus, plate is fixed on peroneal surface, but the wedge osteotomy is done depending on the final desired shape at the appropriate location on upper border of fibula **(Figs. 16A to C)**.
- Prior to the final osteotomy on the donor fibula, recheck the anatomical position, check for the midline with maxillary teeth **(Fig. 17)**.
- Rule out prognathism or retrognathism on lateral view. The mandible should lie just behind the upper teeth. Mark exact mandible cuts on the fibula for good contact with the native mandible.
- If teeth are present, temporary intermaxillary fixation can be done. Once fibula is fixed to native mandible

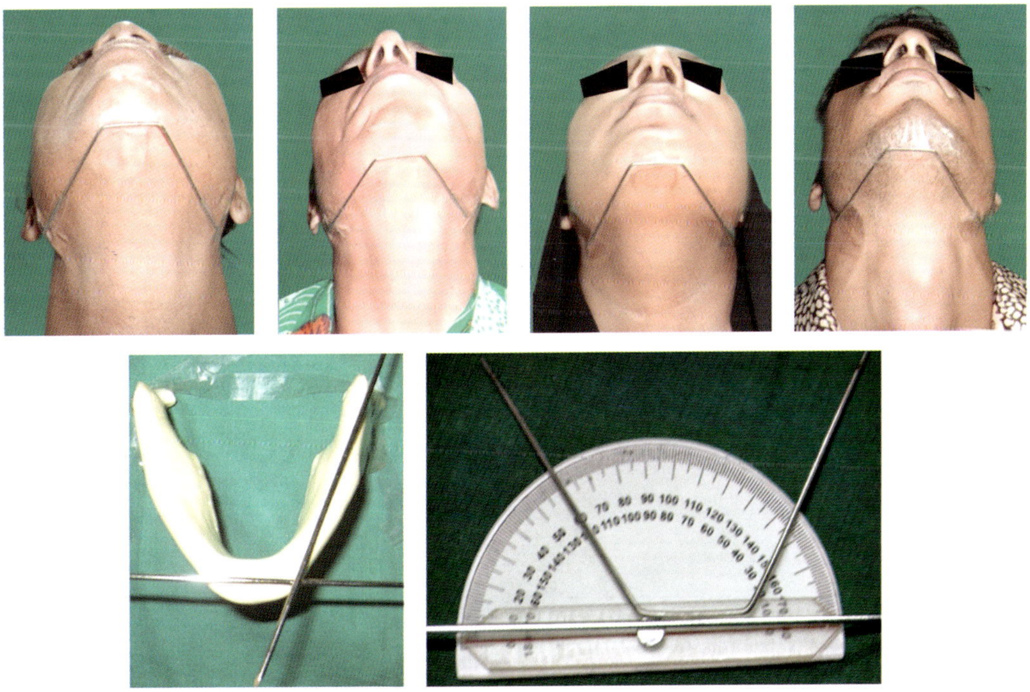

Fig. 14A: K wire template with angle measurements

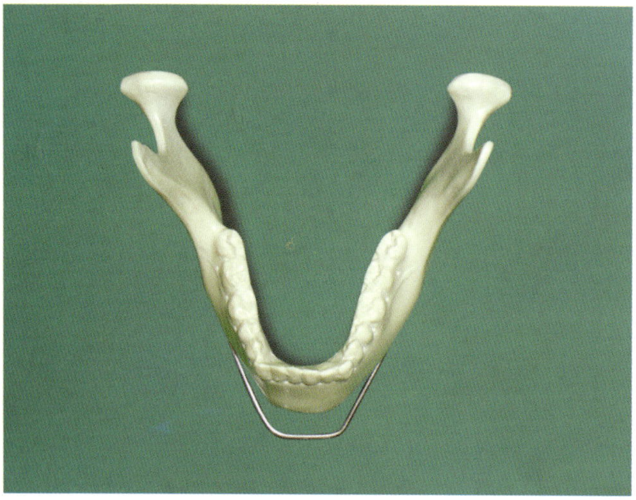

Fig. 14B: K wire template

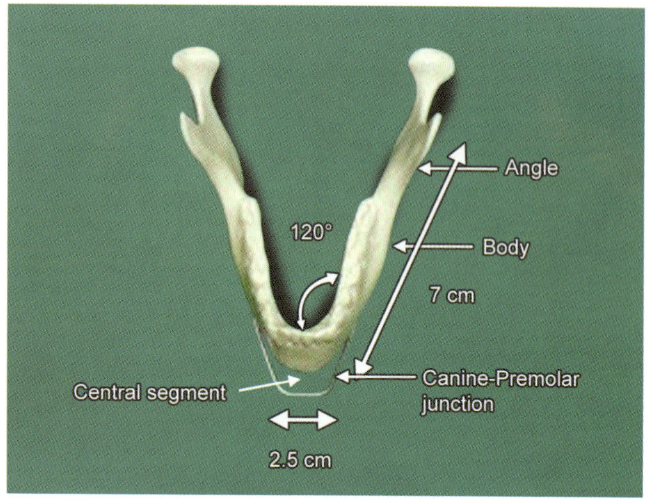

Fig. 15: Intercanine distance

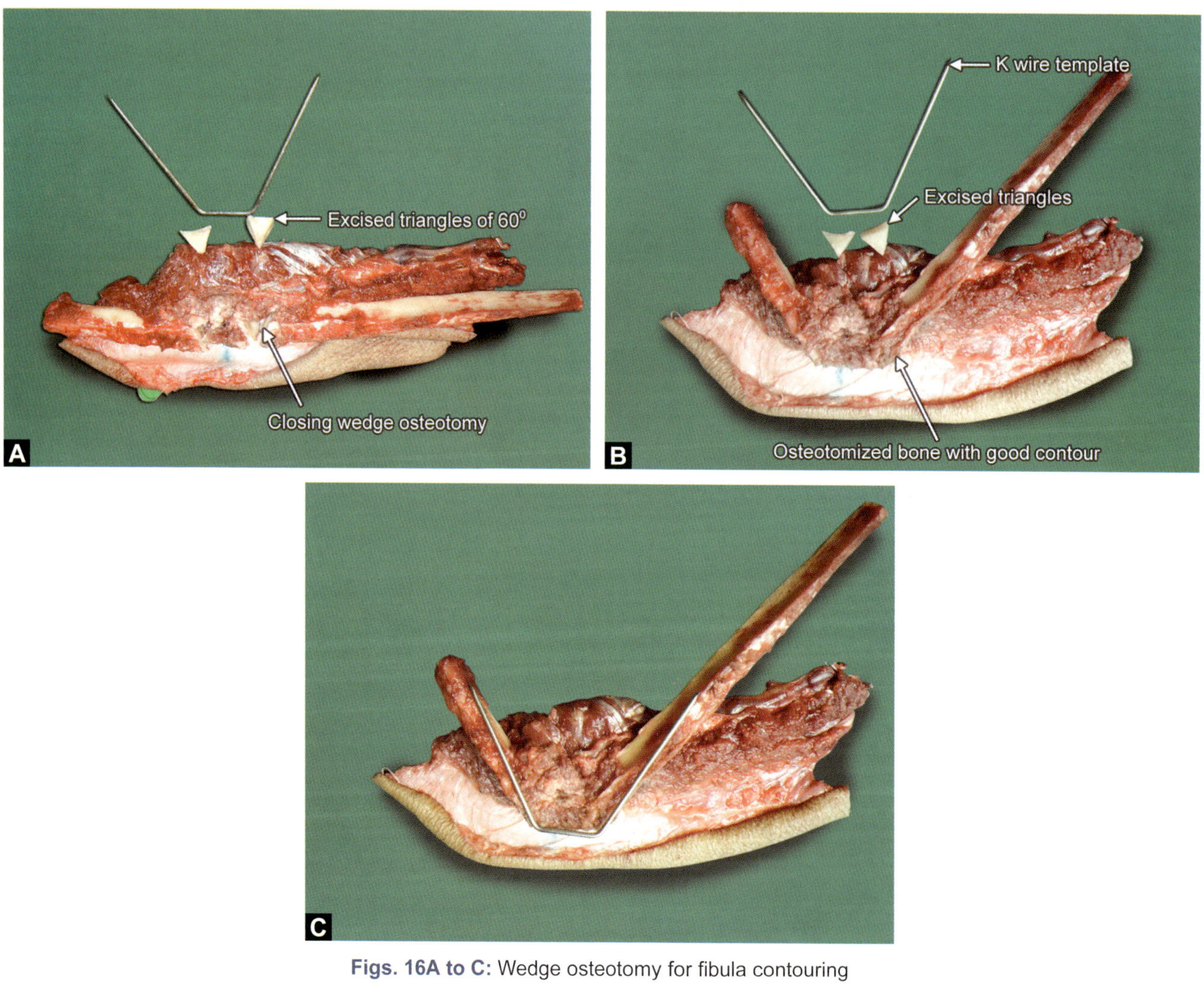

Figs. 16A to C: Wedge osteotomy for fibula contouring

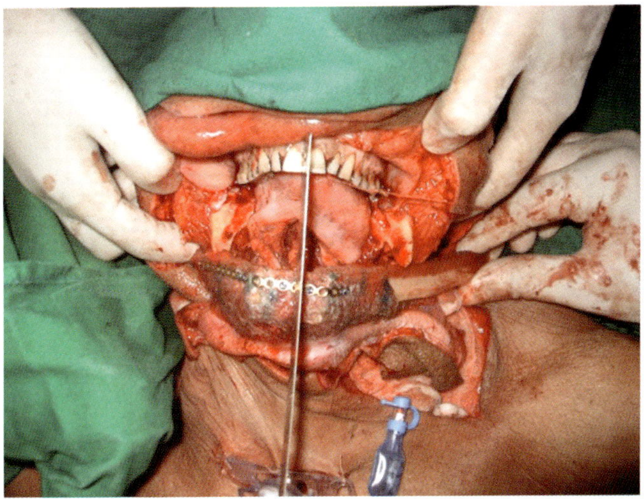

Fig. 17: Checking for alignment

undo intermaxillary fixation. If the occlusion is not perfect, the fixation should be readjusted immediately as it is very difficult to correct occlusion after radiotherapy.

- In presence of an external skin defect, the skin paddle is divided based on two or more separate perforators if available or it is de-epithelized and rotated in continuity for inner lining and outer cover. When this is not possible, either a pedicled or another free flap is used for the outer skin defect **(Figs. 18A and B)**.
- After bony fixation, inset of inner lining is done, followed by vascular anastomosis. Routinely the vein is anastomosed first, either end to end with a tributary of the internal jugular vein or end to side with the internal jugular vein. Recipient artery used is facial artery or superior thyroid artery.
- Blood circulation in the flap in confirmed. Lie of the pedicle is rechecked and inset is completed. At our center left fibula is harvested for logistic reasons.
- There is no side specificity of fibula for mandible reconstruction exceptions:
  1. Associated floor of mouth or tongue defect
  2. Defect reaching beyond upper gingivobuccal sulcus
  3. Excessively thick skin paddle.

MAXILLA RECONSTRUCTION

The maxilla can be compared to a box with the orbit as the roof, nasal septum medially and alveolus inferiorly. It supports the nose and forms basic foundation of the midface. Depending upon the extent of resection reconstruction options vary.

Factors which decide reconstructive option:

1. Size of alveolar and palatal defect
2. Orbital floor support loss
3. Oro or nasocranial communication
4. Remnant dentition
5. Orbital exenteration
   - If orbital exenteration is done and skull base is removed, soft tissues reconstruction with good filler is required. Free anterolateral thigh flap is preferred.
   - If ipsilateral canine is preserved, bony reconstruction is not required.
   - If remaining maxillary teeth are present, it is treated with an obturator prosthesis.
   - If adequate teeth which can retain the prosthesis are not present, it is reconstructed with a soft tissue flap.
   - When maxillary defect crosses the midline, it needs to be reconstructed with a bone flap to provide support to midface skin and lip. It also helps in eating, swallowing and maintaining esthetics of face.
   - When associated with an orbital floor defect is present eye support is provided with a vascularized bone when possible, or with a non-vascularized bone graft.

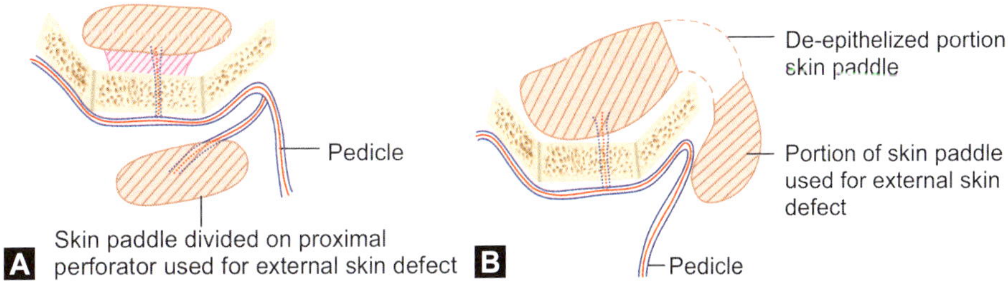

Figs. 18A and B: Fibula divided paddle; (B) fibula de-epithelized paddle

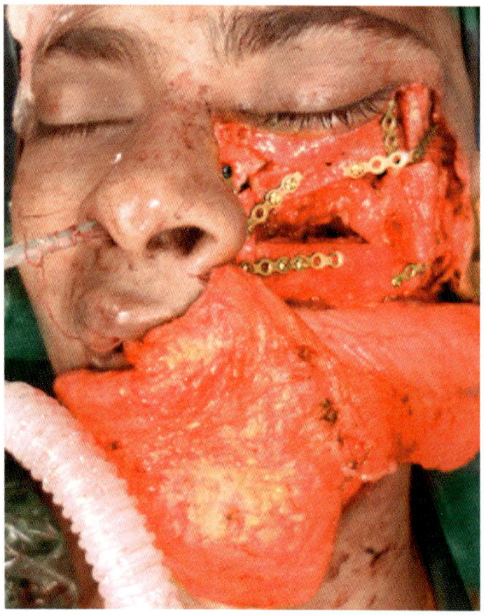

Fig. 19: Comparing eyeball position after fixation of orbital segment

- Osteotomy planning is similar as for mandibular reconstruction. The peroneal surface of the fibula is used for plate fixation, required bone segments are marked from distal end of fibula to proximal end preserving the best perforator for the skin paddle. Bone discarded proximally adds to the vascular pedicle length. Osteotomies are done as per bone segment requirement. Care is taken to avoid prognathism or retrognathism.
- A subcutaneous space or tunnel is created over the angle of the mandible connecting the maxillary defect to the neck incision for passing vascular pedicle of flap into the neck for anastomoses. The tunnel should be about two finger breadth wide so that the pedicle will not get compressed. Bony fixation is done to the remaining alveolus or to the zygomatic bone with miniplate and screws once pedicle is passed. The orbital bone segment is fixed to the zygoma laterally. Eyeball position is compared with the opposite eye to avoid exophthalmos or enophthalmos **(Fig. 19)**.
- The skin paddle is sutured intraorally beginning from posterior margin of the defect. Vascular anastomosis is done once intraoral inset is complete. After confirming flap circulation, the external inset is done. Before neck incision closure, anastomosed vessels must be rechecked for any twist or kink.
- For unilateral maxillary reconstruction FFOCF from the same side as the defect is harvested. For bilateral maxillectomy defect, FFOCF is harvested from the side same as the side of which the neck vessels are chosen for anastomoses.

FOR EXTREMITY RECONSTRUCTIONS

- For extremity bone reconstruction free fibula flap is used as such.
- Bone reconstruction with vascularized free fibula bone graft is required in case of failure of prosthetic implant or extracorporal radiation therapy (ECRT) bone as limb salvage procedure.
- For humerus, radius or ulna reconstruction, it is used as a vascularized bone flap with or without a monitoring skin paddle.
- For femur or tibia reconstruction, it is used along with an allograft. Half the cortex of the allograft is removed along its length, except at the ends, where its tubular structure is preserved as slotted rings. Within this allograft, the harvested fibula is inserted taking care to avoid pedicle compression. Fibular ends are passed through the rings preserved at both ends and then pegged into the remnant native bone. This assembly is fixed rigidly to the native bone with a long plate spanning its entire length. This is Capanna's technique. Vascularized bone graft, coupled with allograft and rigid plate fixation allows for early rehabilitation **(Fig. 20)**.
- In case of an associated skin defect, it can be used as an osteocutaneous flap. It may also be used as a pedicled flap for tibial defects. If segment to be reconstructed is small, fibula can be used as double barrel configuration to give additional strength.

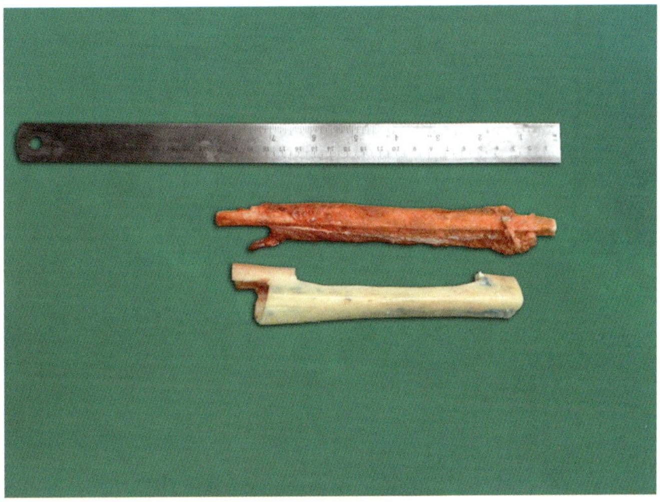

Fig. 20: Capanna's technique

CASE SERIES OF PATIENTS RECONSTRUCTED WITH FIBULA (FIGS. 21 TO 35)

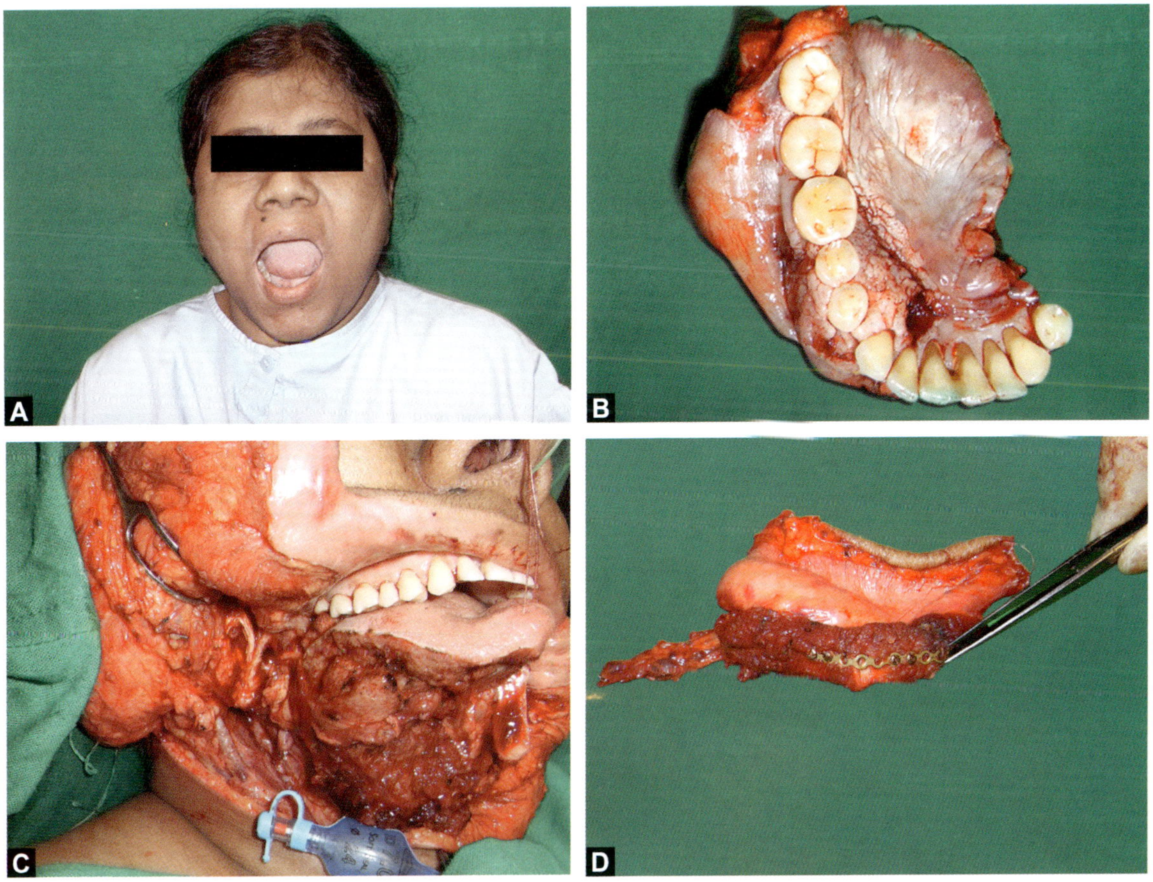

Figs. 21A to D: Fibula for mandible reconstruction without outer skin defect. (A) Preoperative; (B) excised specimen; (C) defect; (D) contoured fibula

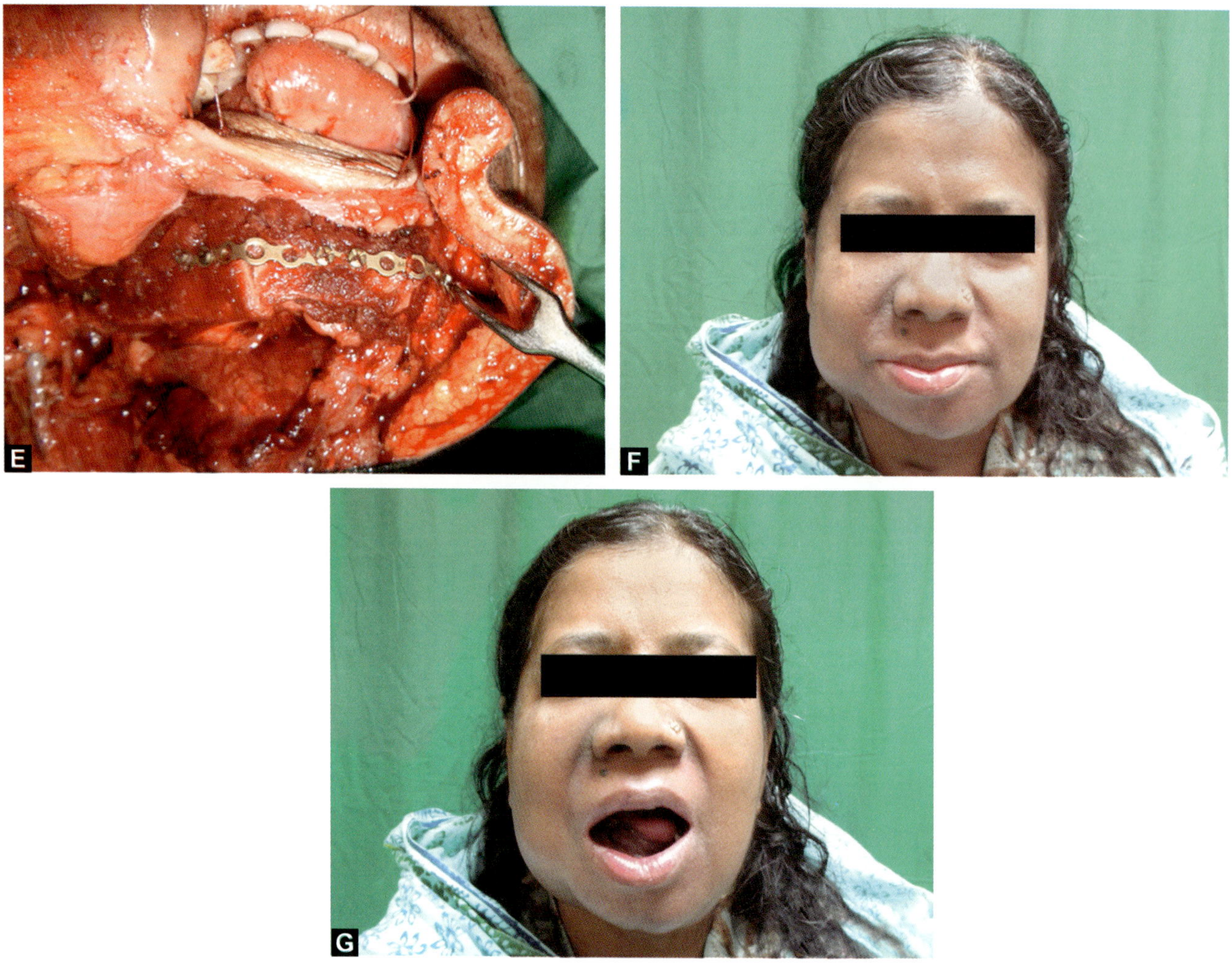

Figs. 21E to G: Fibula for mandible reconstruction without outer skin defect. (E) After fixation; (F) post-radiation; (G) good mouth opening

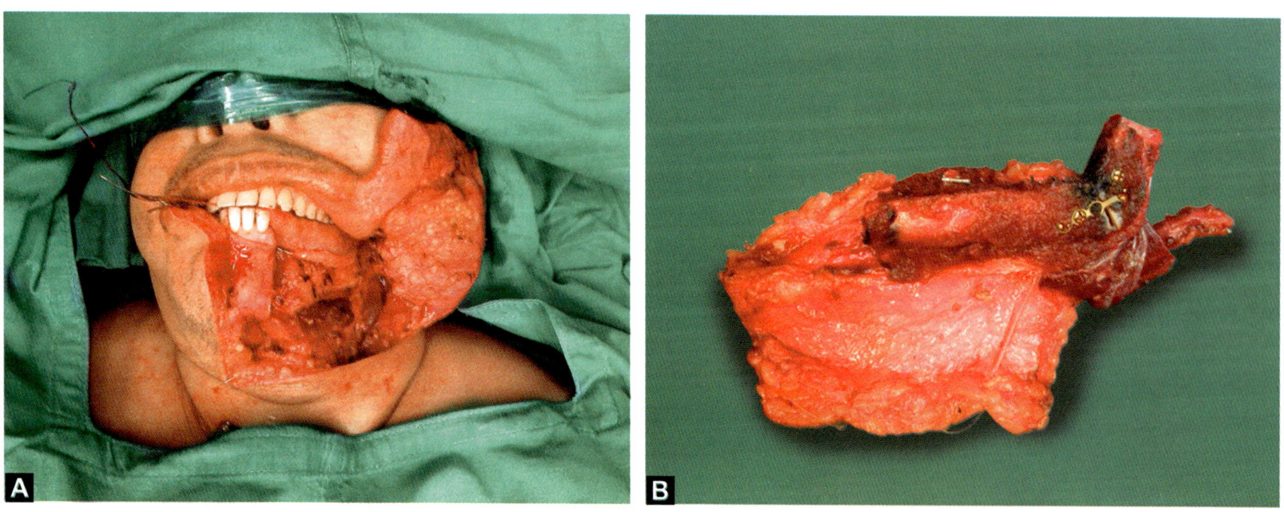

Figs. 22A and B: Fibula for mandible reconstruction with ramus. (A) Defect; (B) contoured fibula

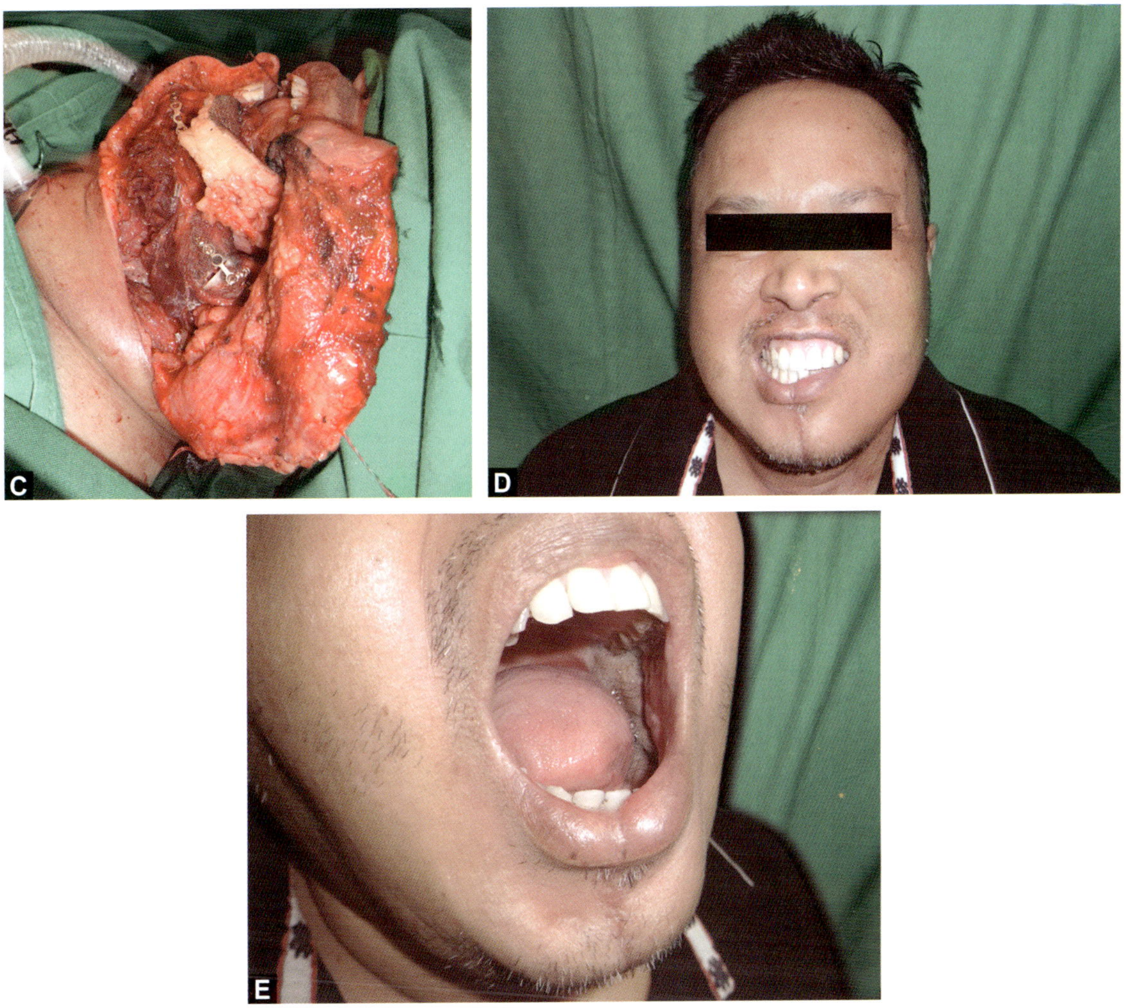

Figs. 22C to E: Fibula for mandible reconstruction with ramus. (C) After fixation; (D) postoperative photograph showing maintained occlusion; (E) postoperative photo showing well-settled fibula skin paddle

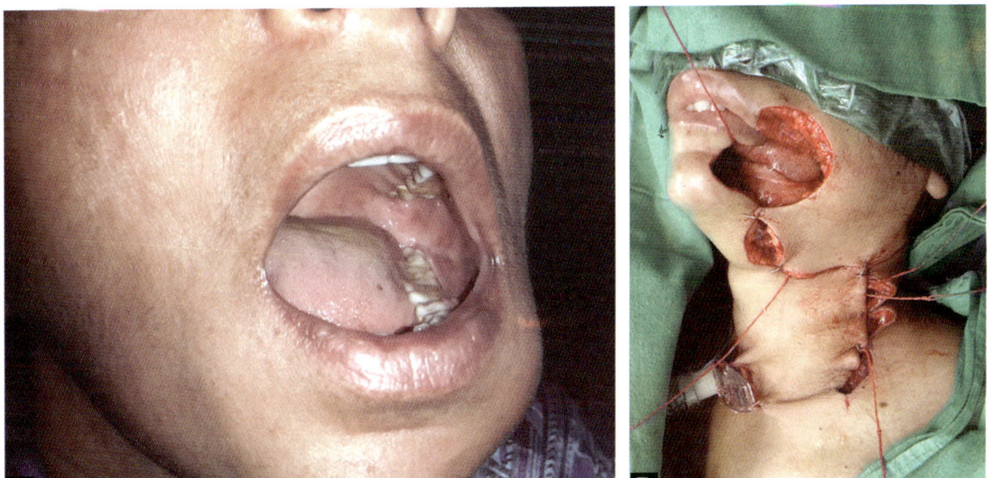

Figs. 23A and B: Fibula for mandible reconstruction with outer skin defect using divided paddle. (A) Preoperative photograph showing tumor; (B) intraoperative photograph showing external skin defect

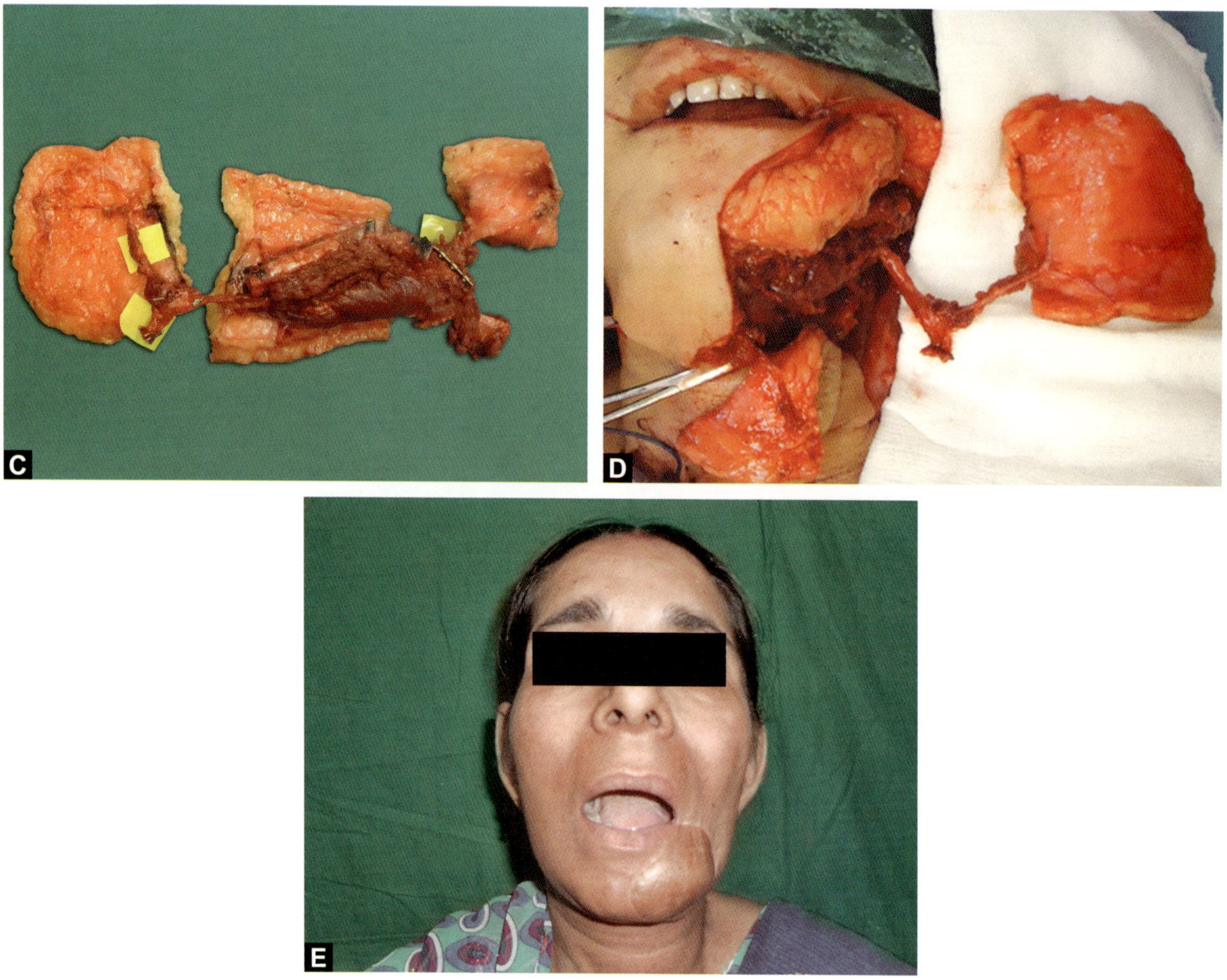

Figs. 23C to E: Fibula for mandible reconstruction with outer skin defect using divided paddle. (C) Contoured fibula with divided skin paddle; (D) after fixation and intraoral inset, (E) postoperative photograph

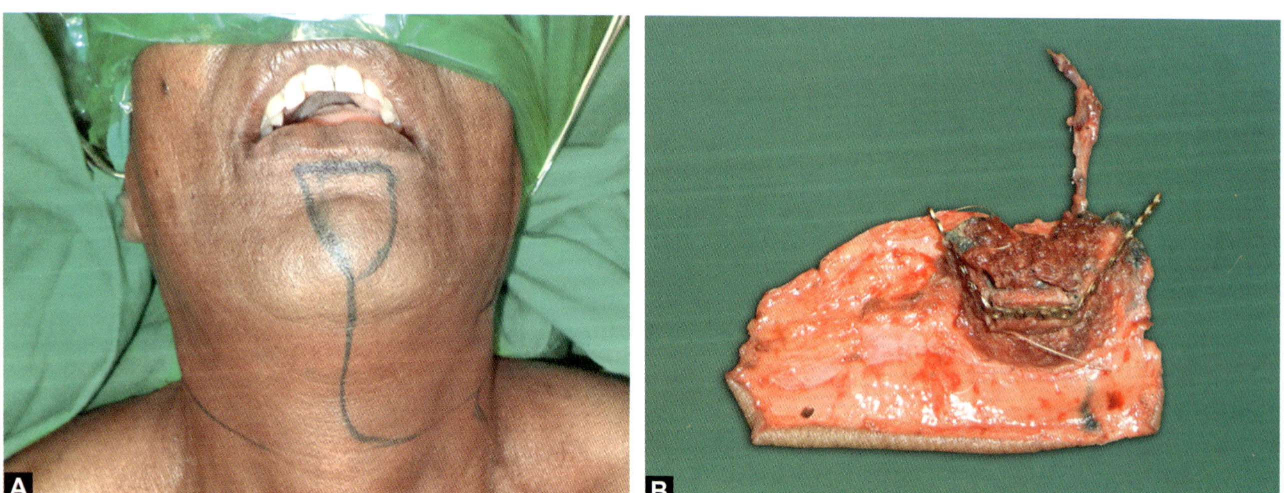

Figs. 24A and B: Fibula for mandible with outer skin defect using de-epithelized paddle. (A) Marking of external skin defect;(B) contoured fibula

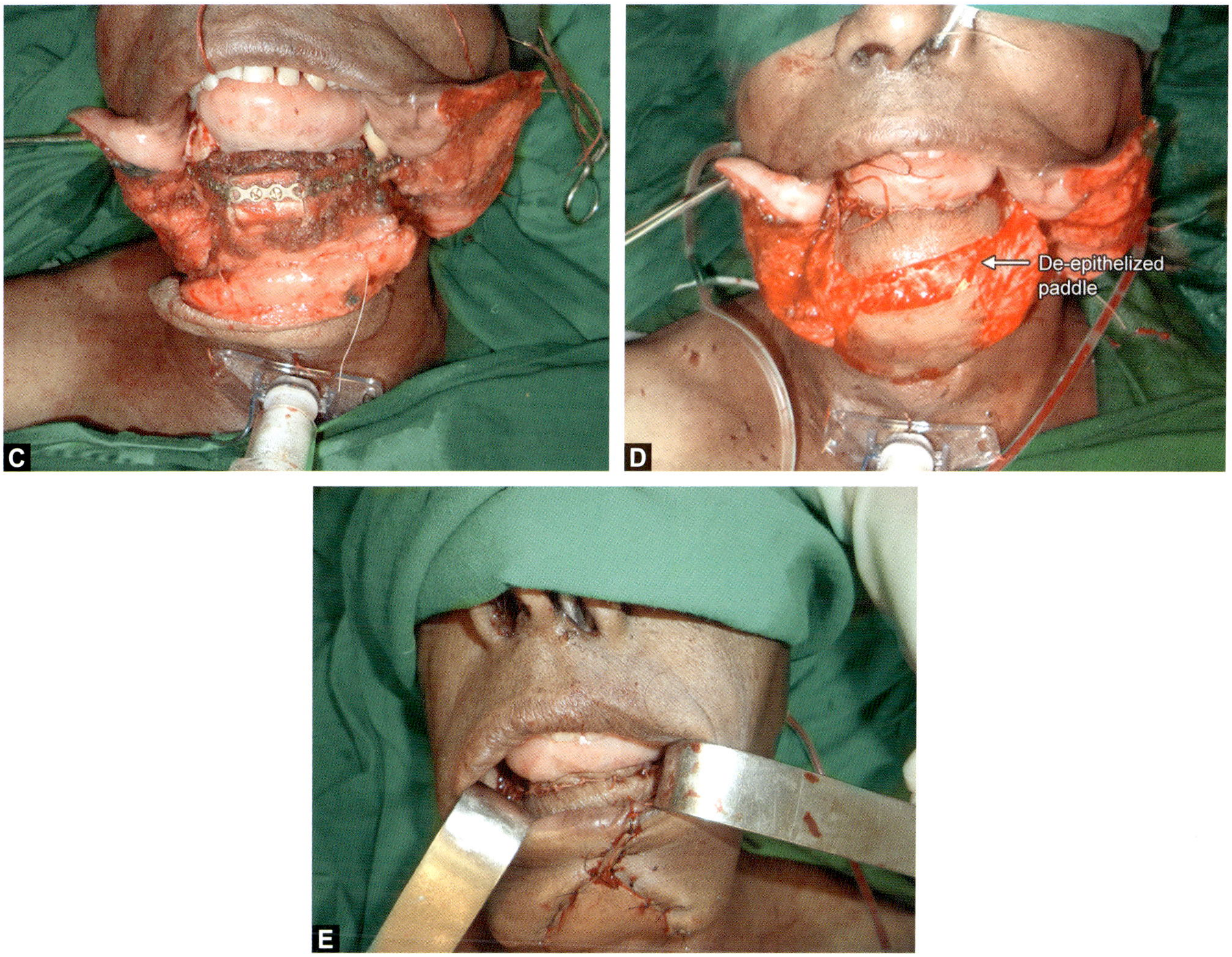

Figs. 24C to E: Fibula for mandible with outer skin defect using de-epithelized paddle. (C) After fixation; (D) showing de-epithelized skin paddle before inset, (E) after skin closure

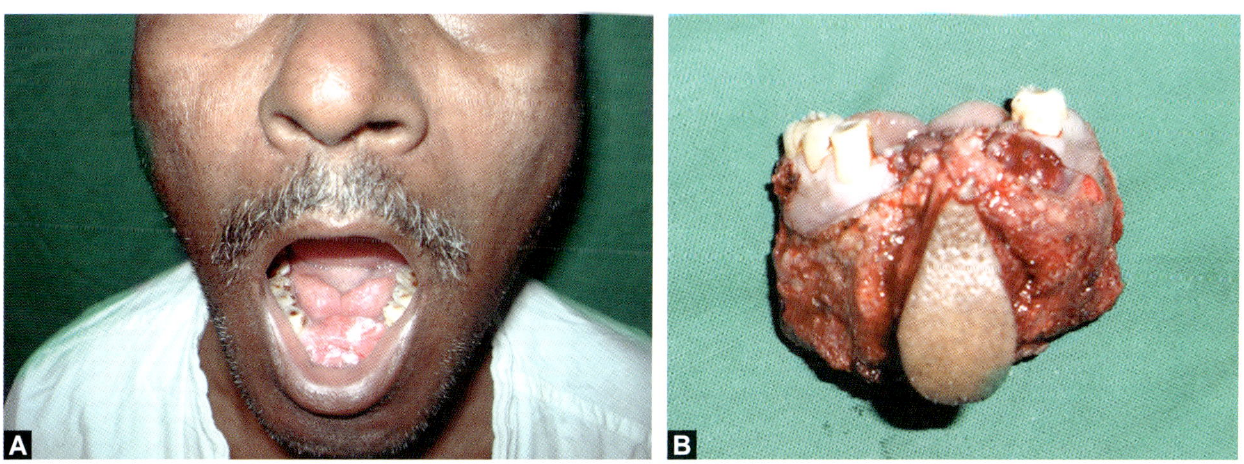

Figs. 25A and B: Fibula for mandible with outer skin defect closed primarily. (A) Preoperative photograph; (B) excised specimen with outer skin

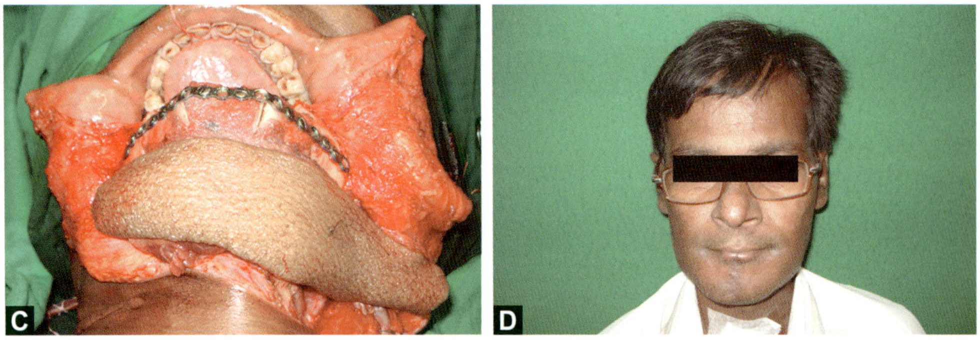

Figs. 25C and D: Fibula for mandible with outer skin defect closed primarily. (C) After contouring and fixation; (D) postoperative result

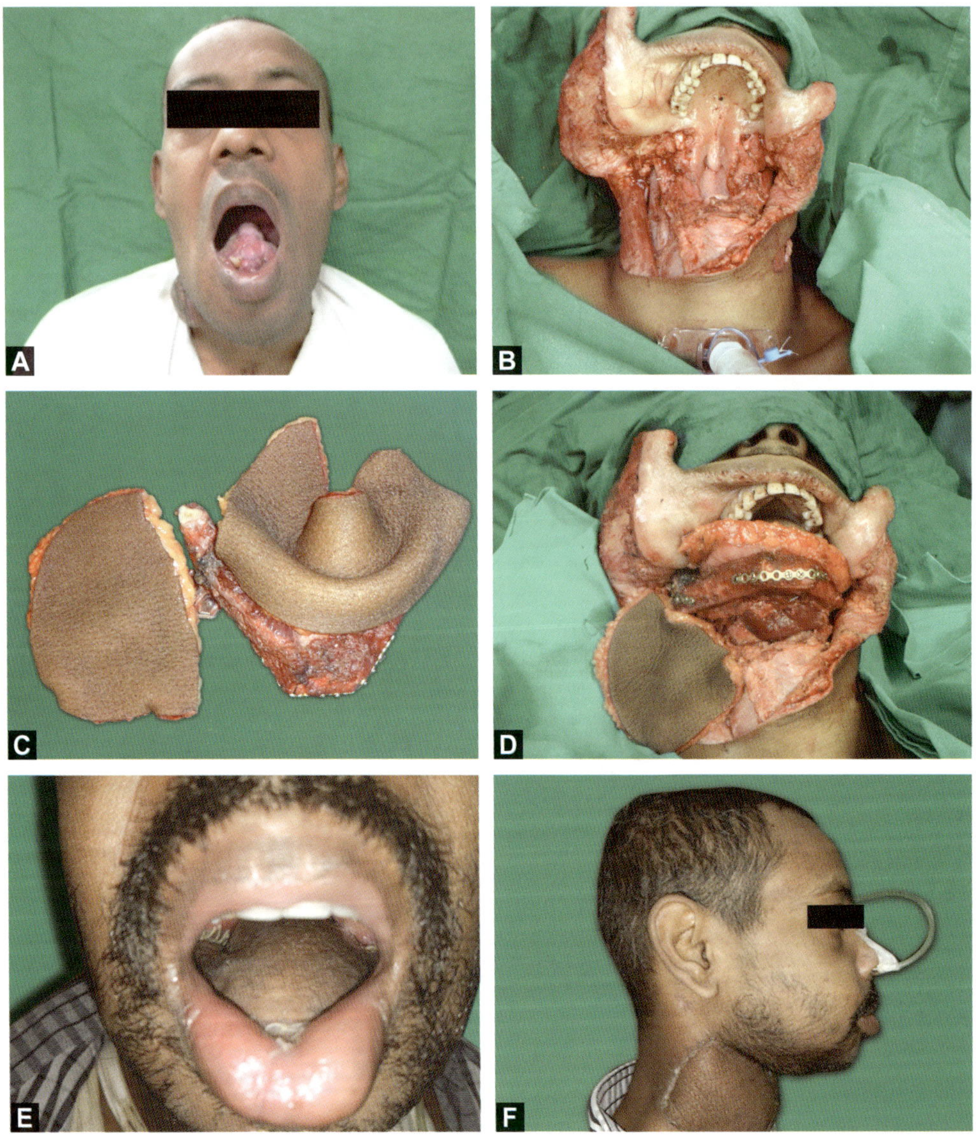

Figs. 26A to E: Fibula for mandibular reconstruction with tongue and neck skin defect. (A) Preoperative photograph; (B) post excision; (C) contoured fibula with skin flap sutured to create tongue mound; (D) after fixation and intraoral inset showing divided skin paddle for neck skin defect; (E) immediate postoperative result; (F) postoperative photograph

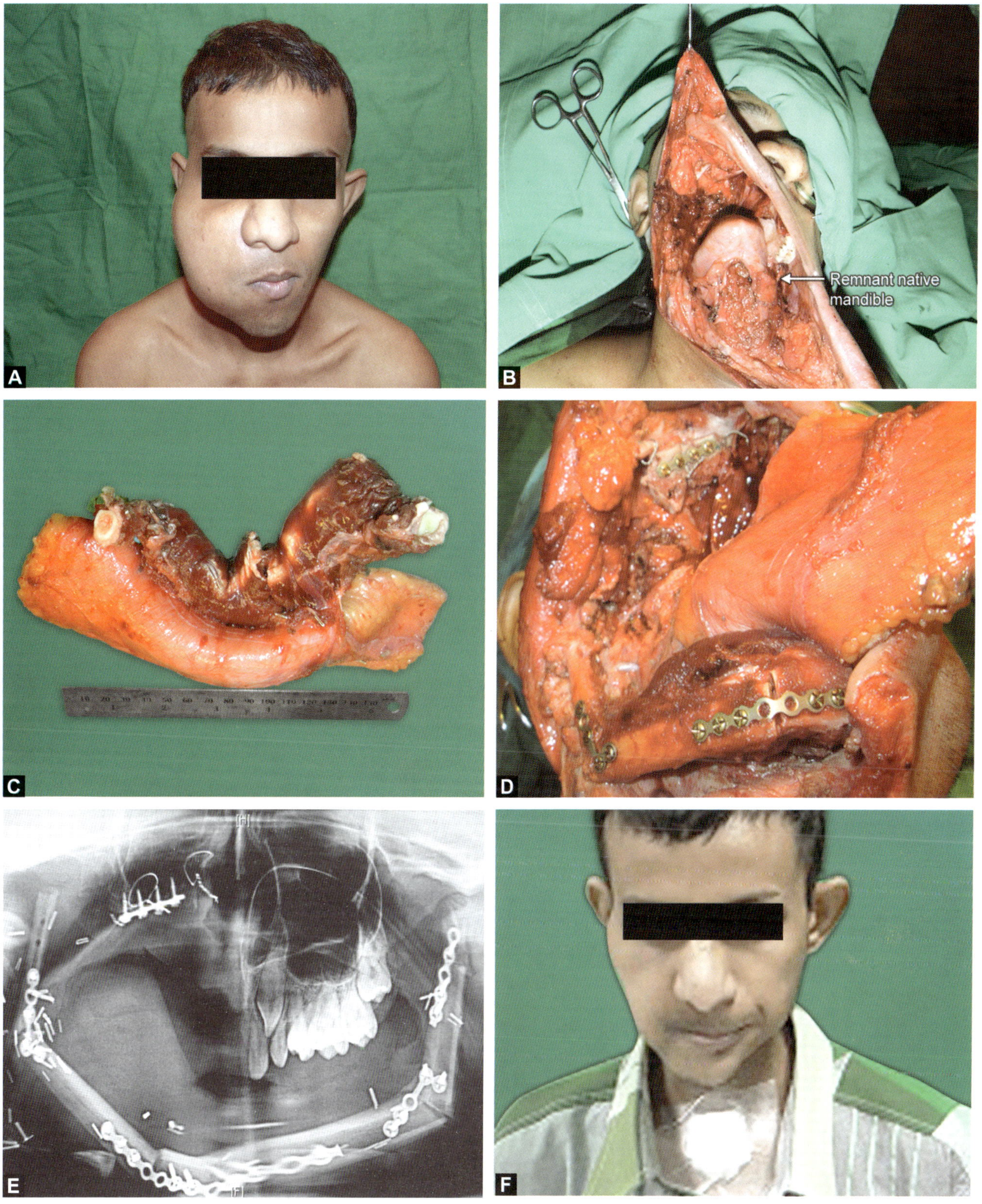

Figs. 27A to F: Fibula for mandibular and maxillary defect. (A) Preoperative; (B) defect; (C) contoured flap; (D) after fixation; (E) postoperative OPG showing reconstructed mandible and orbital floor; (F) postoperative result

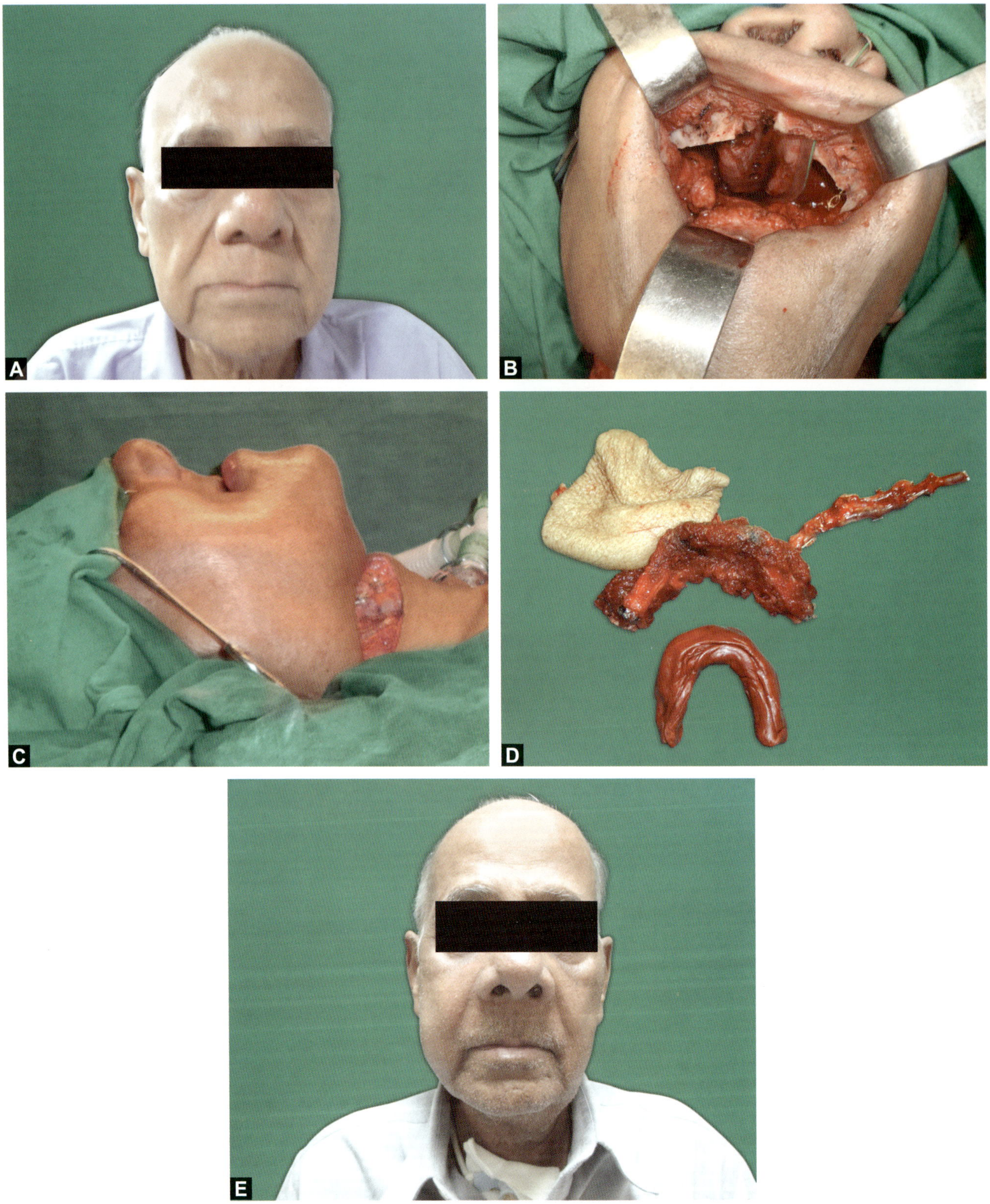

Figs. 28A to E: Fibula for palatal defect. (A) Preoperative; (B) defect; (C) retrusion of maxilla without reconstruction; (D) dental compound used for contouring; (E) postoperative result

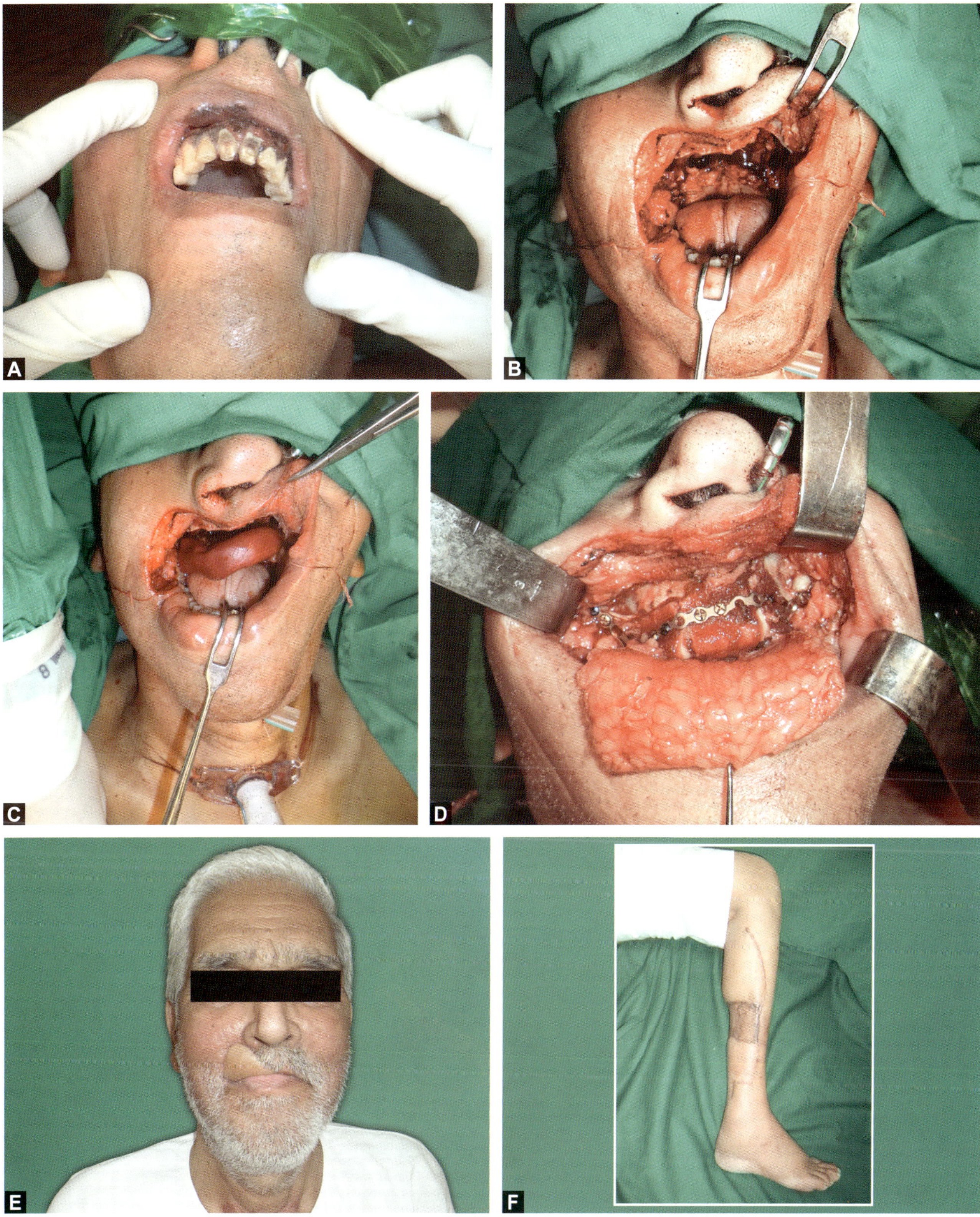

Figs. 29A to F: Fibula for palatal defect with outer skin. (A) Preoperative photograph; (B) defect; (C) dental compound used for contouring; (D) postfixation; (E) postoperative result; (F) well-settled donor site

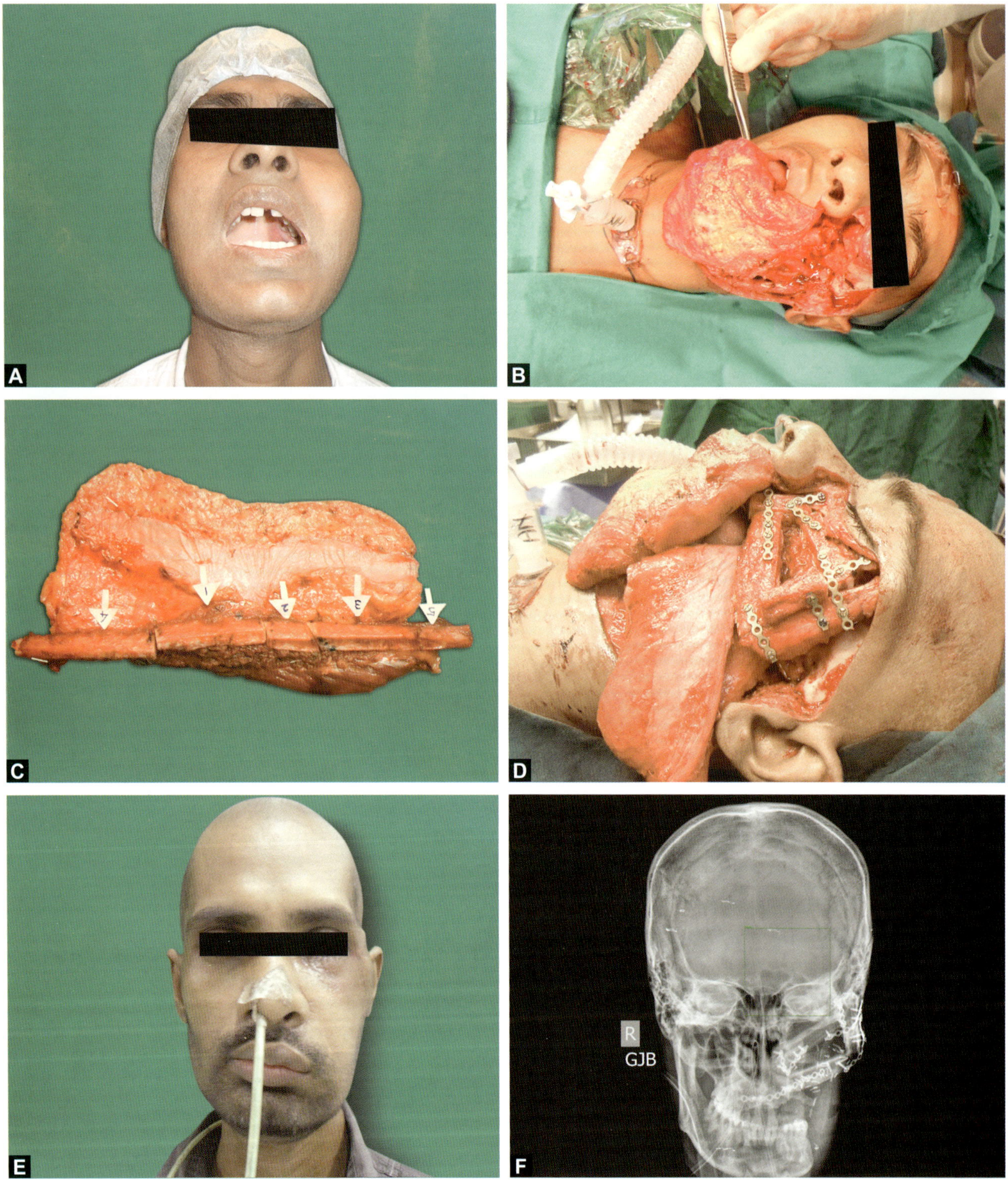

Figs. 30A to F: Fibula used for orbital floor reconstruction. (A) Preoperative; (B) defect; (C) fibula osteotomy; (D) postfixation; (E) postoperative; (F) postoperative X-ray

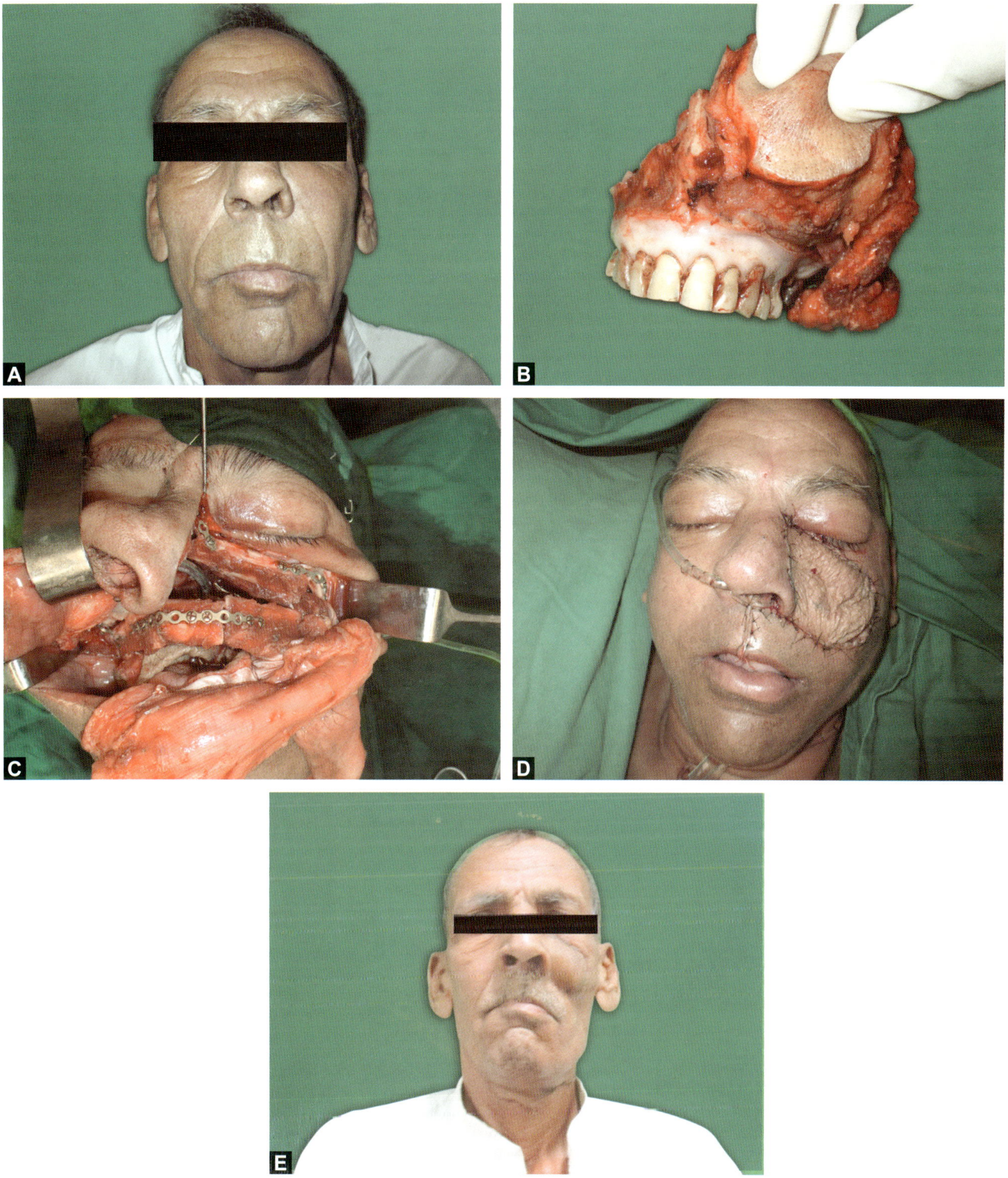

Figs. 31A to E: Fibula for orbital floor reconstruction with outer skin defect. (A) Preoperative; (B) excised specimen; (C) post osteotomy and fixation; (D) post skin suturing; (E) postoperative showing well-settled flap

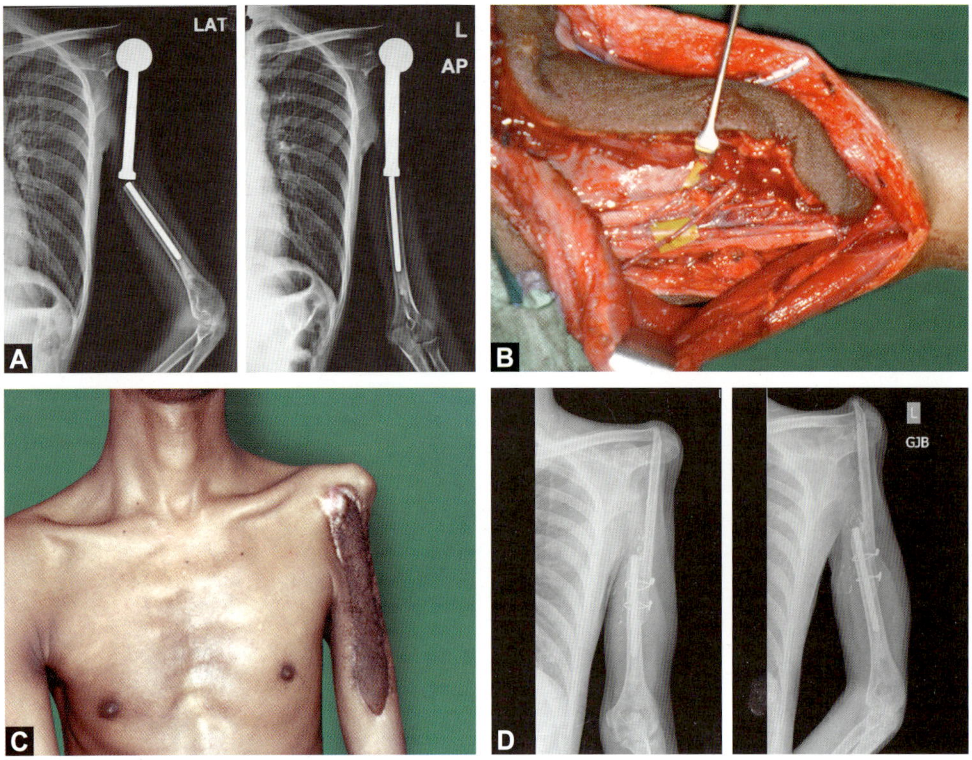

Figs. 32A to D: Fibula for upper limb defect. (A) X-ray showing plate fracture; (B) intraoperative, after anastomosis; (C) postoperative well-settled flap; (D) postoperative X-ray

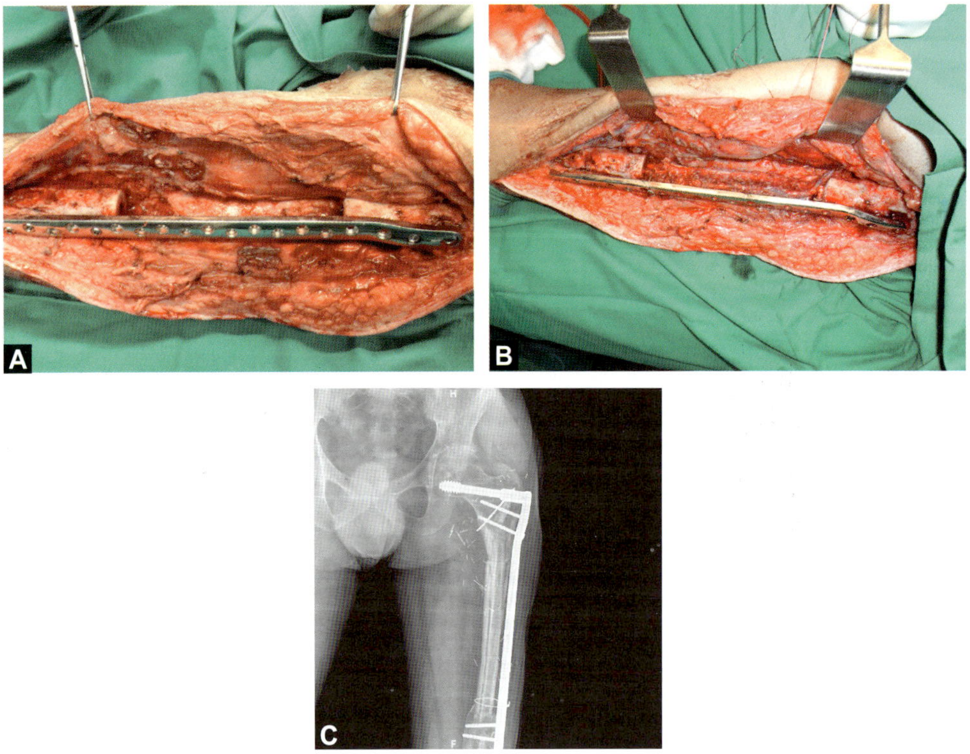

Figs. 33A to C: Fibula for lower limb defect. (A) Intraoperative photograph showing bone defect; (B) after anastomosis and fixation; (C) postoperative X-ray showing well united bone

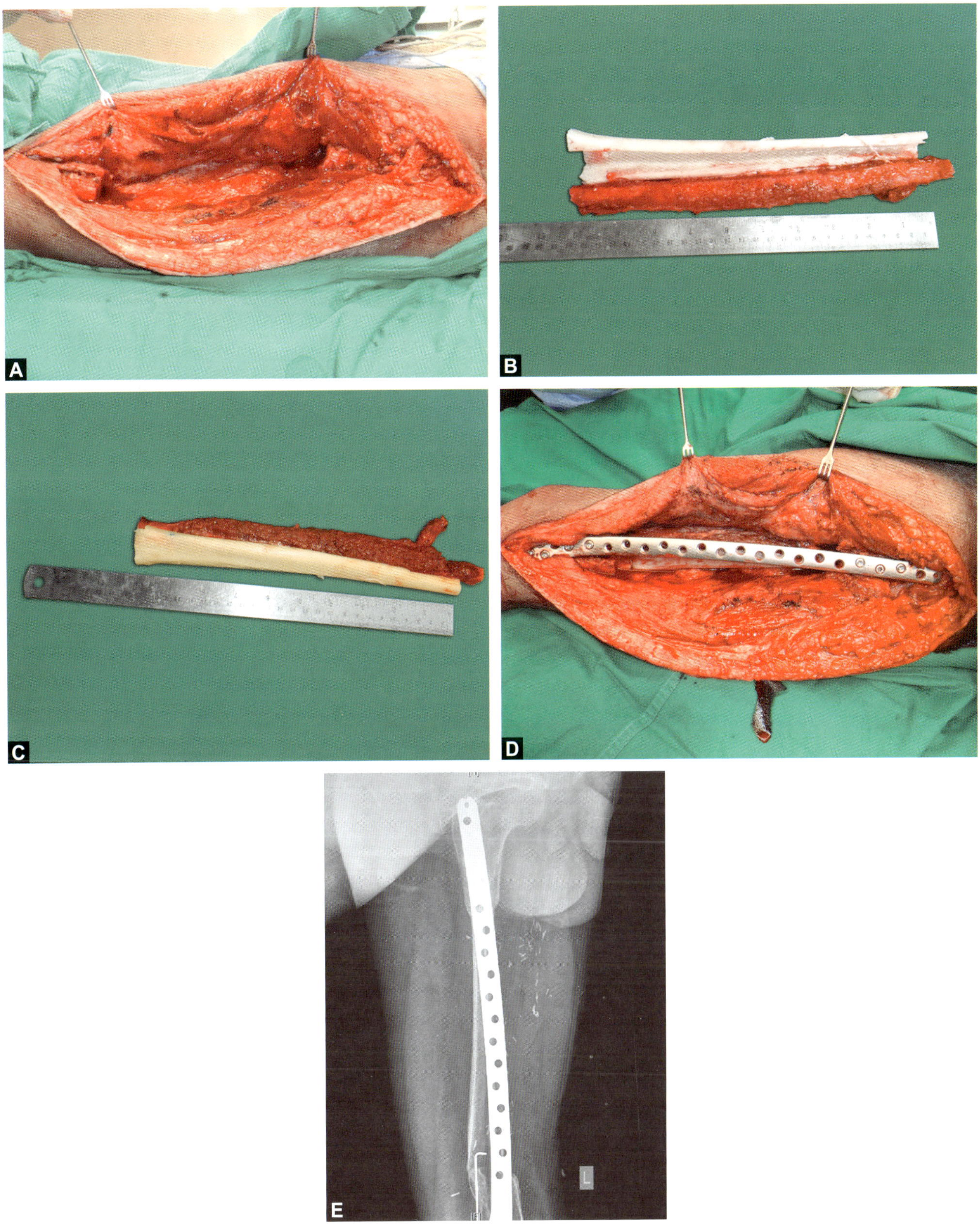

Figs. 34A to E: Fibula for lower limb with allograft—Capanna's technique. (A) Defect; (B) allograft with slot created; (C) bone pegged into slot created in allograft; (D) after plate fixation and anastomosis; (E) postoperative X-ray

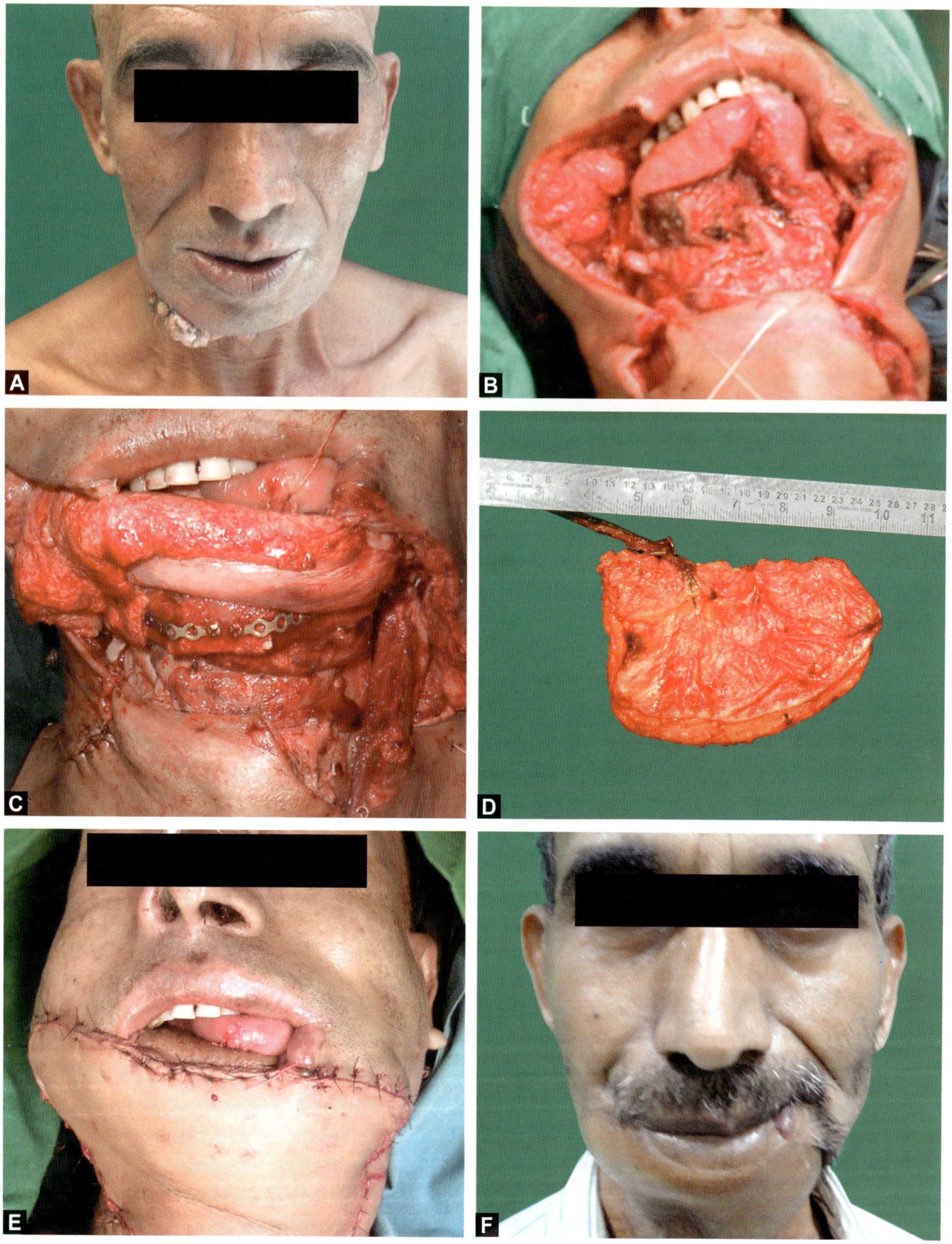

Figs. 35A to F: Double free flap for mandible reconstruction. (A) Preoperative; (B) defect; (C) contoured free fibula flap after fixation; (D) harvested free anterolateral thigh flap; (E) on table after suturing; (F) late postoperative photograph

CHAPTER 8

Radial Forearm Flap

Saumya Mathews, Mayur Mantri, Dushyant Jaiswal

INTRODUCTION

The radial artery forearm flap was first described in 1978 in the anatomical studies by Dr Yang Guofan and Dr Gao Yuzhi.[1] The first clinical series was published in 1980 of 60 cases. The introduction of the flap to the western world happened thereafter. Free radial artery forearm flap (FRAFF) is one of our workhorse flaps at TMC. The defining features of this flap are thinness and pliability. It finds great application in head and neck reconstruction for tongue and buccal mucosa defects. The reliability of the flap is due to its constant pedicle anatomy and numerous perforators.

ANATOMY

The radial artery forearm flap is supplied by the radial artery which is a branch of the brachial artery and arises at approximately 2 cms below the cubital crease. It lies between the pronator teres and the brachioradialis muscle in the proximal forearm and distally between the brachioradialis and the flexor carpi radialis muscle. The radial artery gives off septocutaneous perforators to the overlying forearm skin via the lateral intermuscular septum. The perforators lie superficial to the deep fascia and form an arcade of vessels. This enables the safe suprafascial harvest of the flap. The radial artery is accompanied by two venae comitantes which communicate with each other in a ladder-like pattern and drain into the median cubital vein. The cephalic vein drains the flap via superficial subcutaneous veins. Either system can be used for the venous drainage of the flap **(Figs. 1 and 2)**.

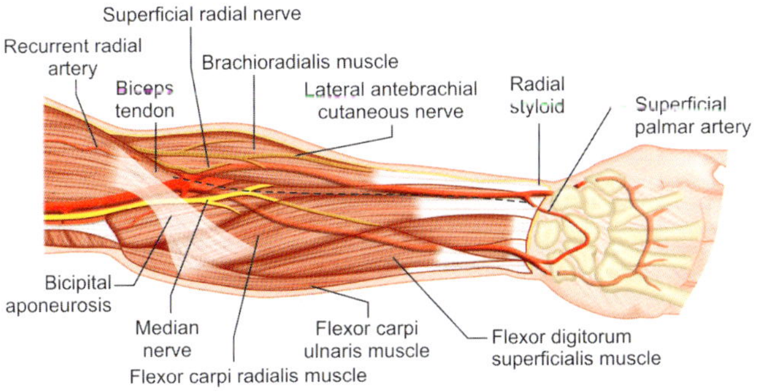

Fig. 1: Radial artery course in forearm

DONOR SITE ASSESSMENT

It includes history of hand dominance, trauma, surgery to upper extremity, and recent injection of chemotherapeutic drugs or intravenous needle pricks through upper limb veins. The physical examination includes a modified Allen's test of the non-dominant hand.

Modified Allen's Test

The patient is asked to clench their fist for 30 secs. The radial and ulnar artery are occluded at the level of the wrist.

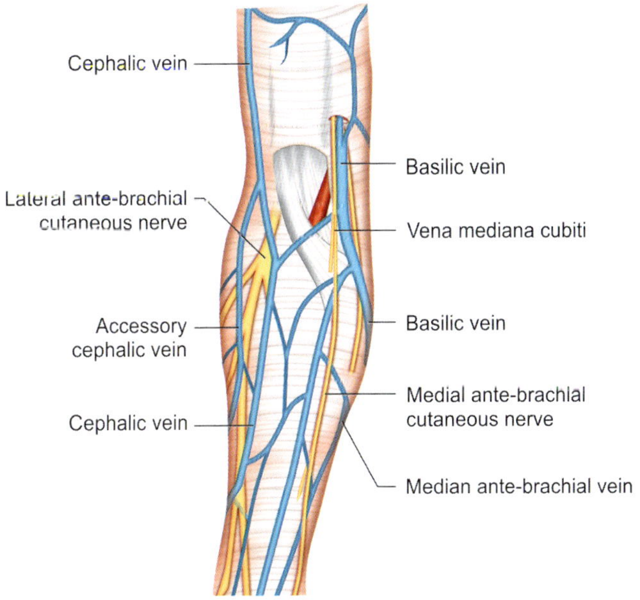

Fig. 2: Superficial veins of forearm

The patient opens his/her wrist and the pallor is observed over the thenar eminence. The return of rubor on releasing the pressure over ulnar artery is noted.

Interpretation: Less than 6 sec – Allen's negative
7–11 secs – Allen's equivocal
Greater than 12 secs – Allen's positive.

On confirmation of both a patent ulnar and radial artery on that side, the patient is advised not to draw blood sample or receive chemotherapeutic injections via that upper extremity.

INTRAOPERATIVE STEPS FOR HARVEST OF FRAFF

The Allen's test is performed again. Patient is placed in supine position with the arm extended at 90°. Pneumatic tourniquet is applied to the arm. The axis of the radial artery and cephalic vein is marked. The flap marking is done based on site, size and shape of the defect **(Figs. 3 and 4)**. Simultaneous harvest with the resection is preferred. A lazy S incision is marked proximal to the flap marking up to 2 cms below the cubital line to coincide approximately with the course off the cephalic vein.

The tourniquet is raised and maintained at 250 mm of Hg. Exploratory incision is taken on the lazy S mark to identify the cephalic vein. The incision is extended to follow the course of the cephalic vein proximally just short of the cubital fossa and distally up to the edge of the flap marking **(Fig. 5)**. The cephalic vein is dissected till the cubital fossa with a cuff of fat **(Fig. 6)**. The skin incision is extended laterally along the flap marking. The superficial radial nerve is identified and preserved **(Fig. 7)**.

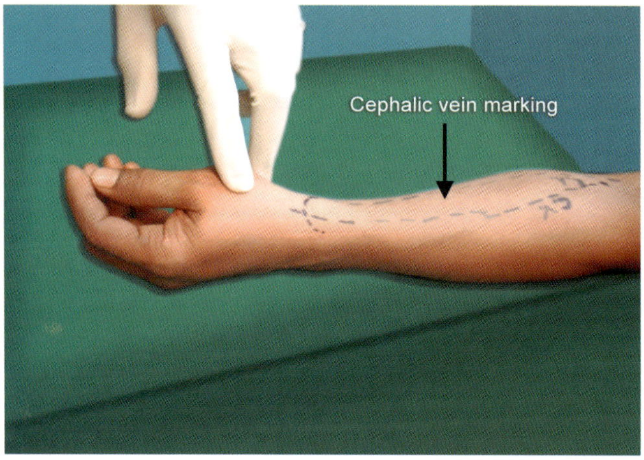

Fig. 3: Axis of radial artery and cephalic vein

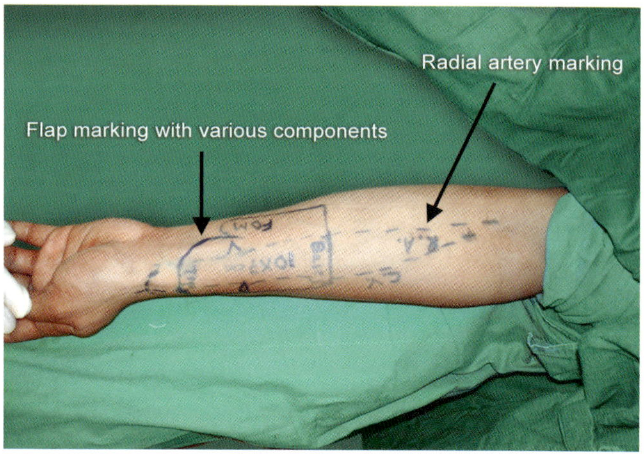

Fig. 4: Flap marking based on site, size and shape of defect, e.g. tongue with floor of mouth defect

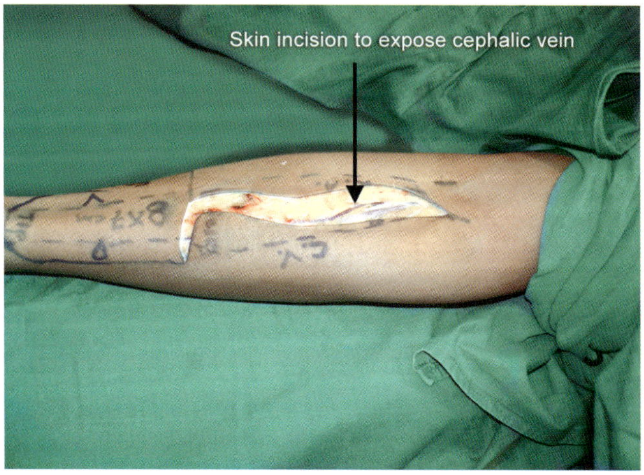

Fig. 5: Exploratory lazy S incision taken to expose the cephalic vein

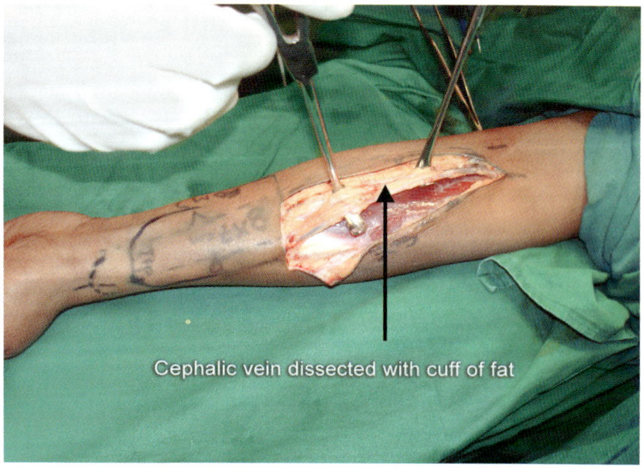

Fig. 6: Cephalic vein dissected with a cuff of fat

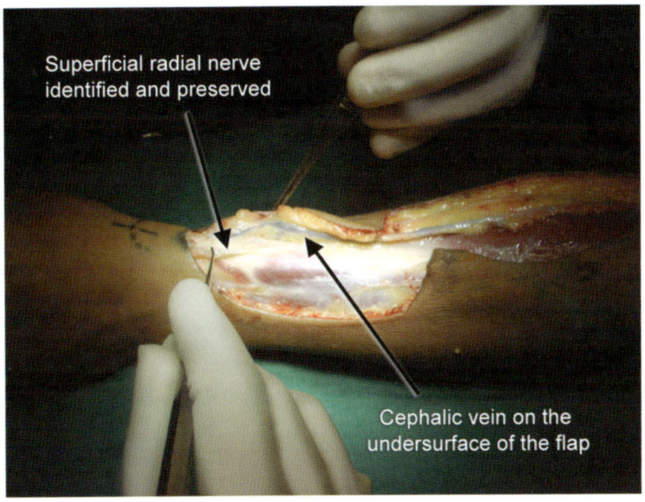

Fig. 7: Identification and preservation of superficial radial nerve

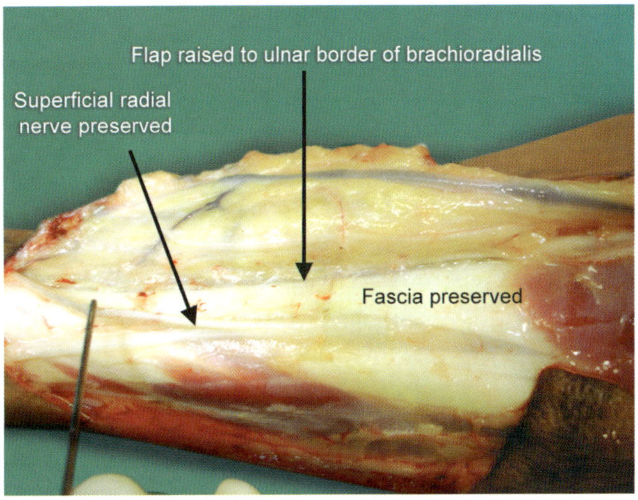

Fig. 8: Flap raised up to ulnar border of brachioradialis

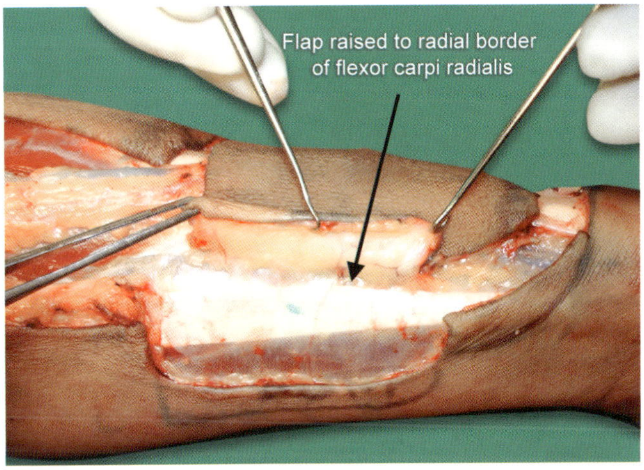

Fig. 9: Flap raised up to radial border of flexor carpi radialis

Suprafascial harvest of the flap is done for better split thickness skin graft (STSG) take, subfascial harvest risks damaging the paratenon and likelihood of graft loss.[2,3] The flap is raised up to the ulnar border of the brachioradialis stopping short of the lateral intermuscular septum **(Fig. 8)**. The skin incision is deepened along the ulnar border of the flap marking. Superficial veins encountered are divided. The flap is raised over the palmaris longus up to the radial border of the flexor carpi radialis muscle **(Fig. 9)**. Incision is now deepened up to subcutaneous tissue over the distal end of the flap. The distal end of the cephalic vein is identified and ligated. The radial artery and venae comitantes are identified clamped and ligated. The tie on the flap end of the vessel is kept long. Using the long end for gentle traction the radial artery is now raised with the flap preserving the deep fascia along its course. Branches supplying the forearm are identified and ligated **(Figs. 10A and B)**. Once

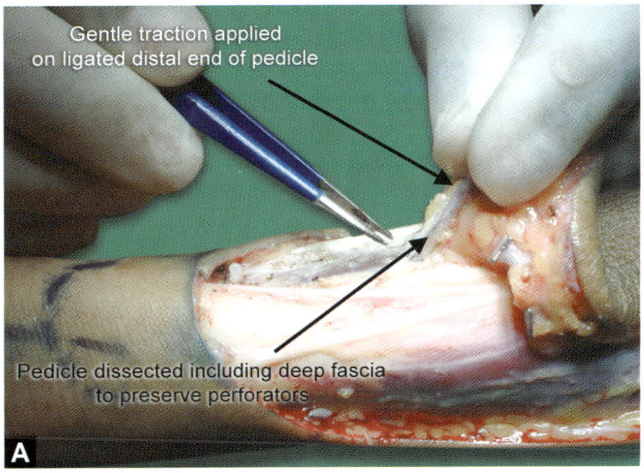

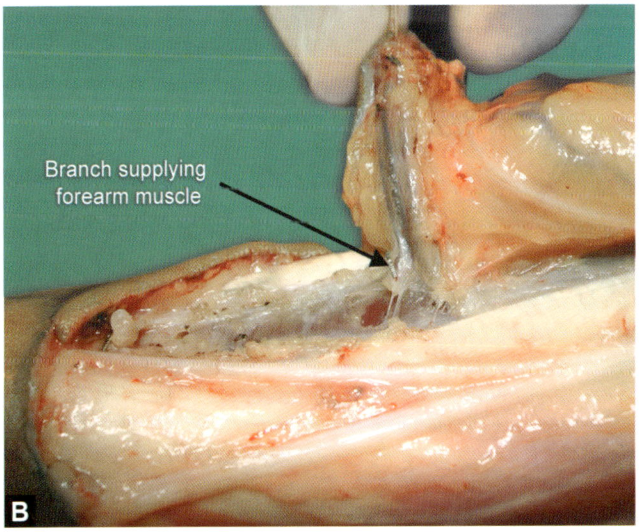

Figs. 10A and B: Gentle traction is given to dissect the radial artery and venae comitantes; (B) Deep branches supplying the forearm muscles are divided

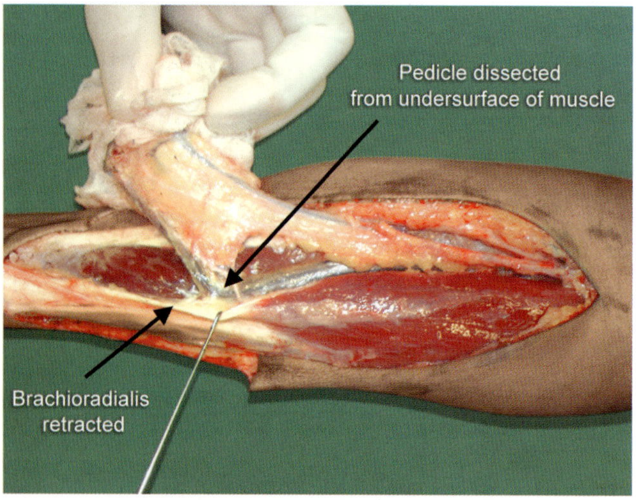

Fig. 11: Belly of brachioradialis retracted for dissection and preservation of proximal perforators

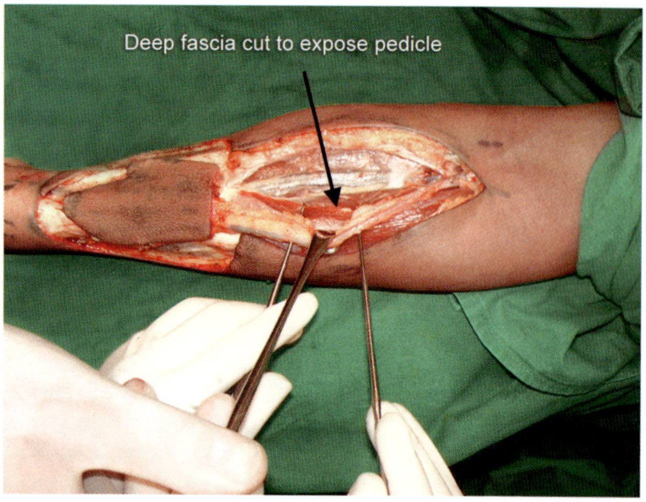

Fig. 12: Intermuscular septum cut to facilitate pedicle dissection

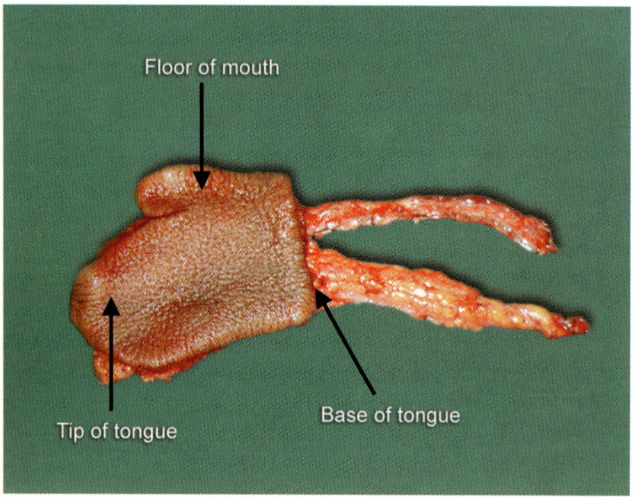

Fig. 13A: FRAFF harvested

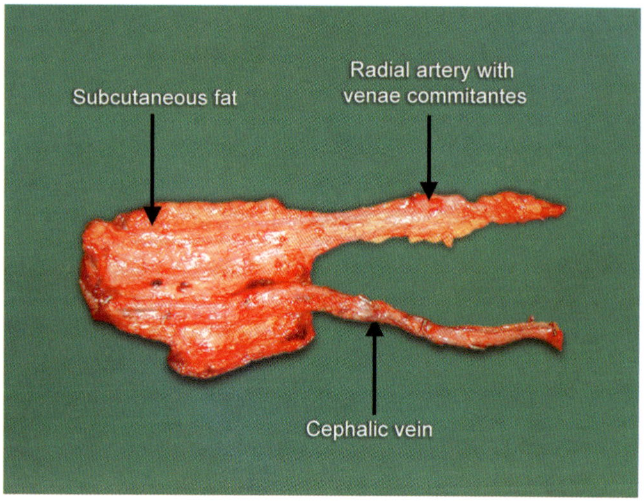

Fig. 13B: FRAFF harvested

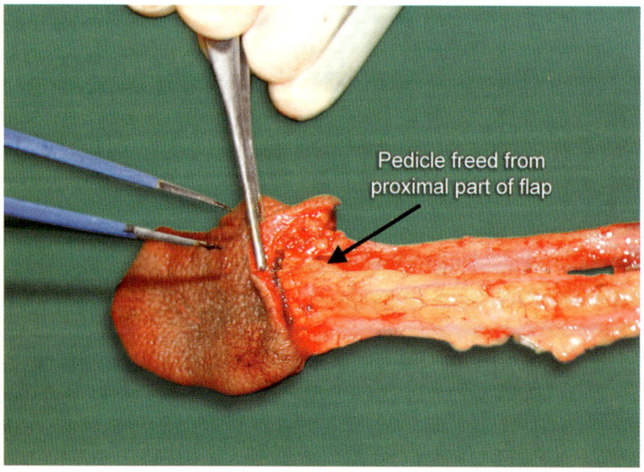

Fig. 14: The pedicle is separated from the proximal end of the flap for approx 1 cm

the belly of the brachioradialis and flexor carpi radialis are encountered, the muscles are retracted to enable the dissection of the vessels with the subcutaneous tissue in order to preserve the proximal perforators **(Fig. 11)**. The intermuscular septum beyond the flap is cut to facilitate easy harvest of the pedicle till the length required **(Fig. 12)**. The tourniquet is released and flap bleed is checked and confirmed before division of the pedicle **(Figs. 13A and B)**. The pedicle is separated from the proximal end of the flap for 1 cm to prevent kinking of the vessel post flap inset **(Fig. 14)**.

How Large a Flap can be Harvested?

The entire circumference of the forearm can be included in the flap preserving a strip of skin 3 cms wide along the ulnar border.

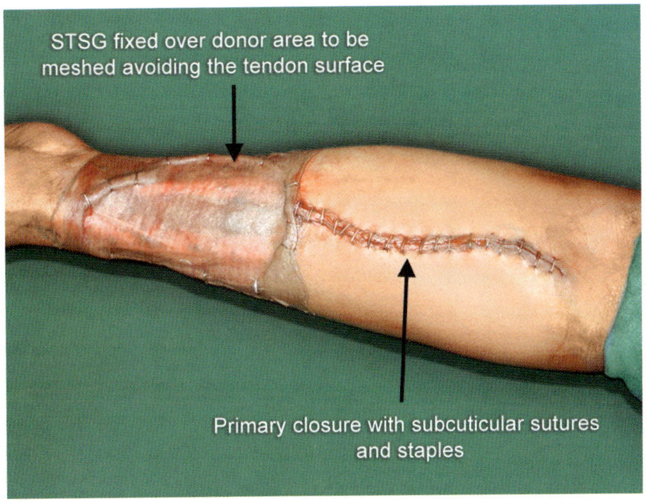

Fig. 15: STSG over FRAFF donor area

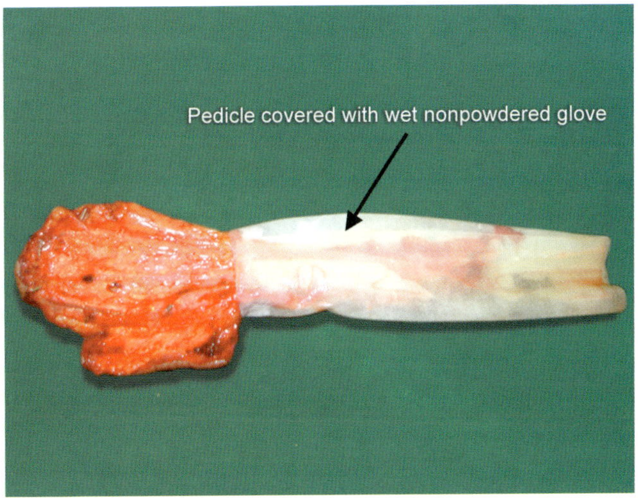

Fig. 16: Pedicle covered in a cut piece of glove

What are the Components that can be Harvested with the Flap?

Osteocutaneous Flap

A wedge of cortical radial bone up to 10–12 cms in an adult can be harvested by preserving the periosteum and raising it along with the flap. Osteotomy can be performed to contour the straight bone after harvest. The remnant radial bone however is prone to fracture due to trivial trauma and needs to be reinforced with a plate. Since the widespread use of the free fibula flap to reconstruct bony defects the osteocutaneous radial flap is rarely used.

Sensate Flap

The flap is harvested with the lateral cutaneous nerve or the medial cutaneous nerve dissection is continued proximally to identify the nerves. The nerve is coapted at the recipient site for a sensate flap.

Prefabrication

The FRAFF can be used for prefabrication with cartilage grafts for reconstruction of nasal and tracheal defects. The flap is partially elevated and the cartilage grafts are placed in the subcutaneous tissue pockets.

Donor Site Management

The donor site of the flap is covered with a split thickness skin graft. Care is taken during flap harvest to preserve the paratenon over the tendons of the forearm to improve graft take. The exploratory incision for pedicle length is closed with subcuticular sutures **(Fig. 15)**. A slab is applied to the forearm with the wrist in extension and the metacarpophalangeal joints in anatomical position.

Safe Passage of the Pedicle

The FRAFF pedicle is covered with a moist cut piece of sterile non-powdered latex glove **(Fig. 16)**. The proximal end of the glove piece is grasped with an artery forceps and passed through the tunnel. The glove piece is gently freed off the pedicle and the final lie of the pedicle is determined **(Figs. 17A and B)**.

Flap Inset

Division of the flap based on perforators or de-epithelization is done to provide two or more paddles if required. Partial flap fixation is done prior to arterial or venous anastomoses. Final adjustments to flap fixation are done post-anastomoses.

INDICATION FOR USE

Head and Neck Reconstruction

Buccal Mucosa

FRAFF is used for reconstruction of isolated buccal mucosa defects and partial buccal mucosa defects involving the retromolar trigone **(Figs. 18A to E)**. In cases where moderate soft tissue replacement is required flaps like anterolateral thigh flap or thoracodorsal artery perforator flap is used as FRAFF results in contour defect due to insufficient bulk.

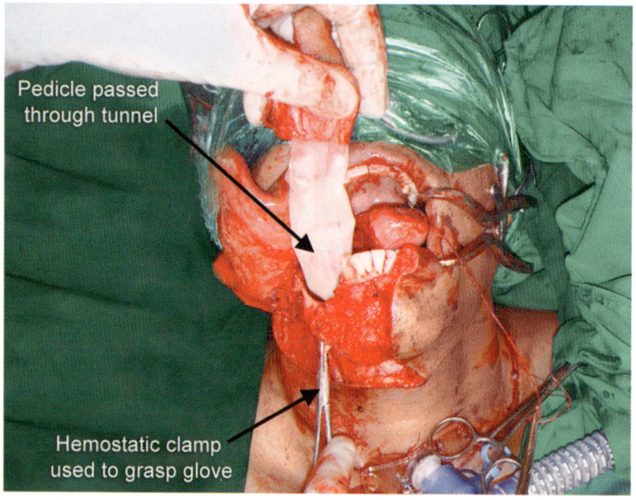

Fig. 17A: The pedicle is passed through the tunnel by grasping the glove with a pair of artery forceps

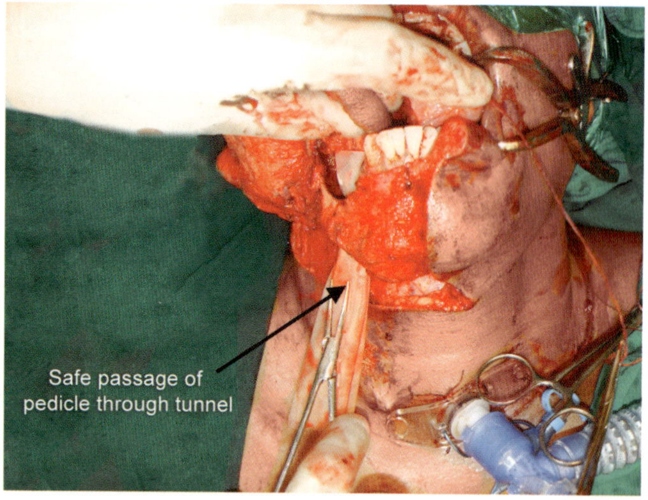

Fig. 17B: The glove is gently withdrawn through the tunnel

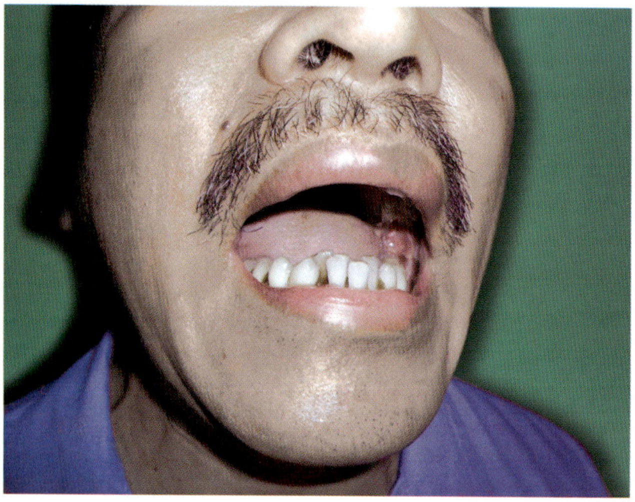

Fig. 18A: Left buccal mucosa lesion

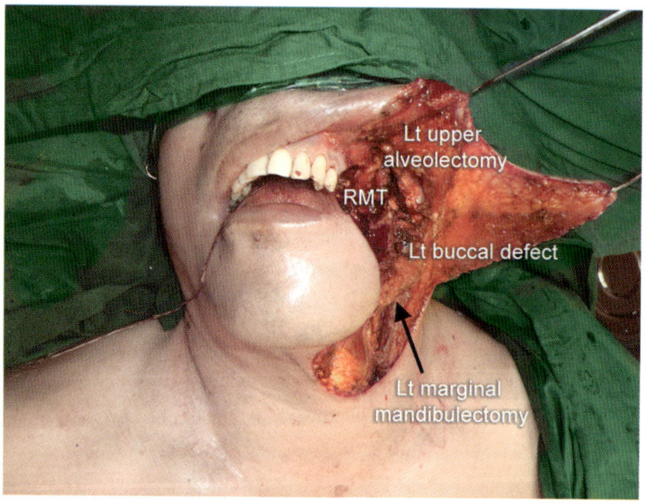

Fig. 18B: Buccal mucosa defect post-tumor resection

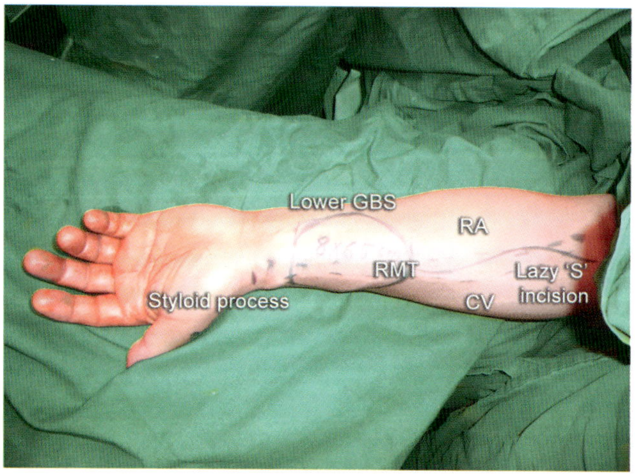

Fig. 18C: FRAFF skin marking

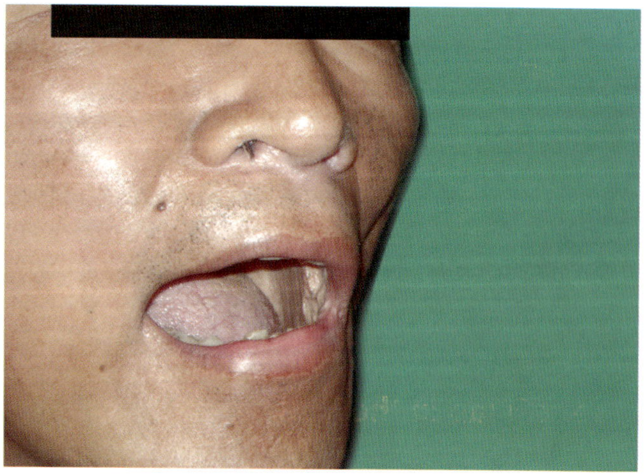

Fig. 18D: Follow-up

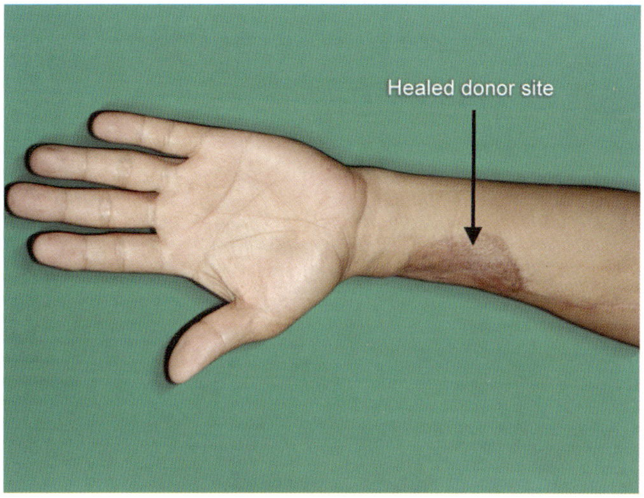

Fig. 18E: Donor site follow-up

Lip

FRAFF proves to be a versatile flap for various lip defects **(Figs. 19A to E)**. The pliability of the flap makes it amenable to be contoured to irregular defects **(Figs. 20A to G)**. When addressing the lip reconstruction, the patient's height of the oral curtain and oral competence must be determined.[4] This determines if a palmaris longus sling should be incorporated into the FRAFF to assist with competence[5] **(Figs. 21A to F)**.

Tongue: Tongue defects less than a hemiglossectomy that require a thin, pliable flap with restoration of tongue function can be treated with FRAFF **(Figs. 22A to G)**.

A combination of all of these defects, lip, tongue, and buccal mucosa, can be treated FRAFF providing a robust and reliable fasciocutaneous flap **(Figs. 23A to F)**.

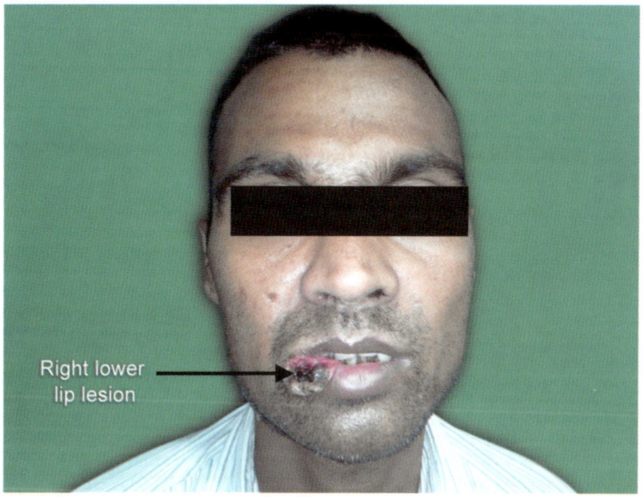

Fig. 19A: Right lower lip lesion

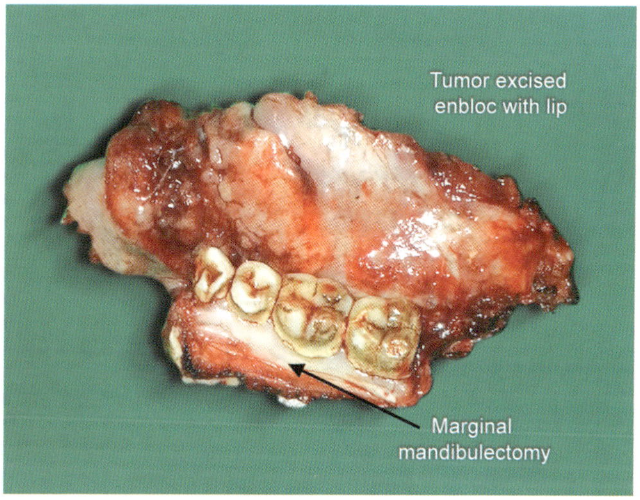

Fig. 19B: Excised lesion

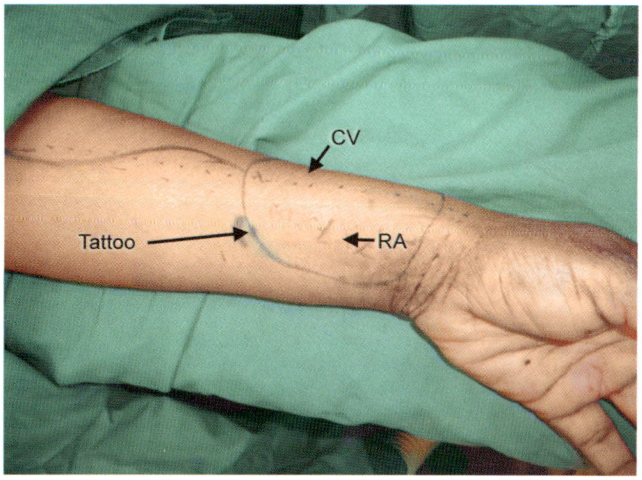

Fig. 19C: Flap marking

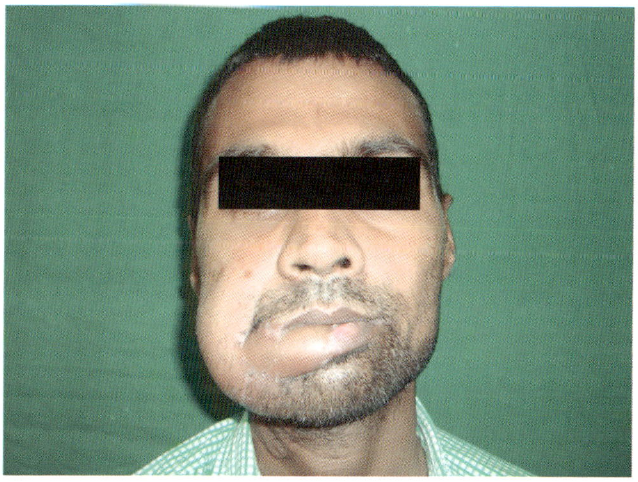

Fig. 19D1: Immediate follow-up

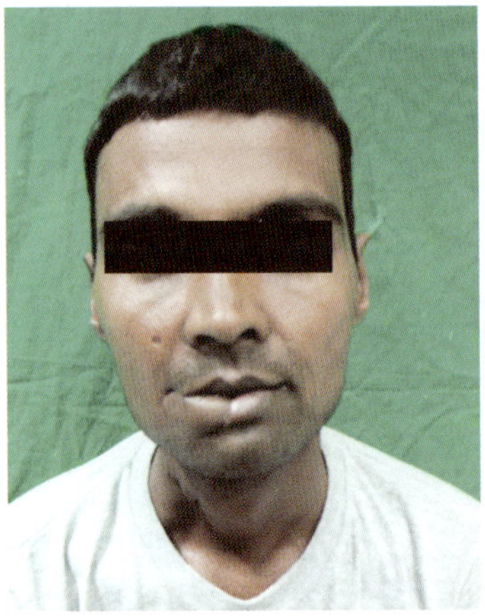

Fig. 19D2: Late follow-up

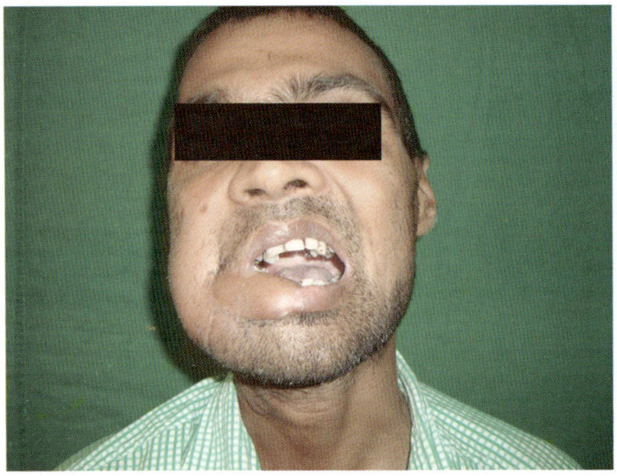

Fig. 19E1: Immediate follow-up mouth opening

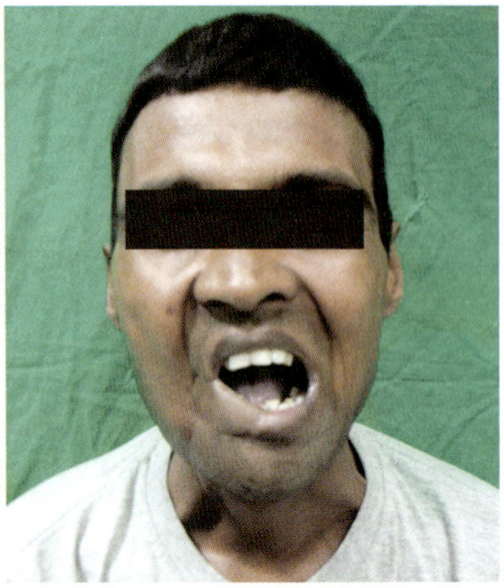

Fig. 19E2: Late follow-up mouth opening

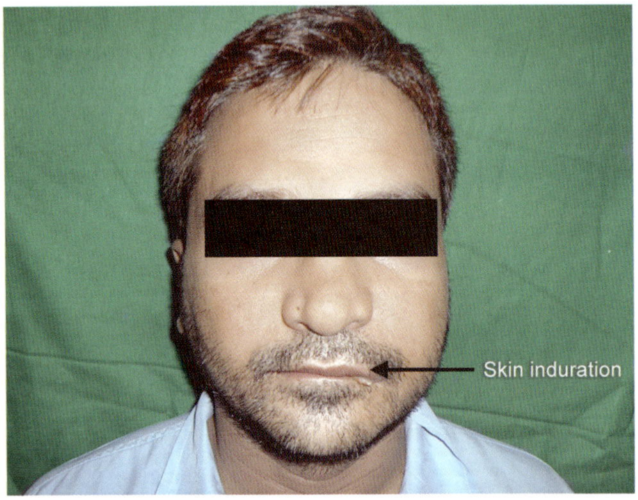

Fig. 20A: Right upper lip lesion with outer skin induration

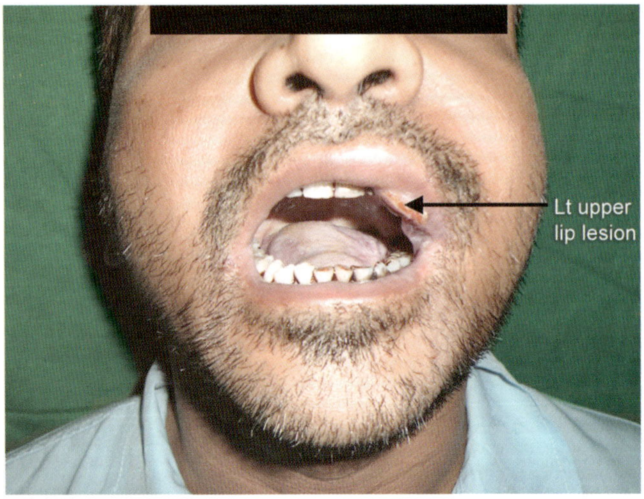

Fig. 20B: Left upper lip lesion

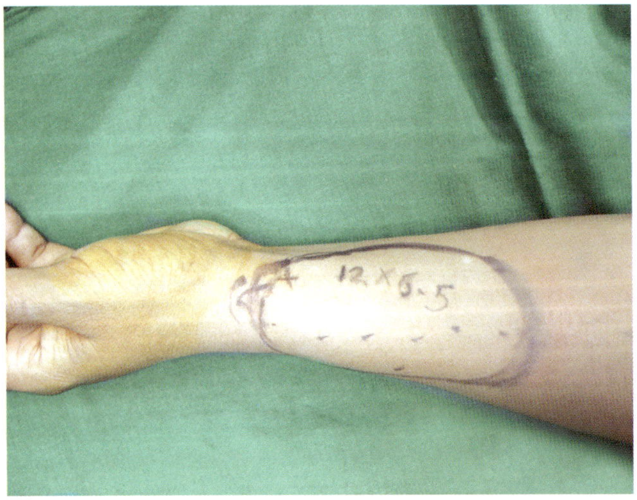

Fig. 20C: Flap marking

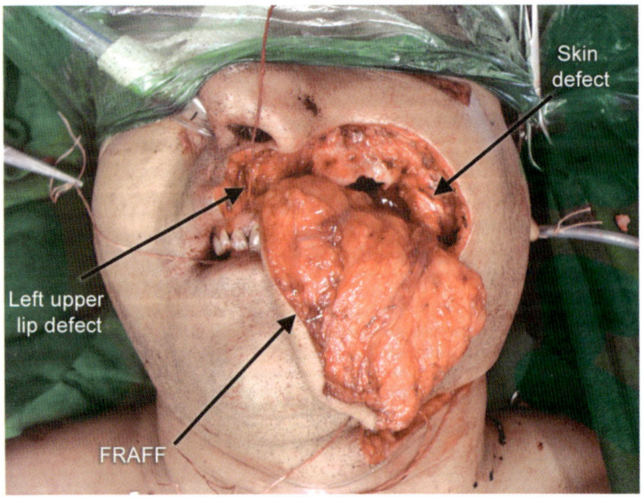

Fig. 20D: Defect post excision with partial flap inset

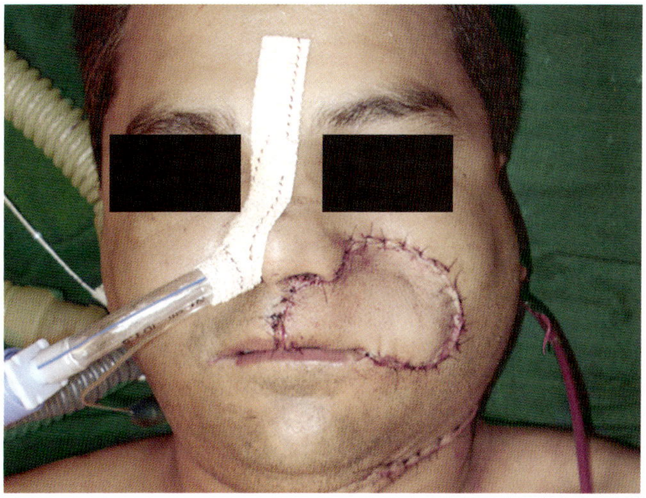

Fig. 20E: Flap inset completed

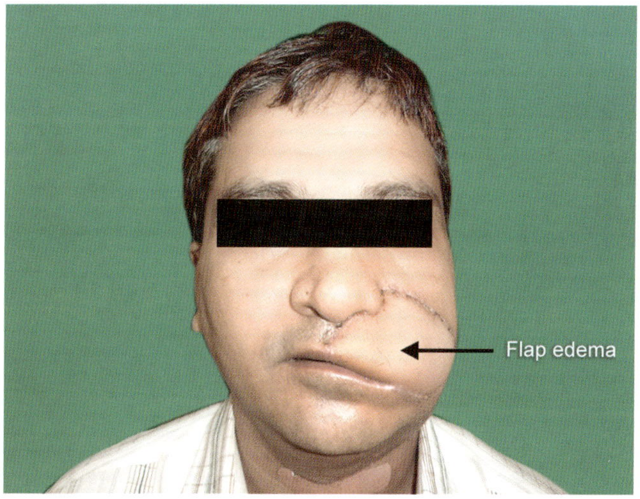

Fig. 20F: Immediate follow-up

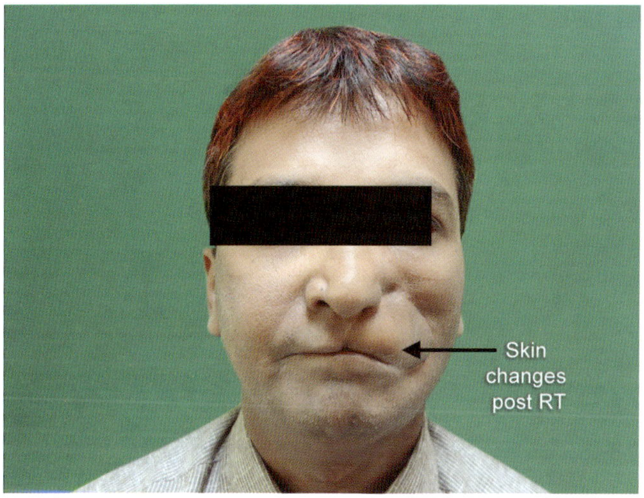

Fig. 20G: Follow-up post radiation

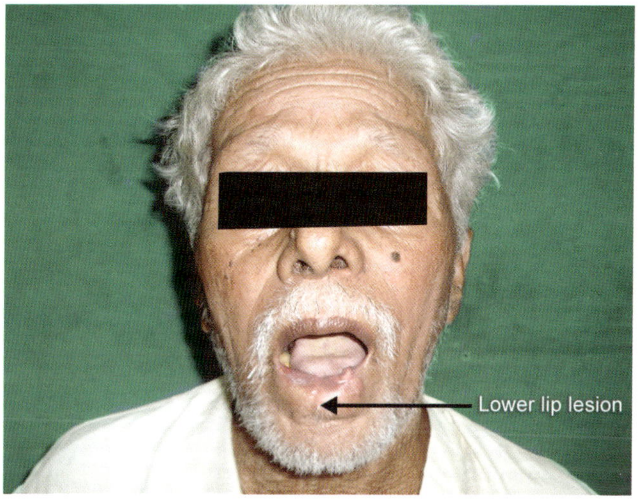

Fig. 21A: Preoperative lower lip lesion

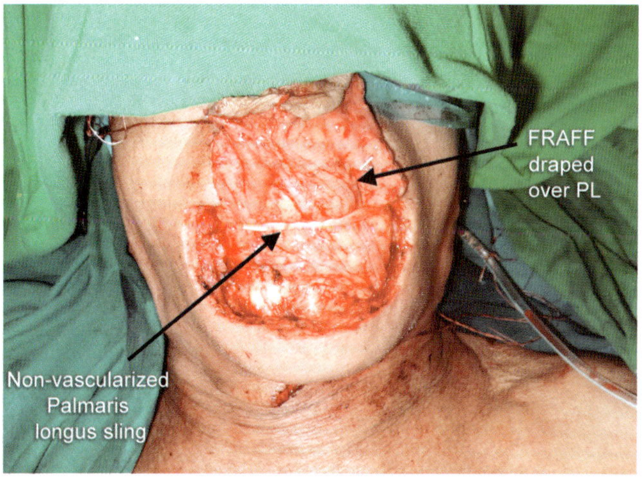

Fig. 21B: Palmaris longus sling

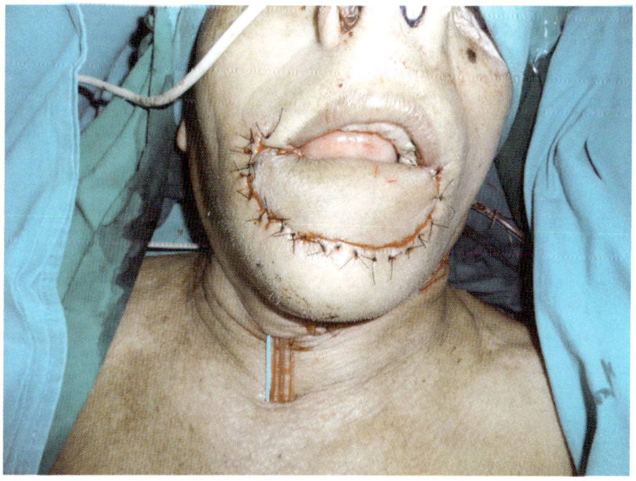

Fig. 21C: Intraoperative flap inset completed

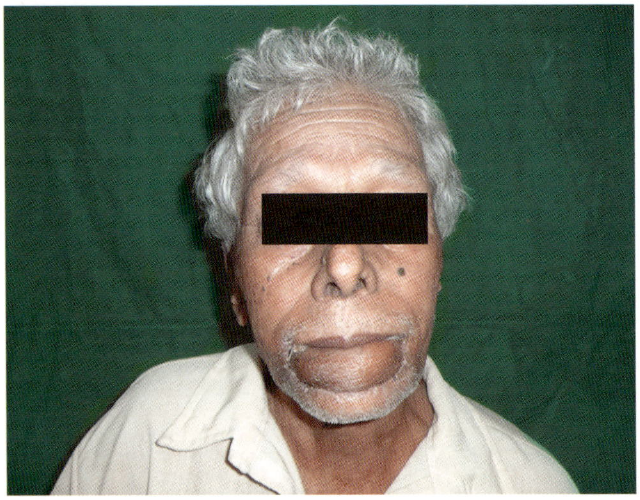

Fig. 21D: Immediate follow-up with lip height maintained

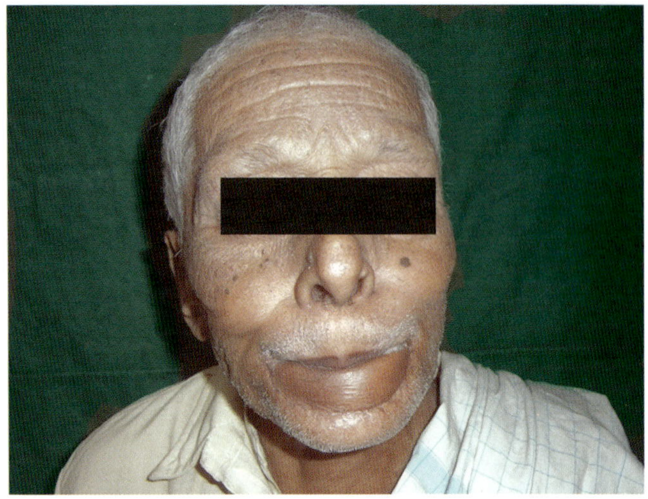

Fig. 21E: Long-term follow-up with lip height maintained

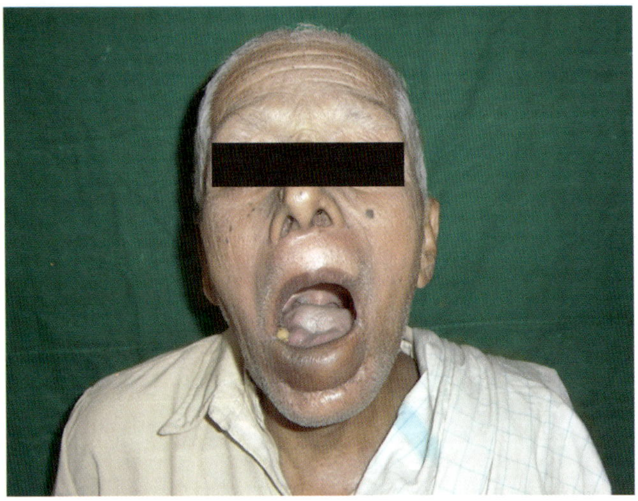

Fig. 21F: Long-term follow-up with oral competence maintained

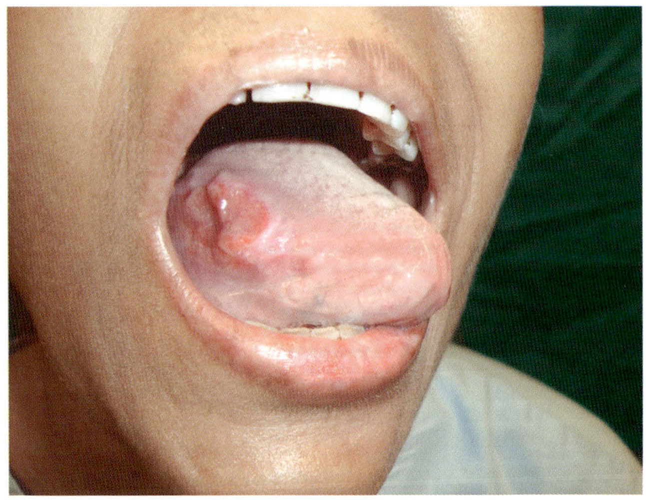

Fig. 22A: Lesion over right lateral border of tongue

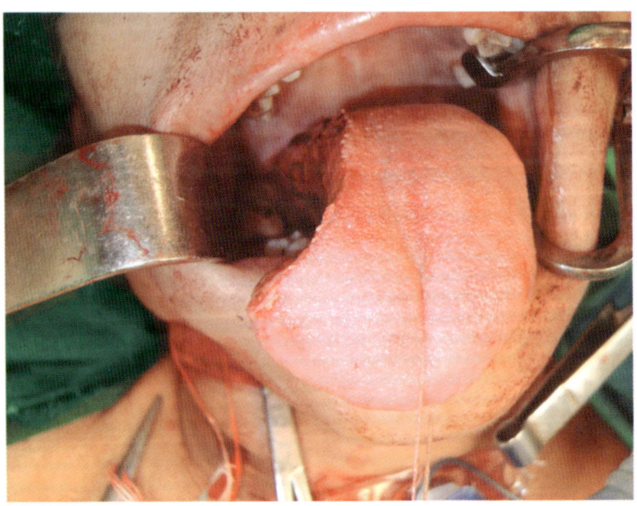

Fig. 22B: Defect post-tumor excision right lateral border sparing anterior two third

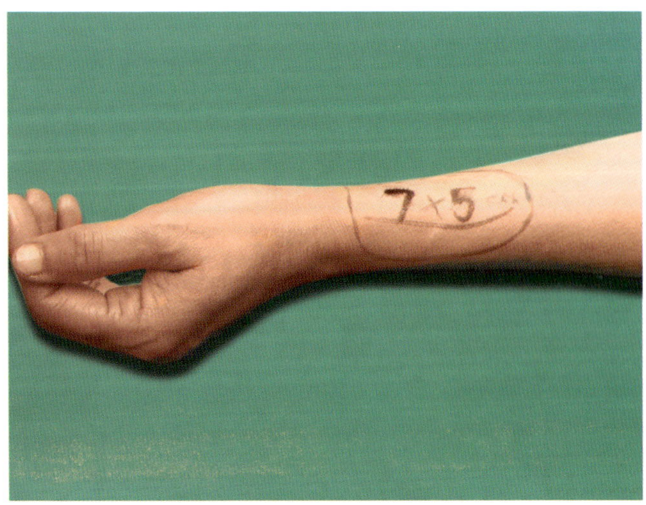

Fig. 22C: FRAFF flap marking

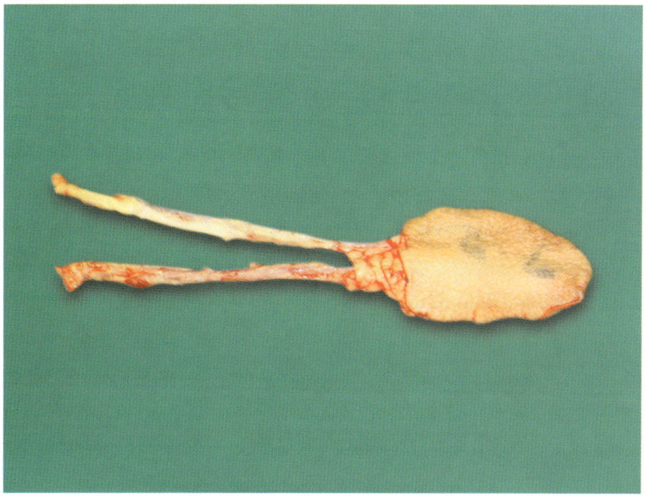

Fig. 22D: FRAFF harvested

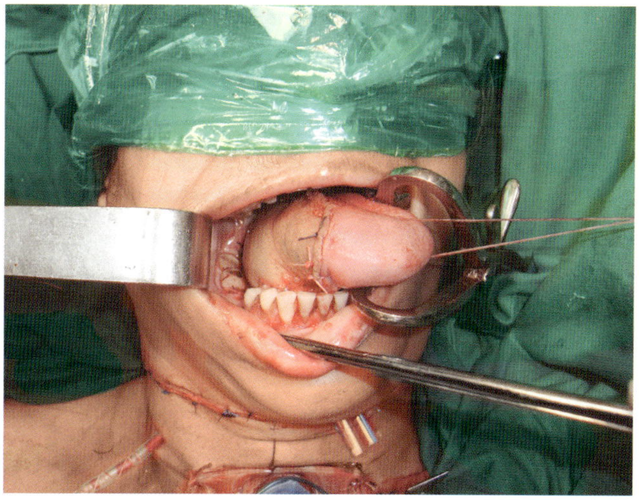

Fig. 22E: Flap completed inset

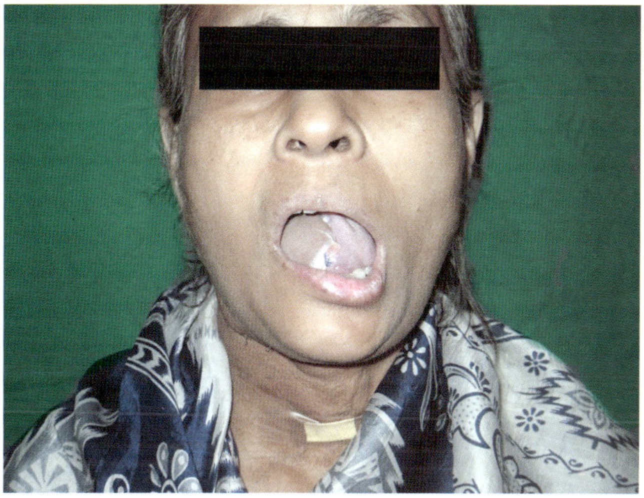

Fig. 22F: Immediate follow-up frontal view

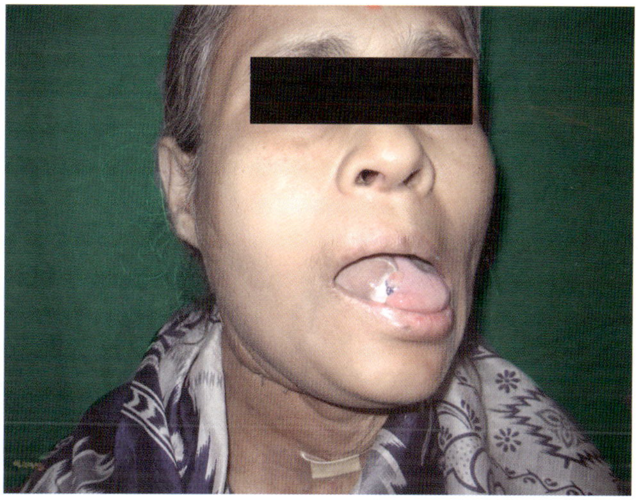

Fig. 22G: Immediate follow-up lateral view

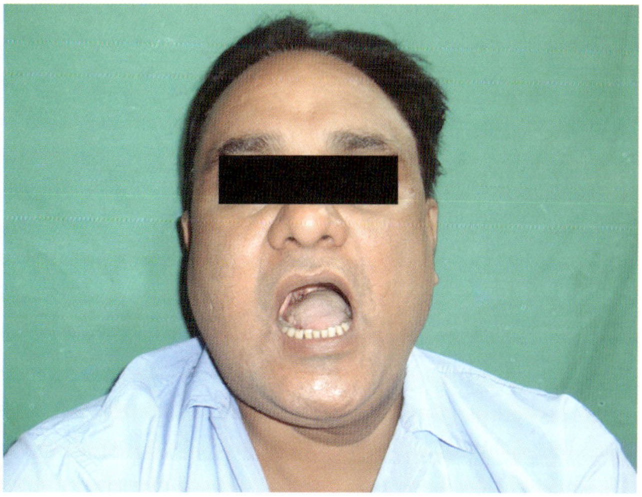

Fig. 23A: Lesion involving tongue mandible and buccal mucosa

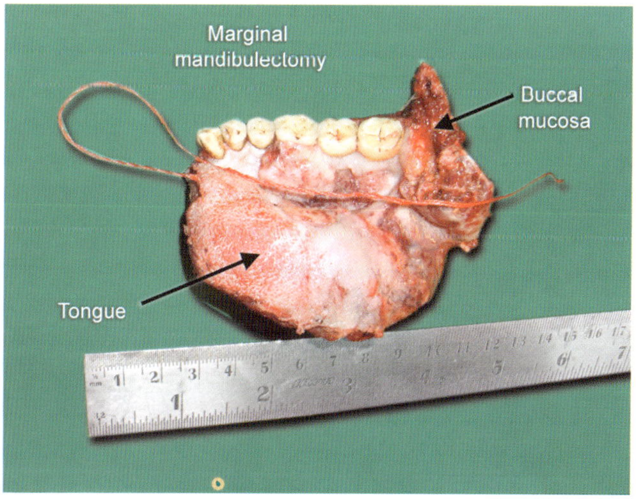

Fig. 23B: Resected specimen

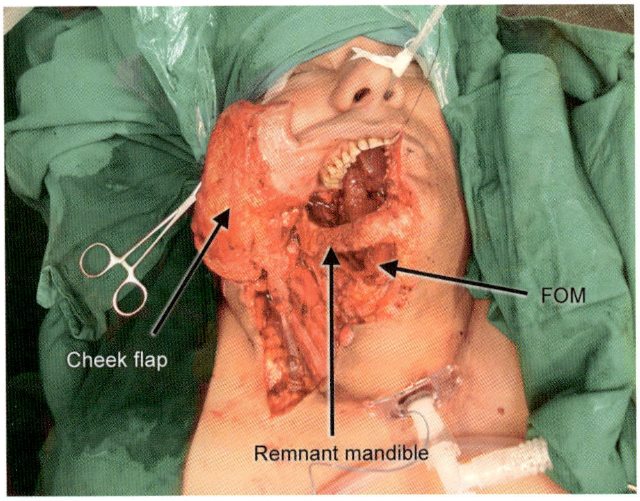

Fig. 23C: Defect involving right lateral tongue

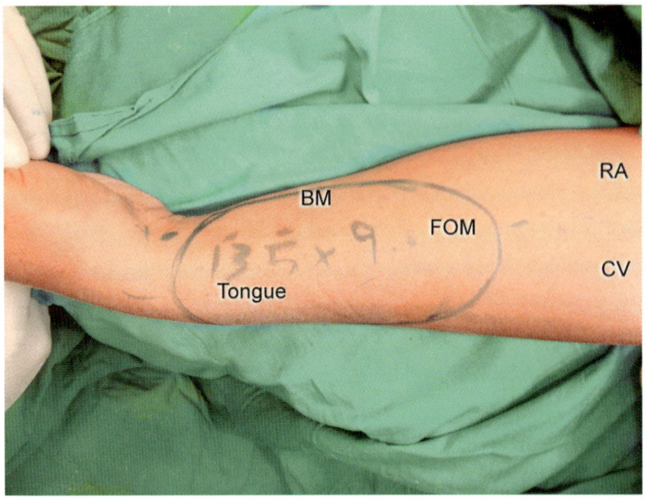

Fig. 23D: Flap marking

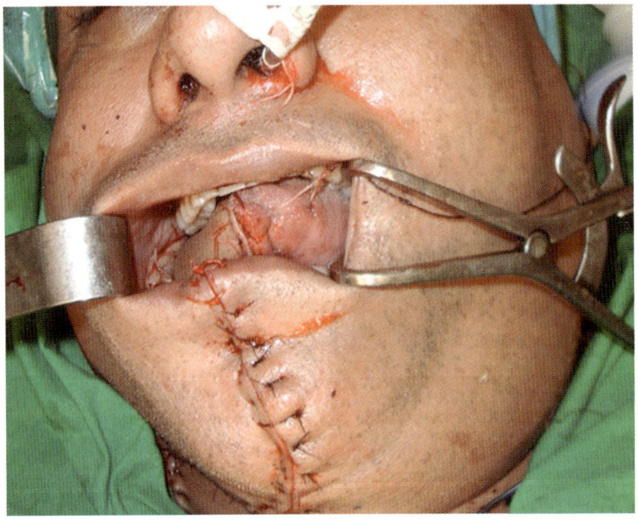

Fig. 23E: Flap inset completed

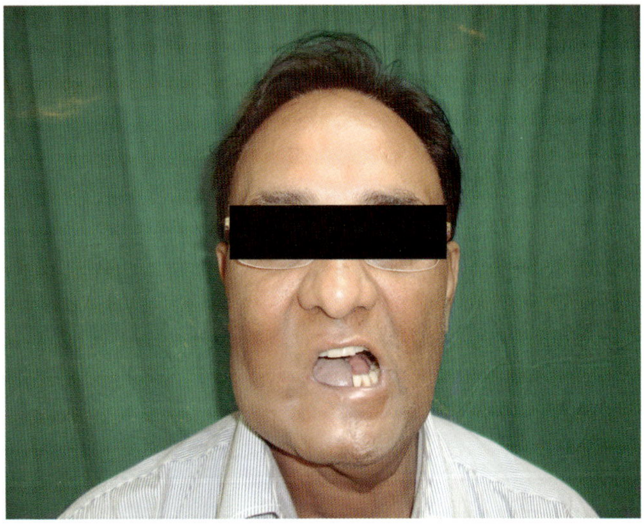

Fig. 23F: Post-radiation follow-up

Pharyngeal Reconstruction

The pharynx is a fibromuscular tubular structure that connects the oral cavity to the cervical esophagus. Pharyngeal reconstruction post-tumor extirpation aims at providing a leak proof food passage and speech normalcy.

Pharyngeal defects can be divided into:[6]

a. Large defects (width of the remnant unstretched mucosa is less than three centimeters): FRAFF can be used when other soft tissue flap options prove to be bulky **(Figs. 24A to D)**.
b. Circumferential defects with lower extent above the thoracic inlet: They are reconstructed using skin or mucosa lined tubed flaps. Tubed FRAFF is used occasionally **(Figs. 25A to E)**.

The thinness and the pliability of the flap makes FRAFF ideal for reconstruction and resurfacing of irregular, small to medium sized soft tissue defects of the head and neck region. The length of pedicle increases ease anastomoses to vessels that are remote to the defect itself. We have used FRAFF for the following:

a. Eye socket reconstruction **(Figs. 26A to E)**
b. Palatal defects
c. Nasal lining and skin cover
d. Post craniofacial resection
e. Salvage option after discarding non-viable FFOCF skin paddle

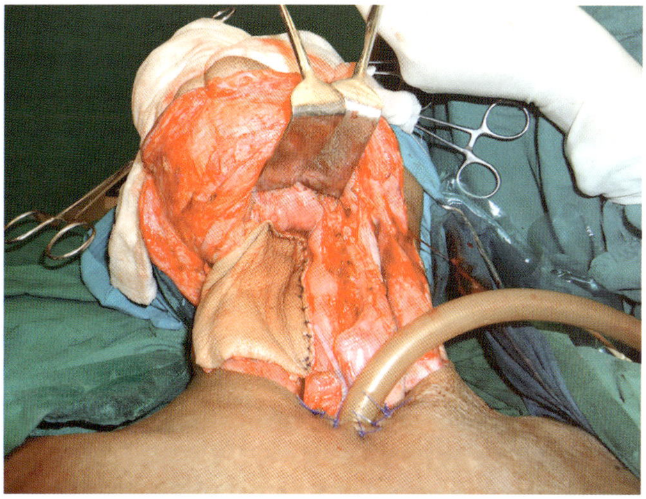

Fig. 24A: Intraoperative partial inset of patch FRAFF to remnant pharyngeal wall

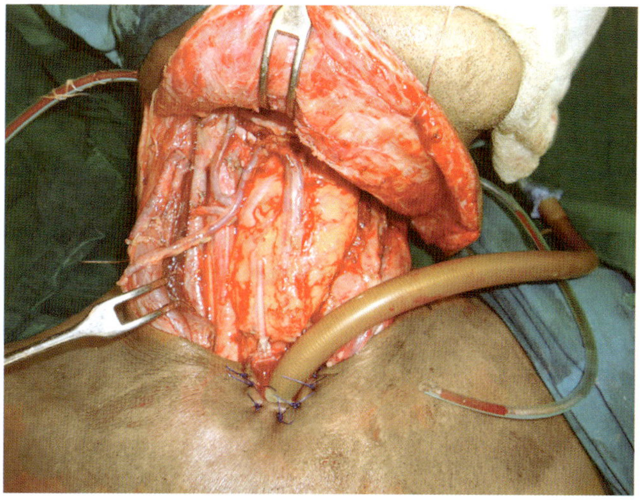

Fig. 24B: Intraoperative flap inset of patch FRAFF completed

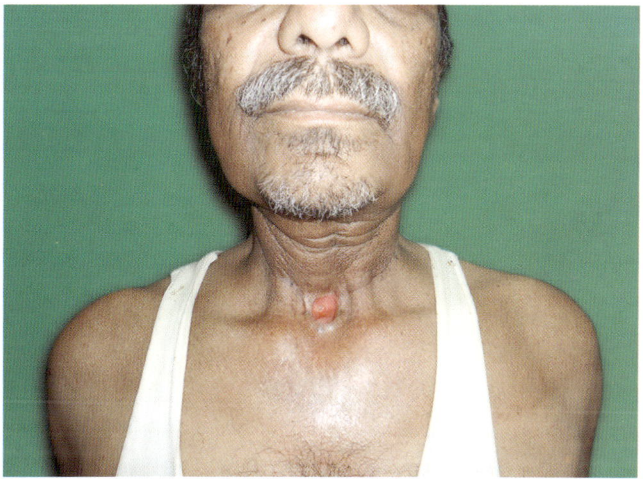

Fig. 24C: End tracheostoma

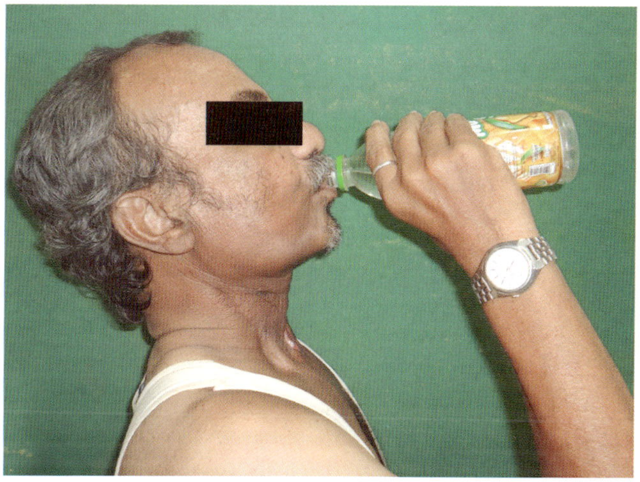

Fig. 24D: Swallowing function maintained post-radiation

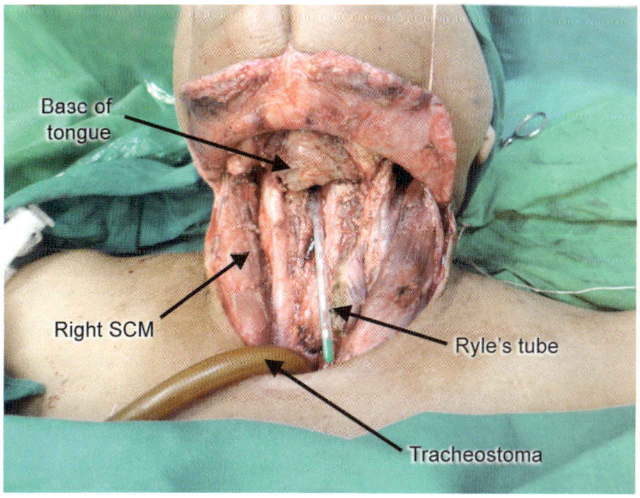

Fig. 25A: Total pharyngectomy defect with end tracheostoma

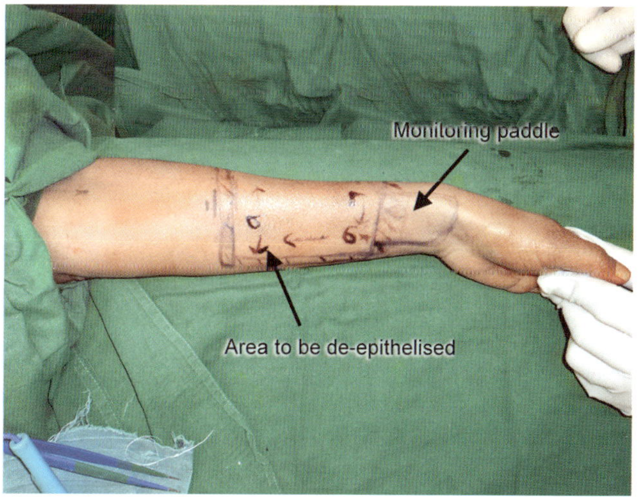

Fig. 25B: Flap marking

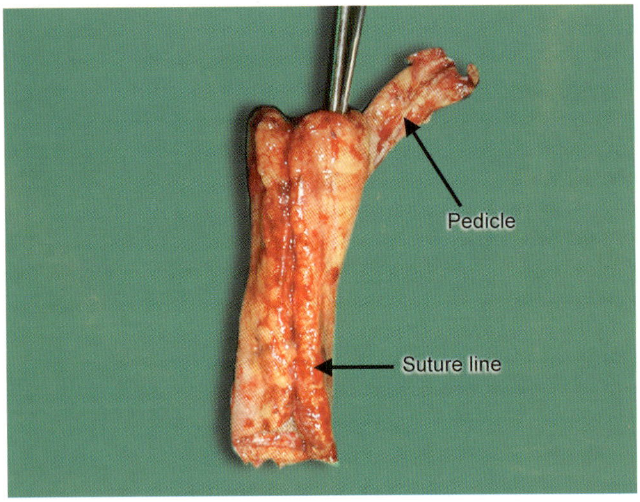

Fig. 25C: Tubed FRAFF with skin surface forming inner lining

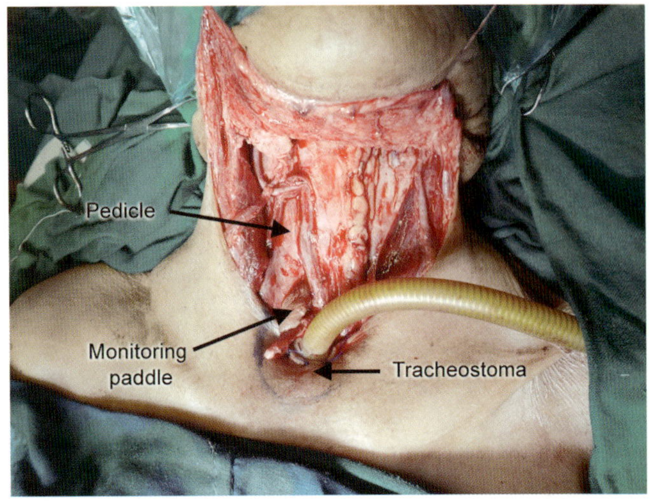

Fig. 25D: Flap inset completed

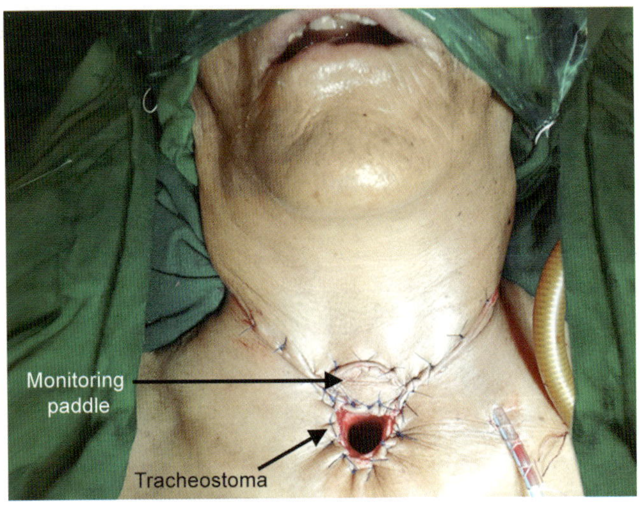

Fig. 25E: End stoma with monitoring paddle

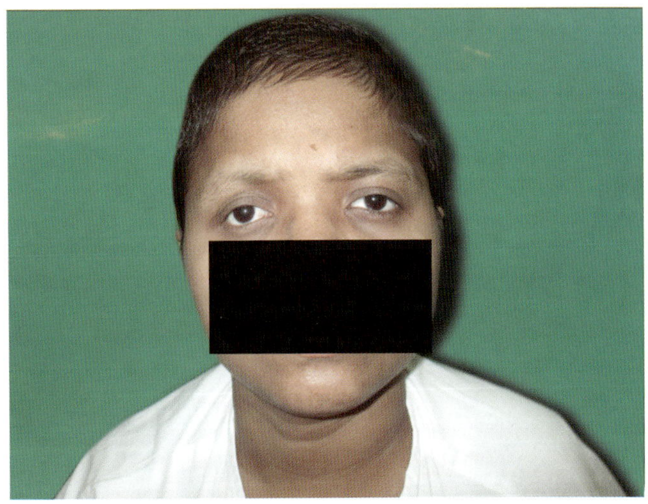

Fig. 26A: Preoperative right retro-orbital tumor

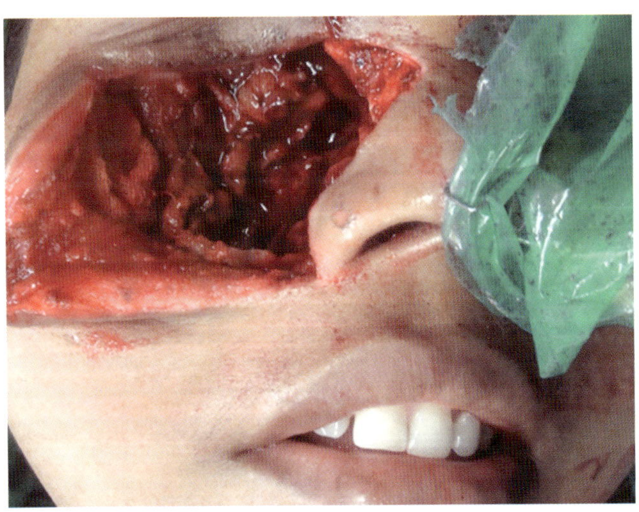

Fig. 26B: Right orbital exenteration defect with eyelids preserved

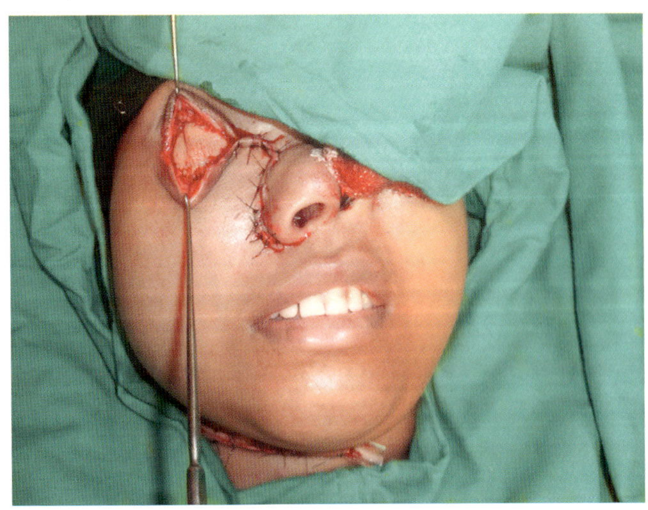

Fig. 26C: FRAFF inset to reconstruct eye socket

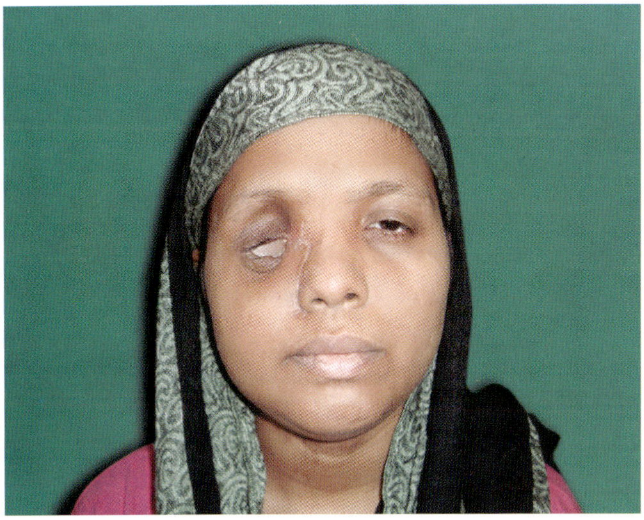

Fig. 26D: Immediate postoperative

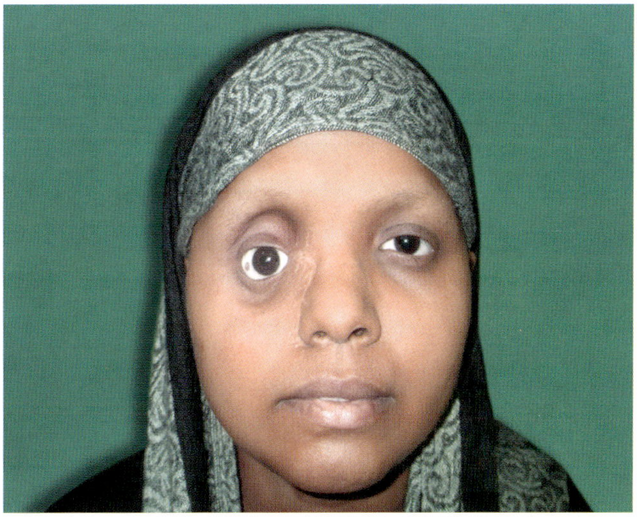

Fig. 26E: Late postoperative with eye prosthesis

Extremity Reconstruction

Upper Extremity

Soft tissue reconstruction of upper extremity can be done with free or pedicled radial forearm flap.

Defects at and Above Elbow Level (Figs. 27A to E)

Proximally-based pedicle RAF is done to cover defects around the elbow.

Defects beyond Wrist Level

Distally based pedicled RAF is done to cover defects over the forearm and hand. Care must be taken to ascertain continuity of the palmar arch prior to flap harvest. The soft tissue over the vessel must be preserved along the length of the flap. The position of the skin paddle should be planned in reverse keeping in mind that the concentration of perforators is the least in the mid forearm. Venous drainage should be ensured in pedicled flaps. If in doubt the vessel should be divided and re-anastomosed in a favorable position **(Figs. 28A to E)**.

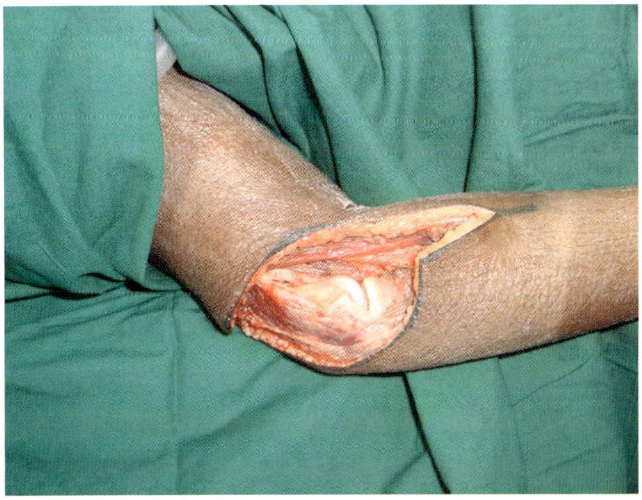

Fig. 27A: Defect at elbow after excision or recurrent soft tissue sarcoma

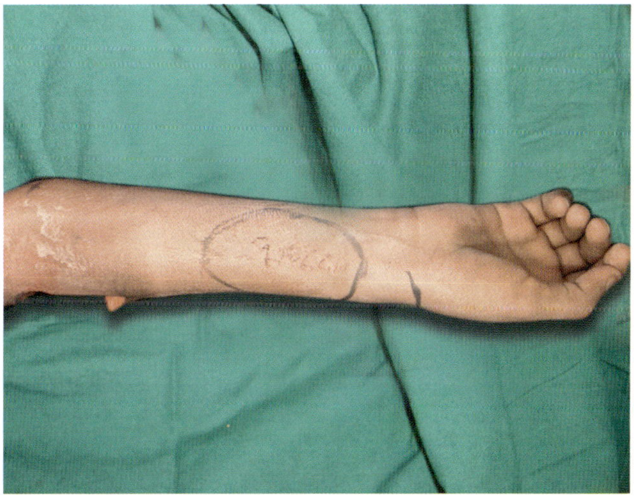

Fig. 27B: Flap marking for proximally based RAF flap

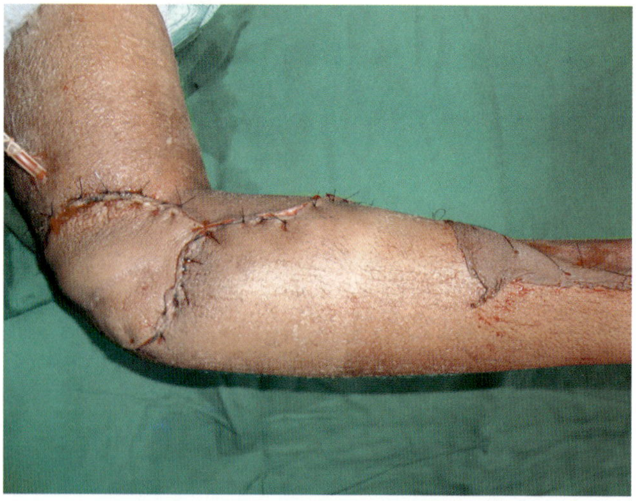

Fig. 27C: Flap inset completed intraoperative

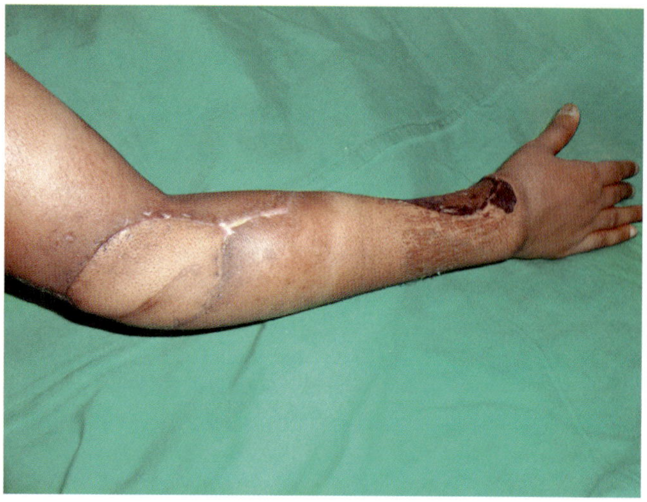

Fig. 27D: Immediate follow-up

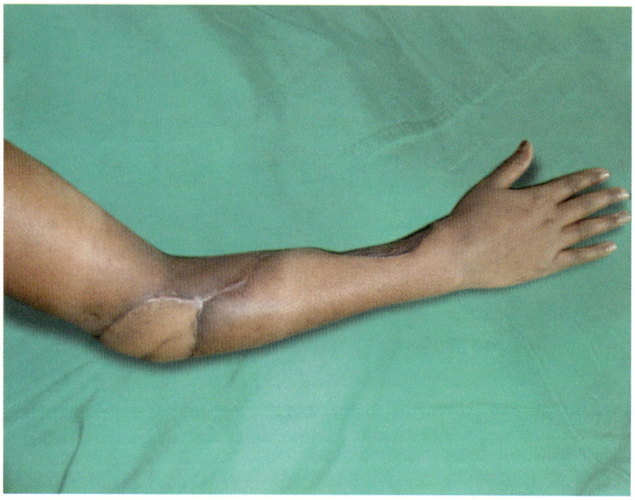

Fig. 27E: Late follow-up

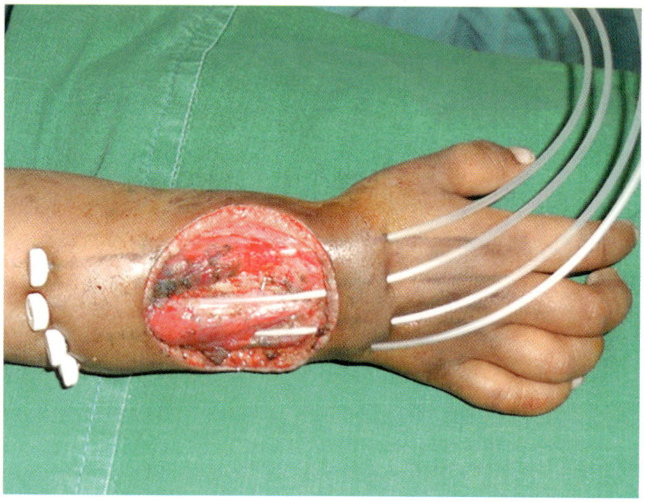

Fig. 28A: Right forearm dorsal aspect defect with brachytherapy tubes in situ

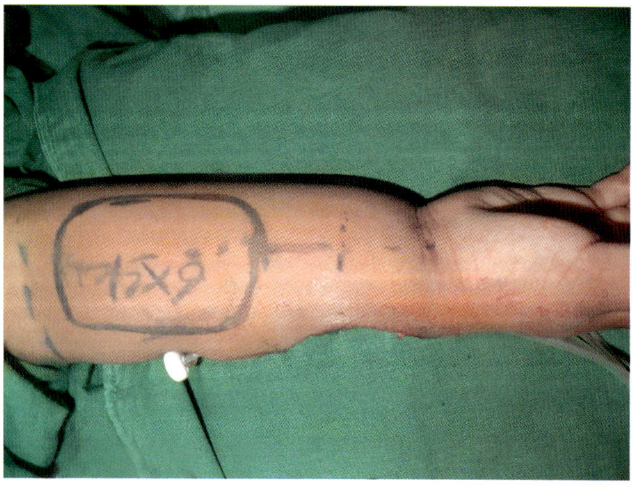

Fig. 28B: Flap marking of distally-based RAF flap

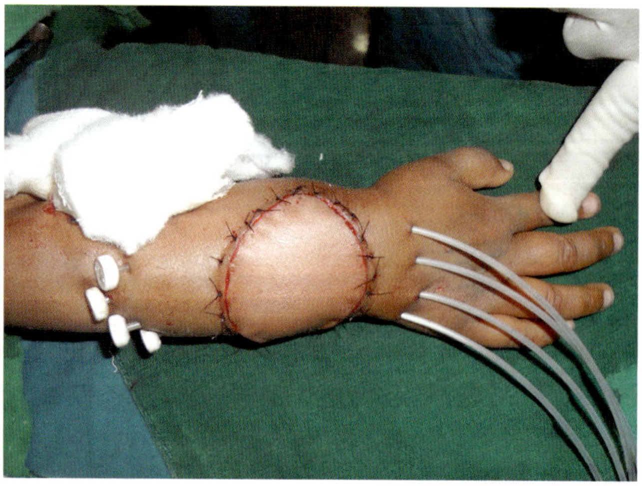

Fig. 28C: Flap inset completed intraoperative

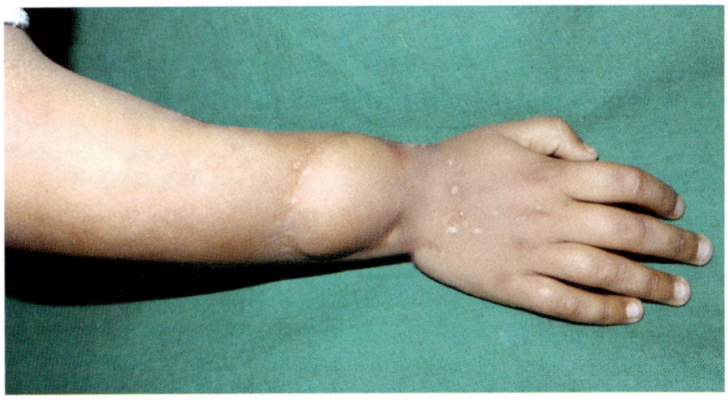

Fig. 28D: Late follow-up

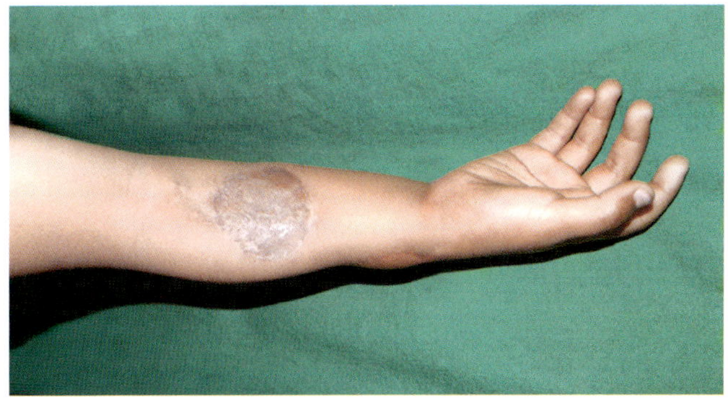

Fig. 28E: Healed donor site STSG

Lower Extremity

Free radial forearm flap is used to cover soft tissue defect where a thin and pliable flap is required e.g. dorsum of foot, shin of tibia,over the tendo achilles etc.

Penile Reconstruction

The radial forearm flap is used in penile reconstruction by double tubing the flap. Various flap designs have been described for the same. However, it results in extensive area of grafted donor site **(Figs. 29A to K)**.

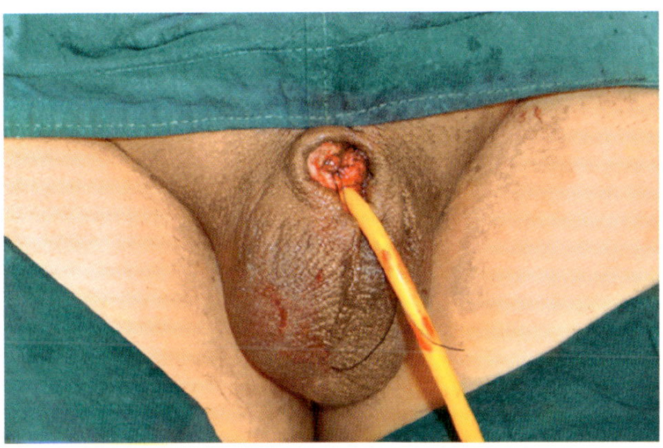

Fig. 29A: Stump of total penectomy

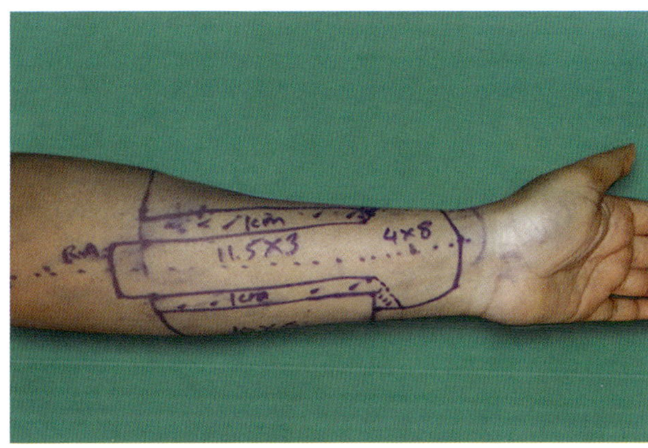

Fig. 29B: Planning of RAFF

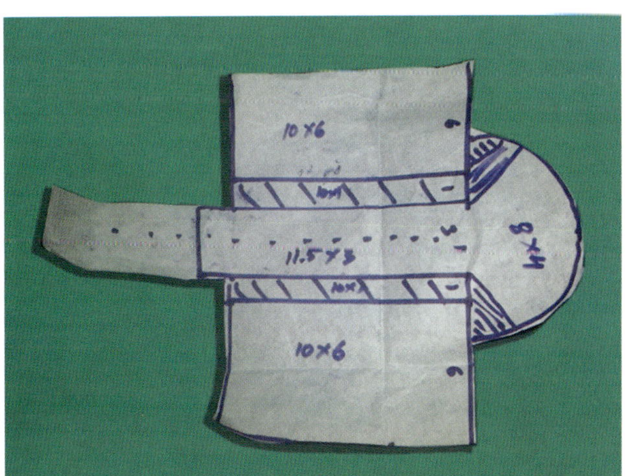

Fig. 29C: Template of plan—Biemer pattern

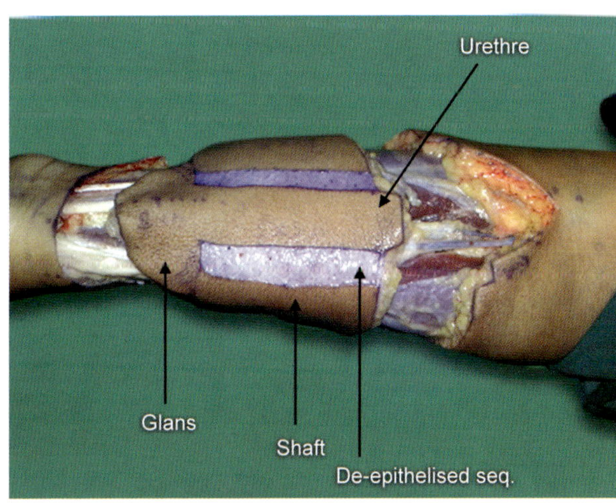

Fig. 29D: Harvested flap

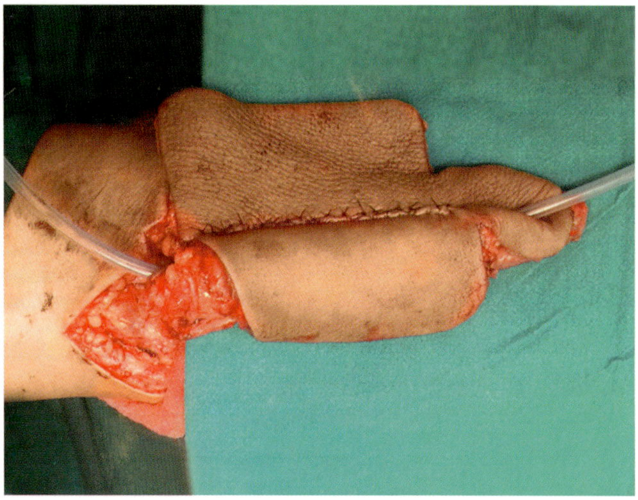

Fig. 29E: Urethra tubed

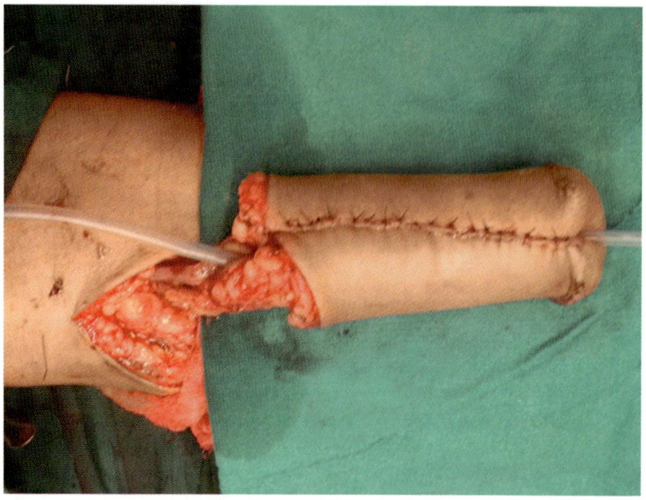

Fig. 29F: Flap ready for transfer

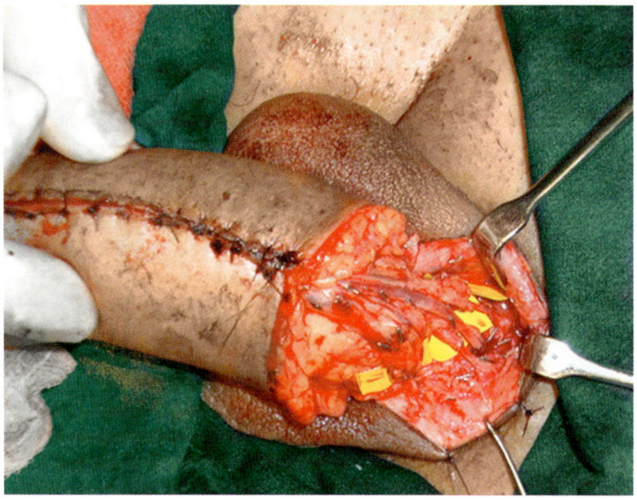

Fig. 29G: Microvascular anastomoses of 1 artery, 3 veins, 2 nerves done

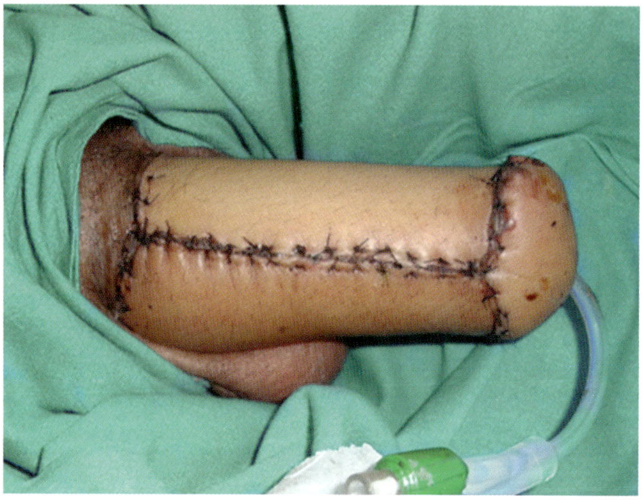

Fig. 29H: Immediate postoperative

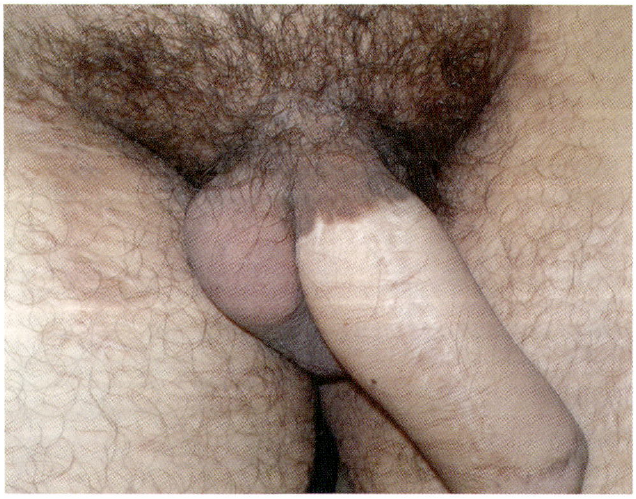

Fig. 29I: 1 year postoperative

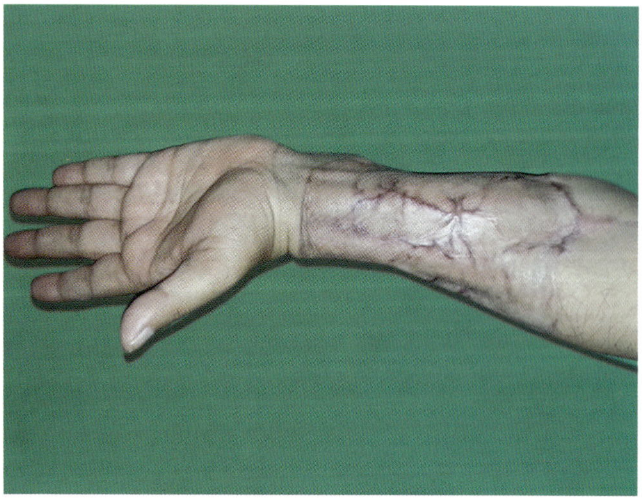

Fig. 29J: Donor site at one year

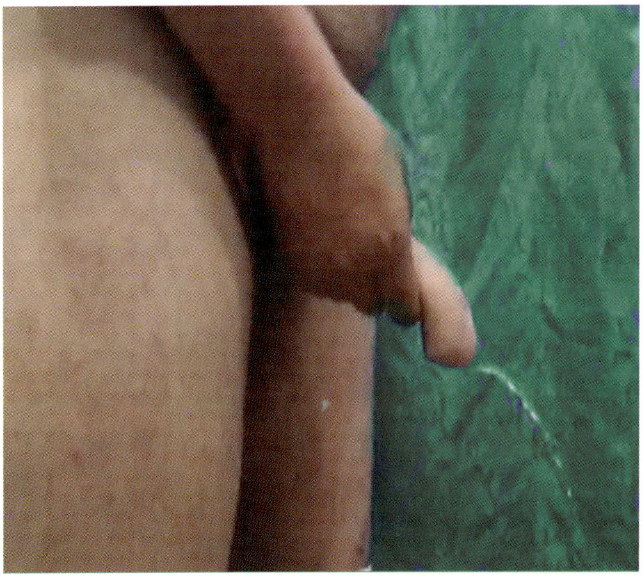

Fig. 29K: Patient micturating in standing position at 1 year

REFERENCES

1. Yang G, Chen B, Gao Y et al. Forearm free skin flap transplantation. Natl Med J China. 1981;61:139-42.
2. Wong CH, JY Lin, and FC Wei. The bottom-up approach to the suprafascial harvest of the radial forearm flap. Am J Surg. 2008;196(5):p. e60-4.
3. Lutz BS, Wei FC, Chang SC, Yang KH, Chen IH. Donor site morbidity after suprafascial elevation of the radial forearm flap: a prospective study in 95 consecutive cases. Plastic and reconstructive surgery. 1999 Jan;103(1):132-7.
4. Wei FC, Tan BK, Chen IH, Hau SP, Liau CT. Mimicking lip features in free-flap reconstruction of lip defects. British journal of plastic surgery. 2001 Jan 1;54(1):8-11.
5. Jeng SF, Kuo YR, Wei FC, Su CY, Chien CY. Total lower lip reconstruction with a composite radial forearm-palmaris longus tendon flap: a clinical series. Plastic and reconstructive surgery. 2004 Jan 1;113(1):19-23..
6. Murray DJ, CB Novak, PC Neligan. Fasciocutaneous free flaps in pharyngolaryngo-oesophageal reconstruction: a critical review of the literature. J Plast Reconstr Aesthet Surg. 2008;61(10):p. 1148-56.

CHAPTER 9

Deep Inferior Epigastric Artery Perforator Flap

Vinay K Shankhdhar, Saumya Mathews, Mayur Mantri

INTRODUCTION

The deep inferior epigastric artery perforator flap (DIEP) is harvested from lower abdomen taking only skin and subcutaneous fat and the rectus muscle is left intact. The DIEP flap was first described for clinical use by Koshima in 1989.[1] It was popularized for breast reconstruction by Robert Allen in 1993.[2] DIEP is a more evolved version of transverse rectus abdominis muscle flap (TRAM) wherein the rectus abdominis muscle was taken for vascularity and muscle sparing TRAM (only a part of muscle harvested). Currently DIEP is the gold-standard for whole breast reconstruction.

ANESTHESIA AND POSITION

The patient is operated in supine position in general anesthesia. Pillow is placed below the knees. Ryle's tube is inserted to decompress the stomach.

VASCULAR BASIS OF DIEP FLAP (FIG. 1)

The deep inferior epigastric artery located on the deep surface of the rectus muscle gives a lateral and a medial row of perforators approximately 3.5 cm and 1.5 cm from the midline. These supply the overlying skin.

Superficial inferior epigastric artery and vein (SIEA) and superficial external pudendal artery and vein (SEPA) also supply the flap.

INDICATIONS

1. Whole breast reconstruction (unilateral or bilateral).
2. Maxillary reconstructions.
3. Reconstruction of any defect requiring large soft tissue flap.

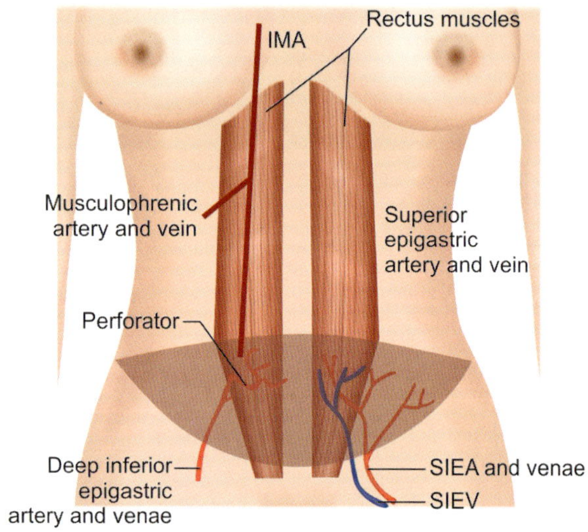

Fig. 1: Vascular network

CONTRAINDICATIONS

1. Insufficient bulk in abdomen.
2. Vascular surgery on the iliac vessels.

PREOPERATIVE EVALUATION

1. Leg raising test: To check amount of extra-abdominal fat.
2. Horizontal or vertical operative scars, incisional hernia or other injury at the flap site.
3. Hand held Doppler and/or CT angiography to identify the dominant perforator.

MARKING (FIG. 2)

The following points are marked:

- Bilateral inframammary crease, anterior axillary fold, umbilicus

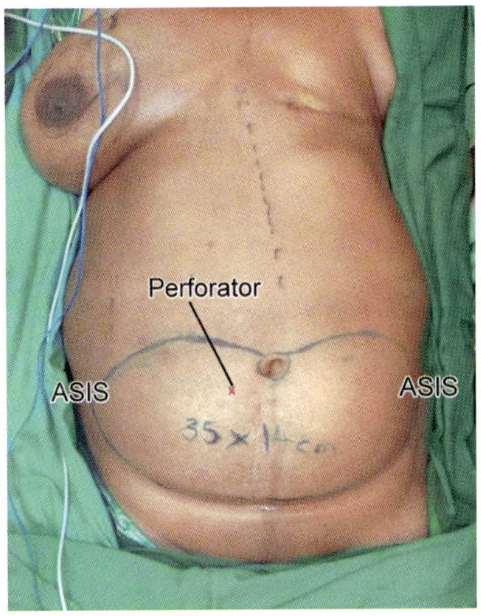

Fig. 2: Skin marking

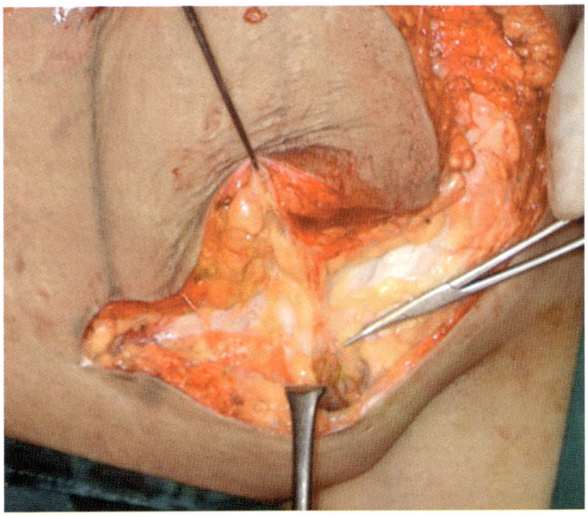

Fig. 3: Dissection of superficial inferior epigastric vein

- Xiphoid, pubic symphysis and a line connecting the two (midline)
- Bilateral anterior superior iliac spine (ASIS), midinguinal points
- Perforator as mapped on audio Doppler or CT angiography marked.

An ellipse is drawn starting adjacent to one ASIS curving gently above the inguinal ligaments and the pubic bone to end adjacent to the other ASIS—this is the lower marking of the ellipse. The upper marking is a gentle curve just above the umbilicus meeting the lower marking on either side and should permit primary closure. Circumumbilical incision is marked as shown in the **Figure 2**. Transverse LSCS scars may or may not be included in incision. Inferior incision given extra curve in midline to ease closure.

SURGICAL TECHNIQUE

Steps

1. Adrenaline infiltration (1:200000) given around flap marking.
2. In case only one breast reconstruction is required only one DIEP vessel is harvested depending on the availability of robust perforator. This side is dissected first.
3. Lower incision is taken first and SIEV lying in the subcutaneous fat is dissected out in the middle one third part of the incision **(Fig. 3)**.
4. Incision is taken along the upper part of the half ellipse and subcutaneous tissue beveled to expose rectus sheath and external oblique aponeurosis **(Fig. 4)**.

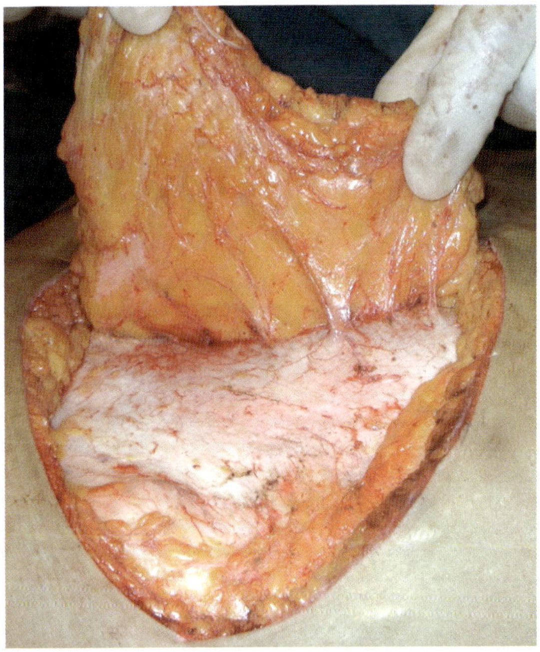

Fig. 4: Lateral row perforators are visible

5. The dissection proceeds from lateral to medial. The lateral row perforators are encountered first **(Fig. 4)**, the dissection now proceeds cautiously to select the perforator from this row or medial row as determined by Doppler or CT angio preoperatively.
6. The selected perforator is now dissected free from the surrounding subcutaneous fat **(Fig. 5)**. This is achieved easily by vascular forceps and mosquito artery forceps. The perforator is visible emerging from the rectus fascia.

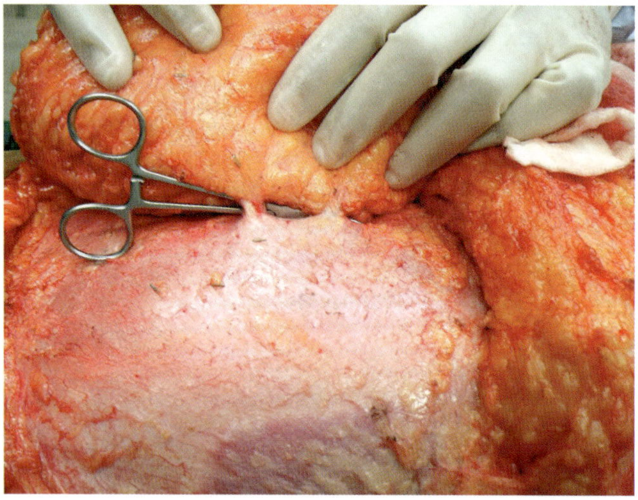

Fig. 5: Perforator dissection

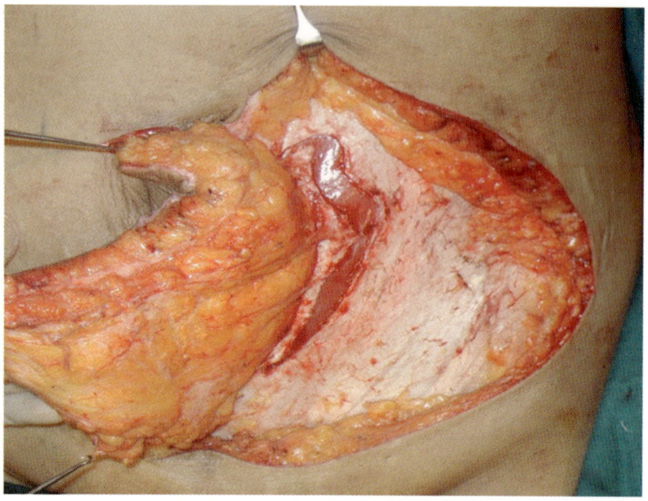

Fig. 6: Rectus sheath incision

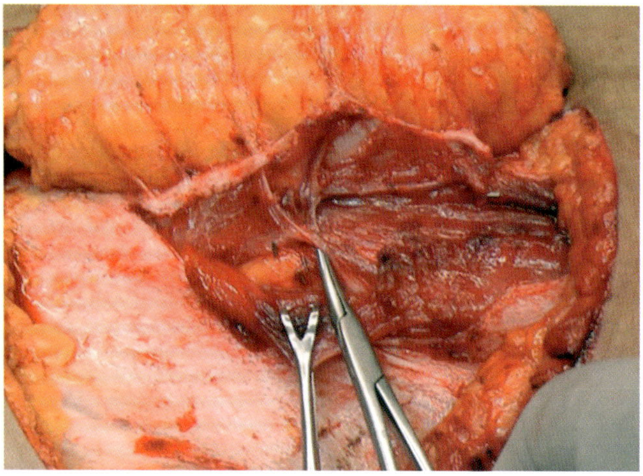

Fig. 7: Perforator dissection

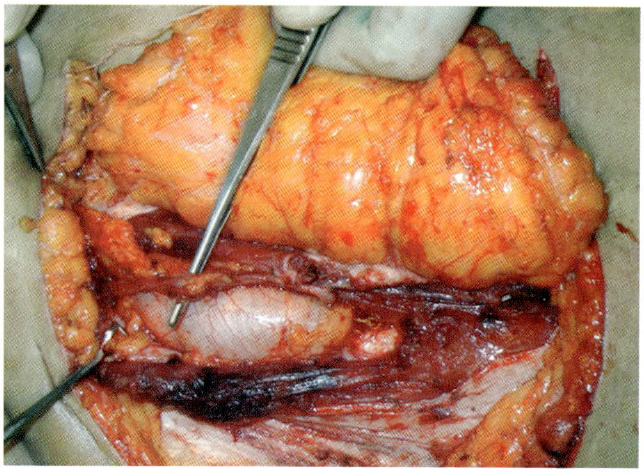

Fig. 8: Dissection of deep inferior epigastric pedicle

7. The flap is elevated to expose the rectus sheath till linea alba (midline) is reached.
8. The rectus fascia is now incised **(Fig. 6)** with a small cuff of sheath around the perforator to expose the rectus muscle underneath. The perforator is dissected free of the muscle **(Fig. 7)**. The technique used is to 'deroof the perforator', meaning, that the muscle above it is carefully removed to expose the perforator. The dissection continues till the point of origin from the deep inferior epigastric vessels is reached.
9. Next step is to dissect out the deep inferior epigastric vessel and separate it from the surrounding tissue **(Fig. 8)**. The distal end of the main pedicle is ligated and divided. The vessel is freed for the desired pedicle length.
10. At this point there are two methods to proceed:
    a. The deep inferior epigastric vessels may be divided at this stage and reverse blood flow in the artery may indicate a good midline cross-over and also the patency of the perforator. At this stage the opposite side vessel and perforators are intact and available as a fall-back option. This is followed by elevating the flap from the opposite side **(Figs. 9A and B)** to expose the rectus sheath. Thus, the flap is now free from all the sides and harvest is complete.
    b. The other method is to divide the vessel after elevation of the opposite half of the flap as described above. The flap is based now only on the perforator **(Fig. 10)** and flap bleeding gives us an idea

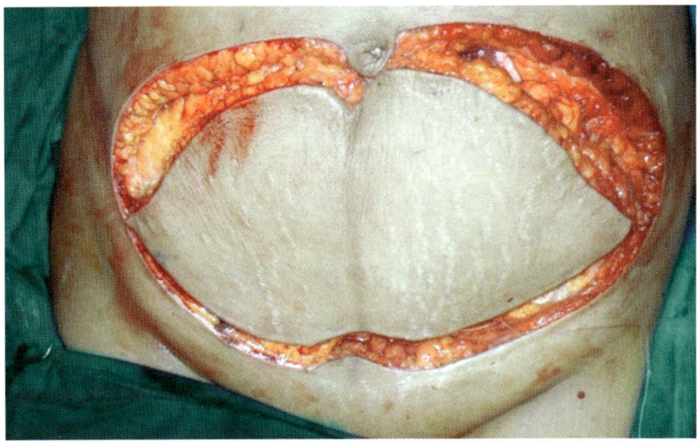

Fig. 9A: Opposite side skin incision

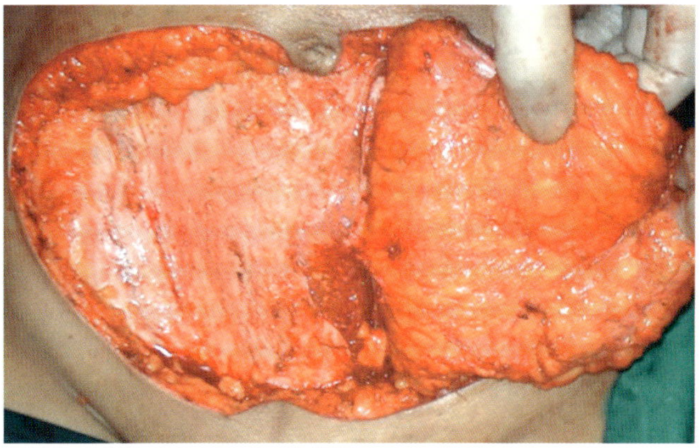

Fig. 9B: Perforator reached from the opposite side

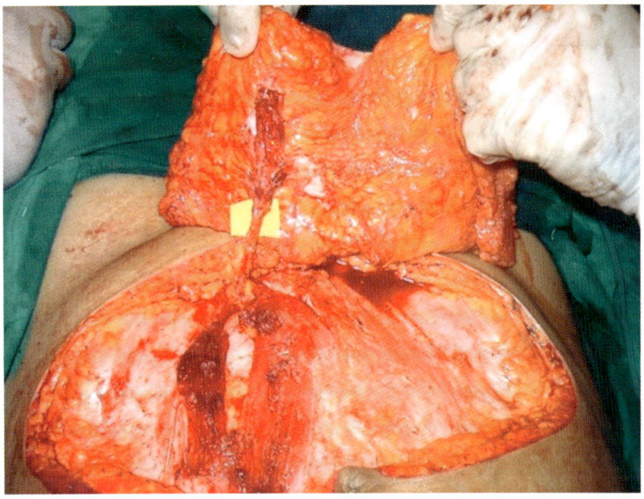

Fig. 10: Flap islanded

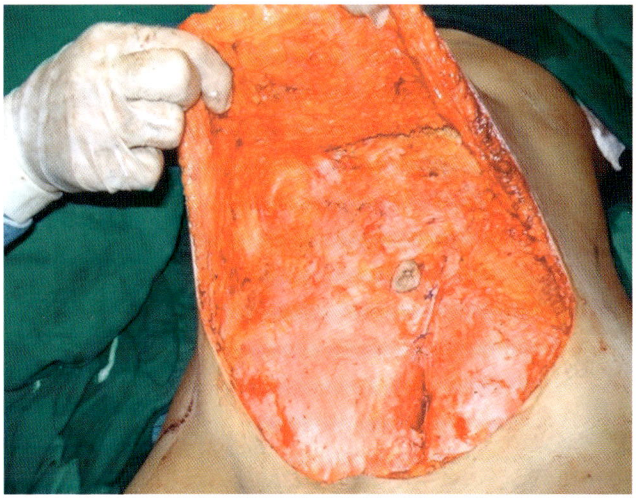

Fig. 11: Rectus sheath closure done and abdominal skin mobilized

of the perforator dominance. The disadvantage in this case is that the opposite side perforators cannot be used as they are already divided.

11. The donor site requires closure of rectus sheath **(Fig. 11)** which is generally possible, however, a mesh should be used, if rectus sheath closure is even under slight tension, to avoid postoperative herniation.
12. Skin closure requires creation of neoumbilicus and abdominoplasty **(Fig. 12)** for primary wound closure. Suction drains are put and wound closed in two layers.
13. Most commonly the internal mammary vessels are used **(Fig. 13)** in the third intercostal space. The third costal cartilage is removed for better access. The internal mammary vessels are high flow vessels and almost always available for anastomosis. Other options include serratus branch of thoracodorsal vessels or the thoracodorsal vessel itself.
14. Finally, the inset of the flap is done after anastomoses **(Figs. 14A and B)**. Zone 4 is always discarded and zone 3 may or may not be used depending on the requirement of the flap and vascularity. The aim is to give bilateral symmetry. The excess skin may be de-epithelized to increase the bulk.
15. In case the superficial inferior epigastric vein looks too full or congested then cephalic may be dissected out in the deltopectoral groove and the two are anastomosed together to provide additional venous drainage **(Figs. 15A and B)**.
16. Methods to increase bulk:
    a. Turbocharging **(Fig. 16)**: Vessels in the flap are anastomosed to each other to improve vascularity

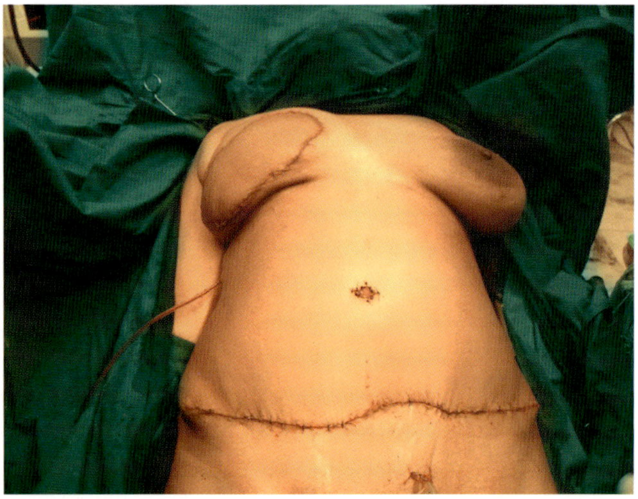

Fig. 12: Abdominal closure and umbilicoplasty

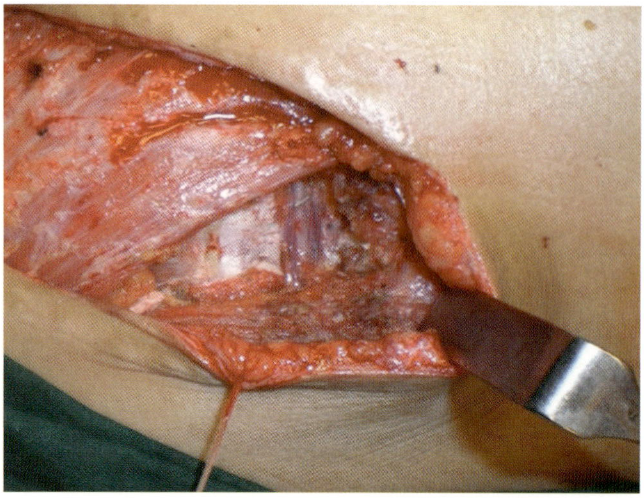

Fig. 13: Internal mammary vessels exposed

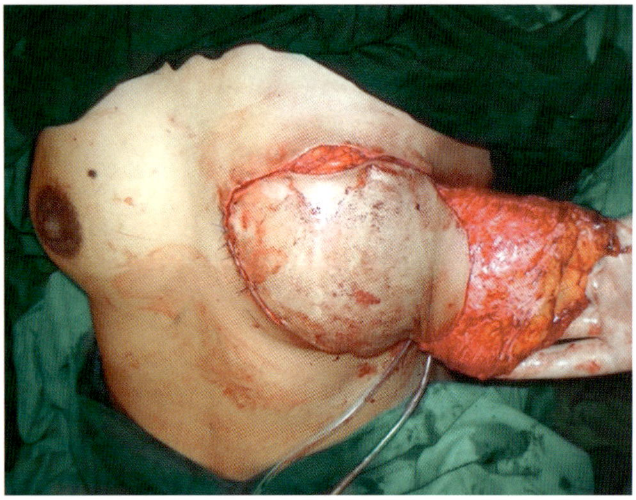

Fig. 14A: Flap inset and anastomosis done

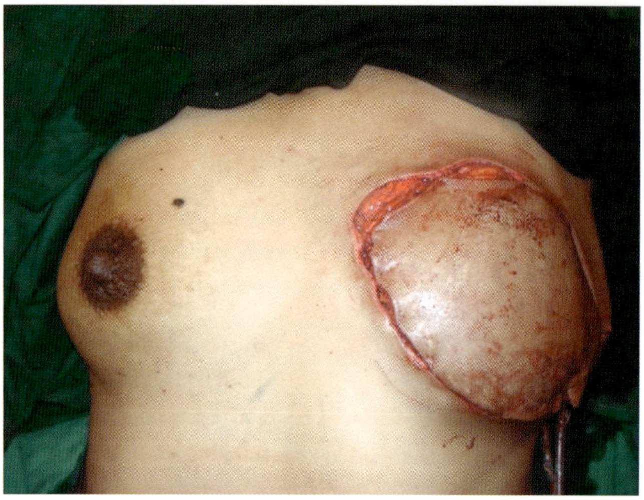

Fig. 14B: Flap contoured and excess flap (zone 4) discarded

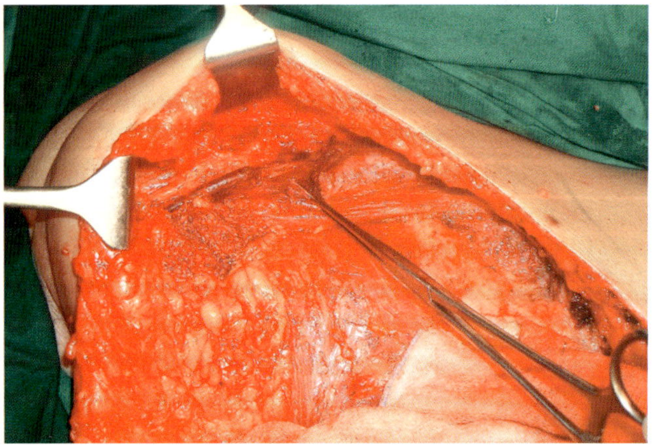

Fig. 15A: Dissection of cephalic vein

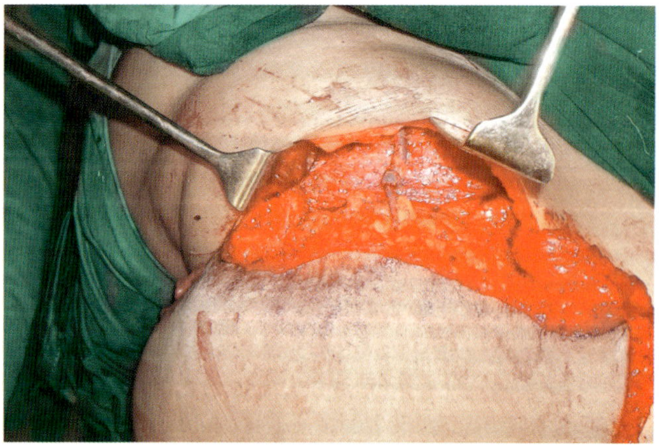

Fig. 15B: Anastomosis of cephalic vein with superficial inferior epigastric vein

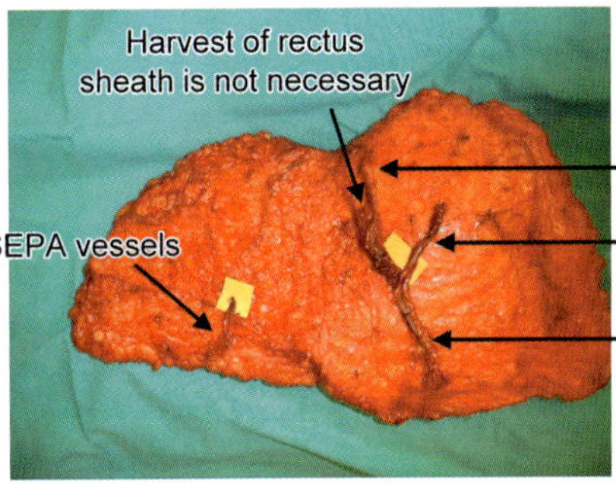

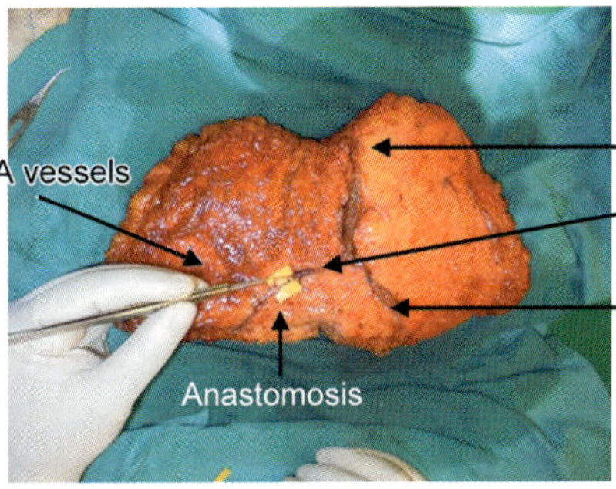

Fig. 16: Turbocharging, the distal end of DIEP vessels is anastomosed with the superficial external pudendal vessels. This thus includes the territory of the SEPA as well

SEPA: Superficial external pudendal artery and vein; DIEP: Deep inferior epigastric artery perforator flap).

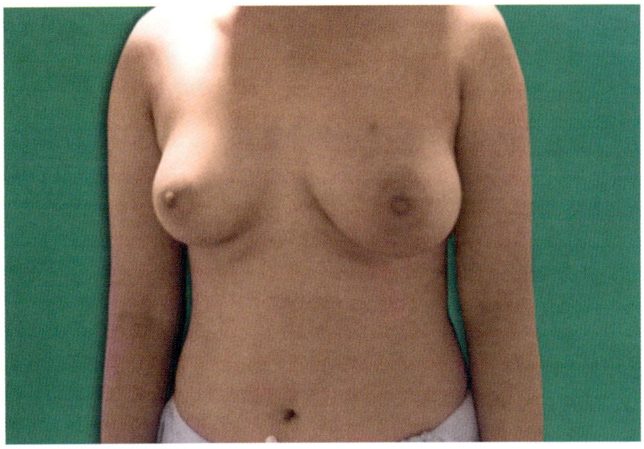

Fig. 17A: Preoperative

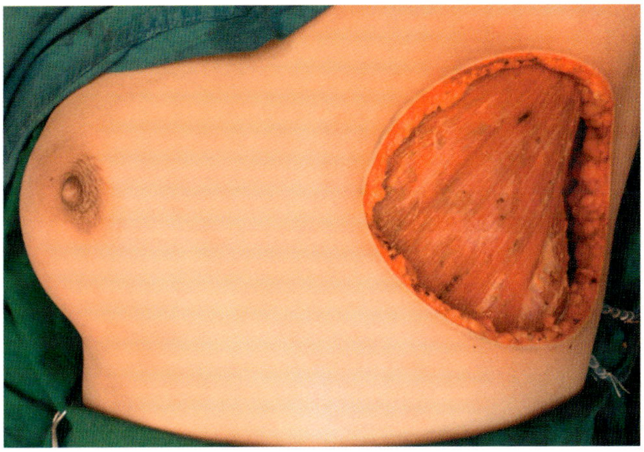

Fig. 17B: Defect post left MRM

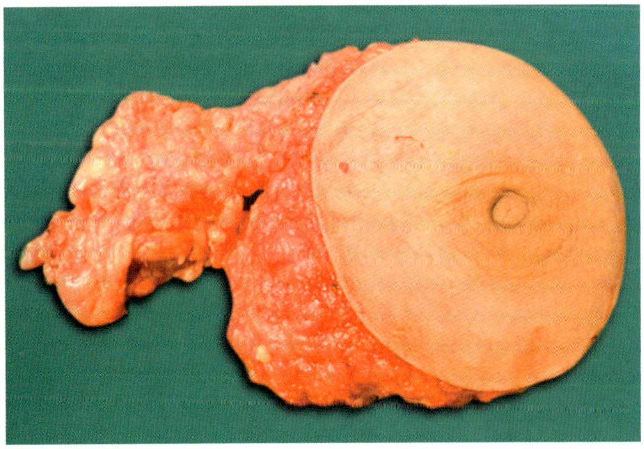

Fig. 17C: Specimen

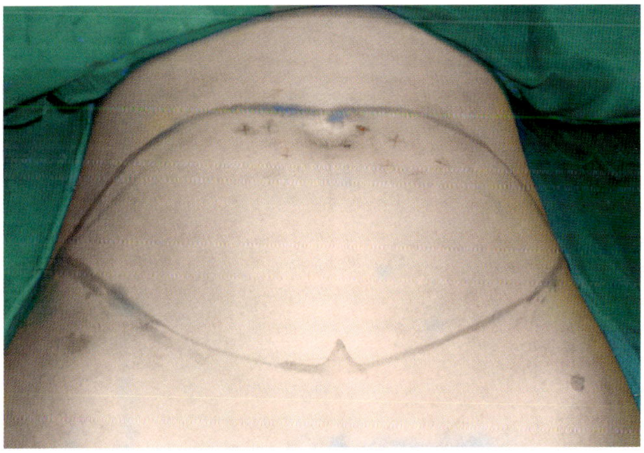

Fig. 17D: Marking of the flap

and recruit additional zones, e.g. the distal end of DIEP vessels is anastomosed with the superficial external pudendal vessels. This thus includes the territory of the SEPA as well.

b. Supercharging **(Figs. 17A to J)**: Two system of vessels are used to augment the blood supply of the flap and thus increase the bulk available, e.g. the other side DIEP vessels along with perforator is harvested

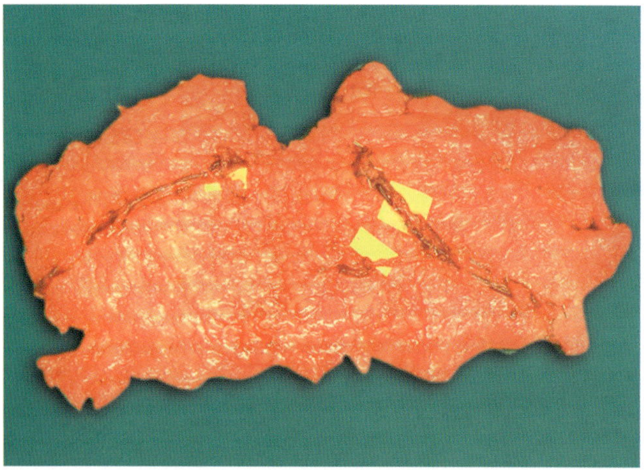

Fig. 17E: Flap with right and left DIEP vessels

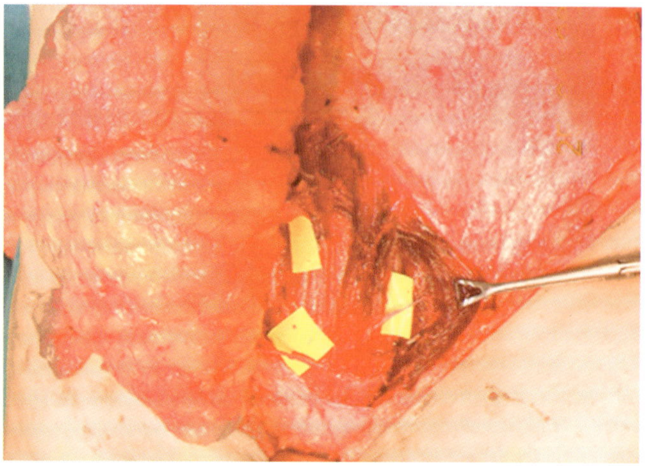

Fig. 17F: Nerve to rectus muscle preserved

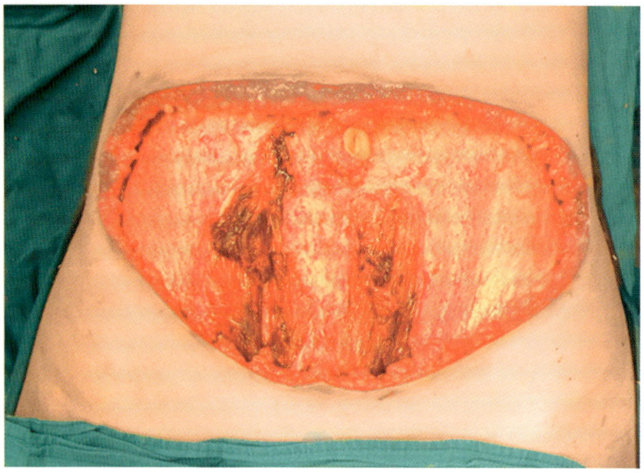

Fig. 17G: Flap harvested without any muscle harvest

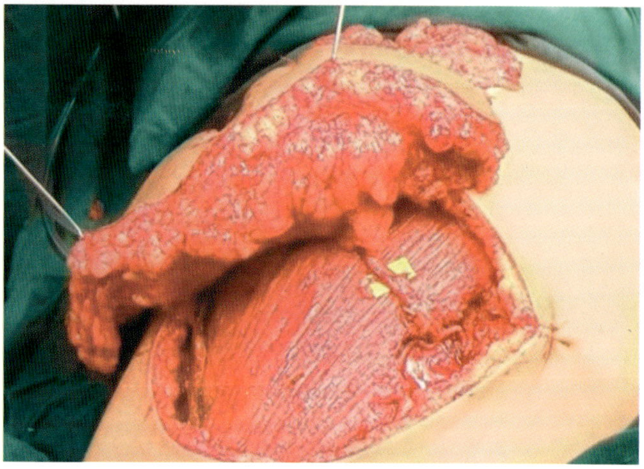

Fig. 17H: Anastomosis to internal mammy and artery to serratus anterior

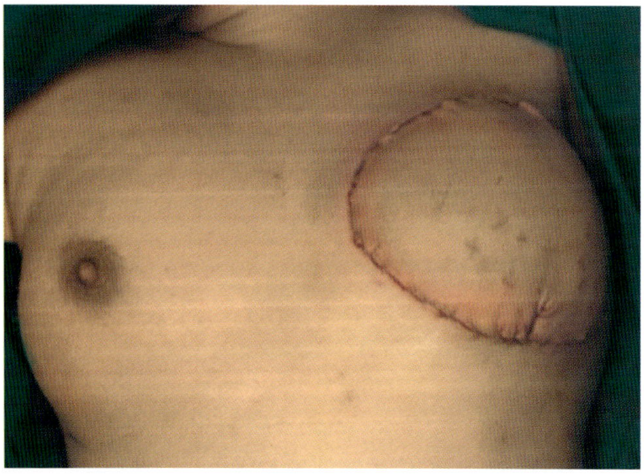

Fig. 17I: Inset of flap

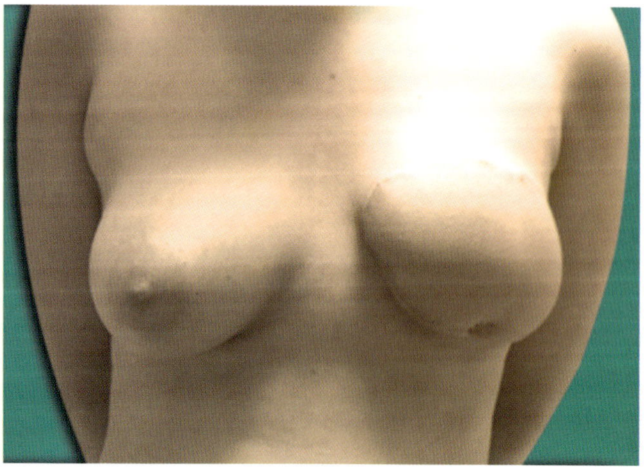

Fig. 17J: Postoperative

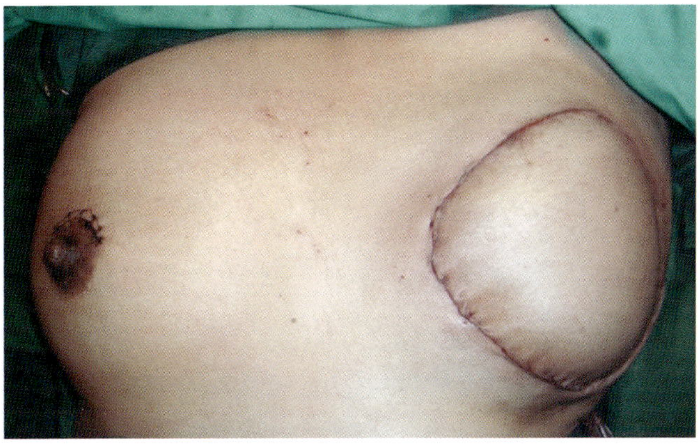

Fig. 18: Stacked DIEP

and both the sets of DIEP Vessels are anastomosed to internal mammary system and serratus vessels.

c. Stacked **(Fig. 18)**: Both sides DIEP flaps are harvested with both the DIEP vessels. The flaps are divided in the midline and stacked one over the other. This helps in improving the projection of the breast.
d. Mosaic arrangement **(Figs. 19A to F)**: The flaps are cut and placed alongside one other. This helps in covering large skin excisions.

17. Postoperative care: Pillows are kept below the thighs to ease tension on the abdominal wound. Wound is checked on the second postoperative day.

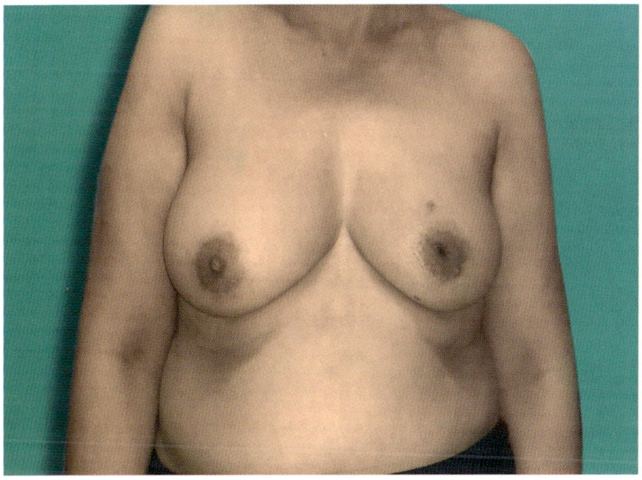

Fig 19A: Preoperative

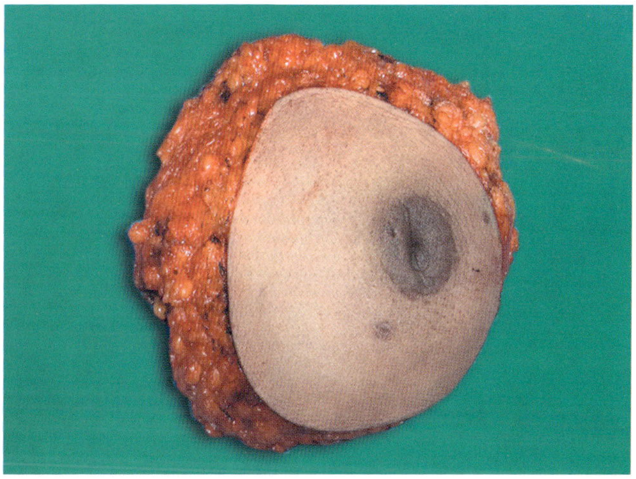

Fig. 19B: Specimen

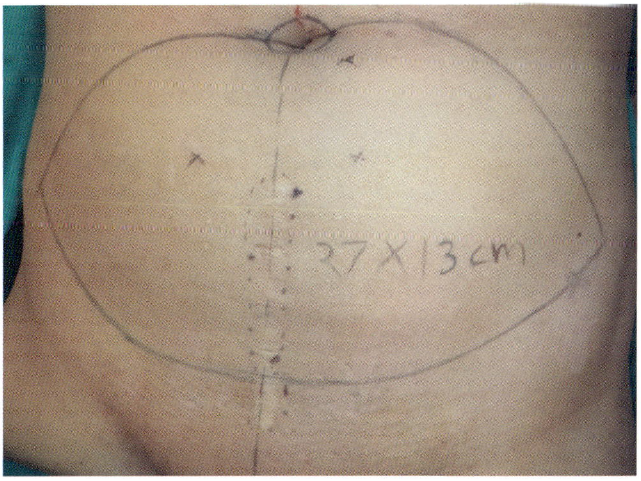

Fig. 19C: Flap marking

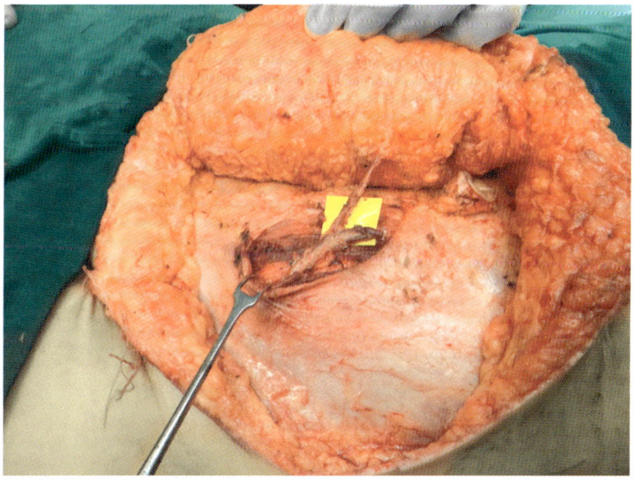

Fig. 19D: Perforator dissection completed

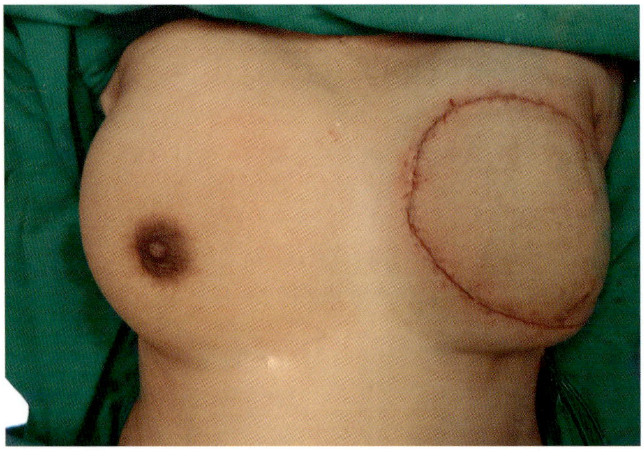

Fig. 19E: Final inset with IMF creation

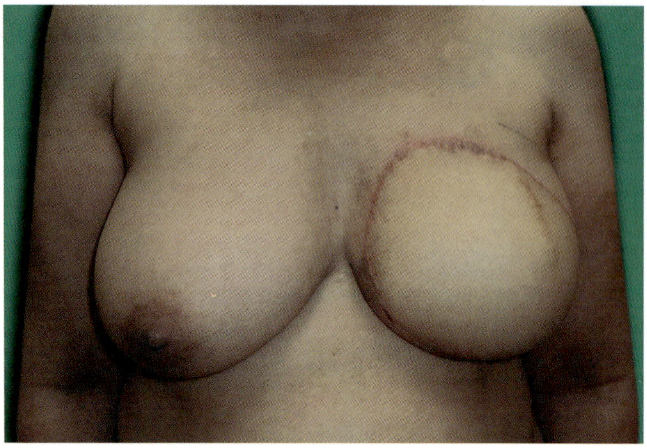

Fig. 19F: Postoperative

REFERENCES

1. Koshima I, Soeda S. Inferior epigastric artery skin flaps without rectus abdominis muscle. Br J Plast Surg. 1989;42(6):645-8.
2. Allen RJ, Treece P. Deep inferior epigastric perforator flap for breast reconstruction. Ann Plast Surg. 1994;32(1):32-8.

CHAPTER 10

Free Jejunum Flap

Amrita Rao, Vinay K Shankhdhar

INTRODUCTION

Siedenberg in 1959 reported the first successful free flap transfer in humans of replacing cervical esophagus with free jejunum flap.

It is the flap of choice at our institute for reconstruction of circumferential defects of the pharynx after total laryngopharyngectomy, as it reestablishes gastrointestinal tract continuity. Free jejunum flap is used when the lower cut end of the esophagus lies above the thoracic inlet. A gastric pull-up or colonic transposition is performed if the resection has gone below the thoracic inlet.

The unique feature of the free Jejunum flap is that it has the least ischemia time of 120 minutes within which arterial flow has to be re-established **(Fig. 1)**.

ANATOMY

Jejunum begins at the duodenojejunal flexure which is suspended from the retroperitoneum by the ligament of Treitz.

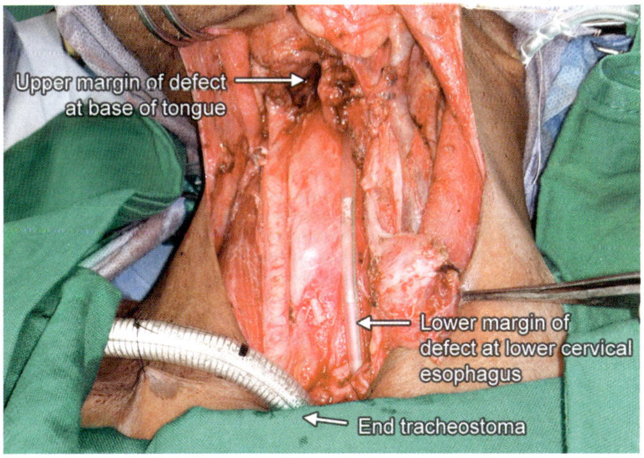

Fig. 1: Defect of total laryngopharyngectomy requiring a free jejunal flap

The jejunum measures approximately 4 cm in external diameter and 2.5 cm in internal diameter matching that of cervical esophagus.

The four layers of the jejunum are *serosa, muscularis externa,* (two distinct layers of smooth muscle: outer thin longitudinal and inner circular) *submucosa* and *mucosa.*

Vascular Anatomy

The superior mesenteric artery, a branch of the abdominal aorta gives off multiple jejunal arteries which enter the mesentery of the jejunum. Each jejunal artery is part of an arcade which in turn communicates with multiple *vasa recti*. The *vasa recta* are end arteries with supply specific segments of the jejunum and hence jejunal blood supply is segmental. Venous drainage follows the arteries.

As we move distally along the jejunum the number of vascular arcades increases and therefore the perfusion pattern becomes less distinct and unsuitable for free flap transfer. The 2nd or 3rd jejunal artery and its corresponding part of the jejunum is the most ideal in terms of vascular pedicle and jejunal length for free flap transfer **(Figs. 2 and 3)**.

HARVESTING THE JEJUNUM FLAP

- The first step of reconstruction is to prepare the recipient vessels in the neck. Any large tributary of *internal or external jugular vein* can be used as recipient for venous anastomosis and in the absence of any such tributaries; end to side anastomosis to internal jugular vein can be done. Either superior thyroid or facial artery can be used as recipient artery. The position superior thyroid artery usually ideal for arterial anastomosis. In the rare event that both these arteries are unsuitable the transverse cervical artery is used.
- A midline upper abdominal incision, extending from the xiphisternum to the umbilicus is taken.

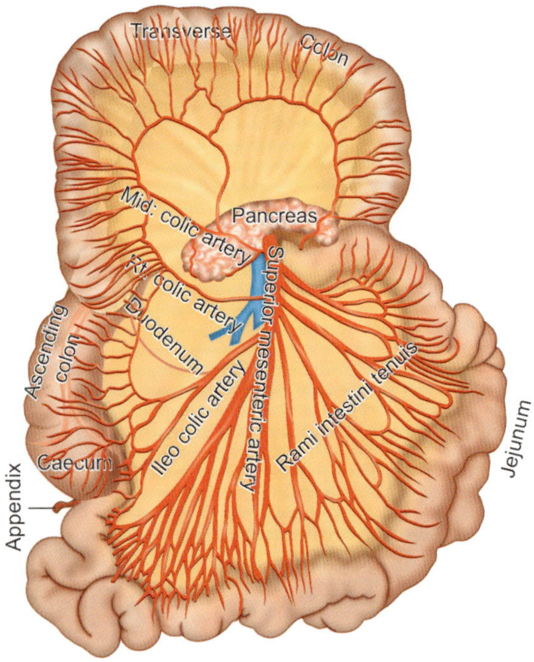

Fig. 2: Vascular anatomy of small bowel

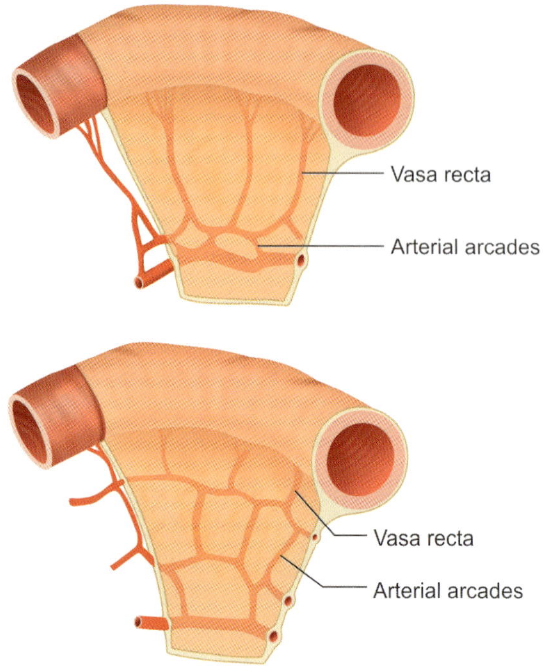

Fig. 3: Jejunal and ileal vascular arcades

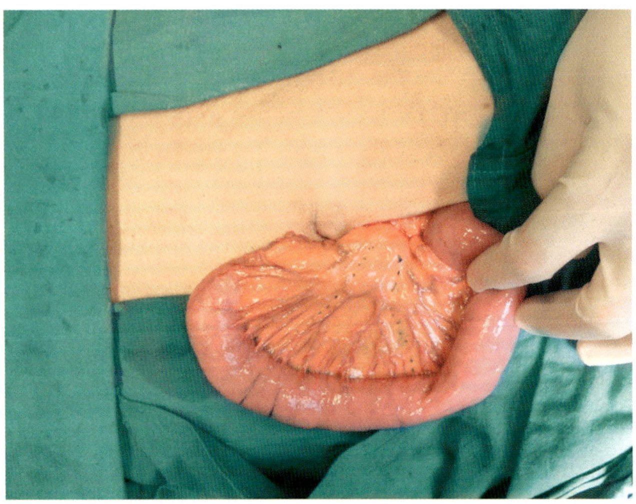

Fig. 4: Appropriate segment of Jejunum selected for harvest

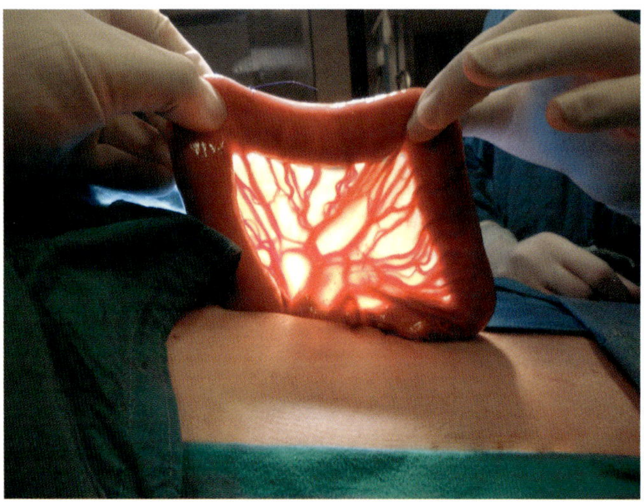

Fig. 5: Transillumination showing vascular arcade

- A jejunal loop at a distance of 25 to 30 cm from the DJ flexure is isolated which is supplied by a single jejunal artery. A simple seromuscular stitch is placed at the proximal end of the jejunal loop to identify it for proper isoperistaltic placement in the neck. Length of segment of jejunum to be harvested is marked **(Fig. 4)**.
- This segment of jejunum is dissected and isolated along with its vascular pedicle up to its origin from the superior mesenteric artery using transillumination technique for proper identification of the course of vessel. Utmost care is required during the dissection of the jejunal vein as the vessel wall is thin and friable **(Fig. 5)**.
- The vessels are completely dissected from the vascular arcade on either side by ligating the communicating vessels **(Fig. 6)**.
- The jejunal segment is isolated and divided (by stapler device) and the perfusion of the divided segment

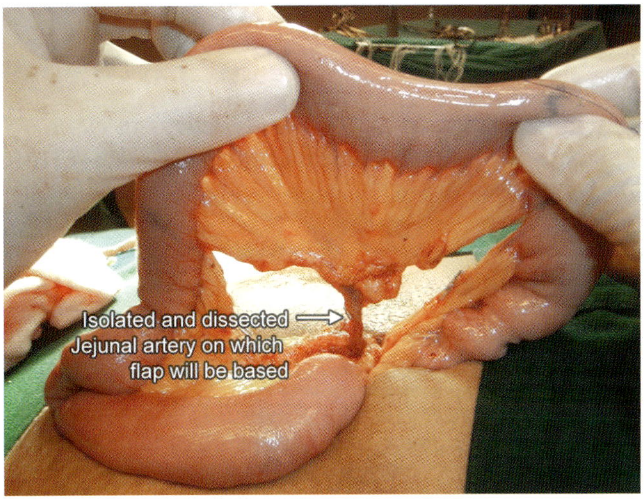

Fig. 6: Completed pedicle dissection before ligating of pedicle

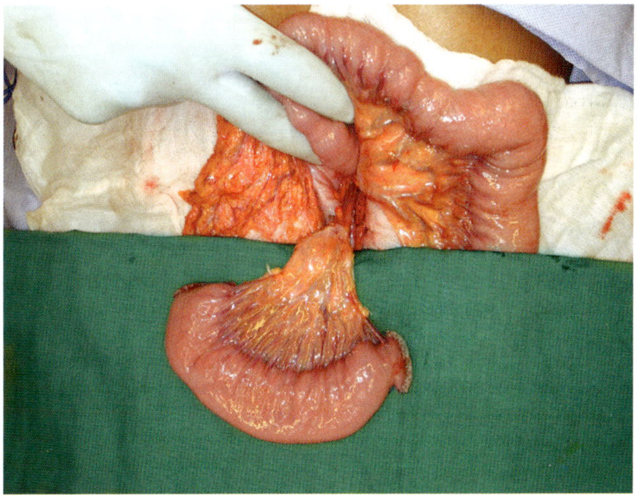

Fig. 7: Jejunal segment isolated for harvest

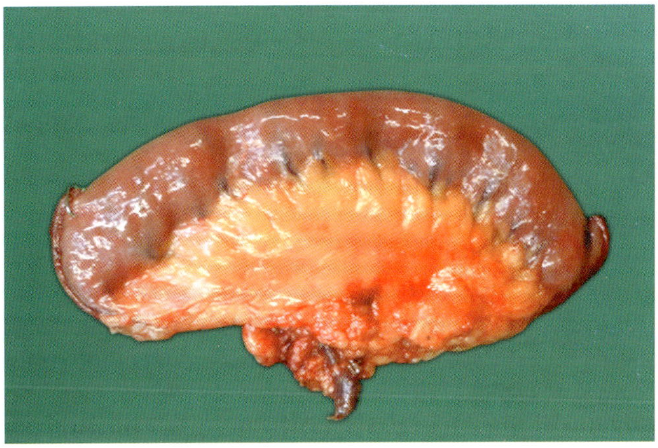

Fig. 8: Harvested jejunal segment

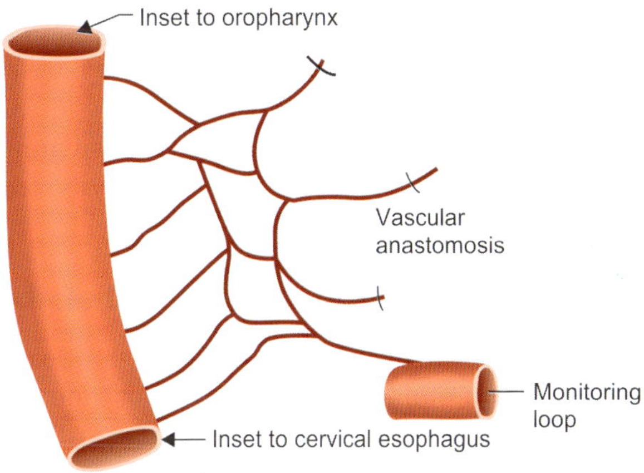

Fig. 9: Monitoring loop with vascular continuity and luminal discontinuity

is confirmed by observing it for a change in color or brisk bleeding from the cut edge for 10 to 15 minutes **(Fig. 7)**.

- Flow in the receipient vessels is confirmed before clamping jejunal vessels as ischemia time is very short approximately 120 mins.
- The jejunal vessels are then clamped and divided and the jejunal segment is transferred to the recipient site ensuring isoperistaltic placement **(Fig. 8)**.
- Anesthetist is asked to note ischemia time.

Inset of Flap in the Neck

- The jejunal segment is stabilized in position with simple anchoring sutures and lie of vascular pedicle is confirmed.
- Vascular anastomoses is performed. Usually venous anastomosis is done first followed by arterial anastomosis. Arterial anastomosis is done first only if ischemia time is increasing due to any intraoperative problem. If arterial anastomosis is done first, the venous anastomosis is troublesome.
- After vascular anastomoses the jejunum distends to its original size and peristaltic movements are observed.
- After deciding the required jejunal segment the remanent flap is divided (usually 2 cm) with vascular continuity and exteriorized for the purpose of monitoring. This segment is stabilized on the skin with 2 simple sutures avoiding any twist on vascular pedicle **(Fig. 9)**.

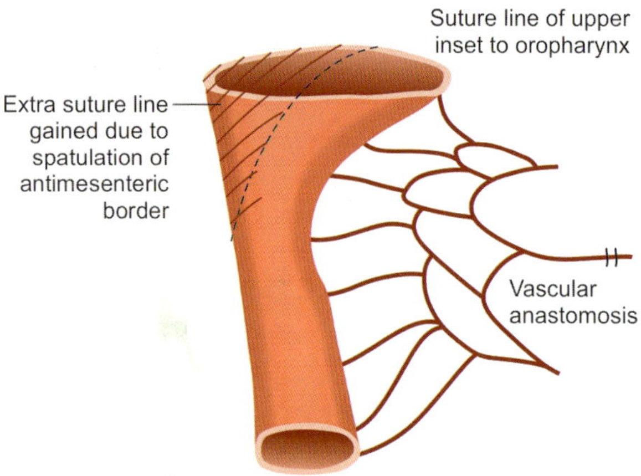

Fig. 10: Spatulation of proximal end of jejunum at antimesenteric border

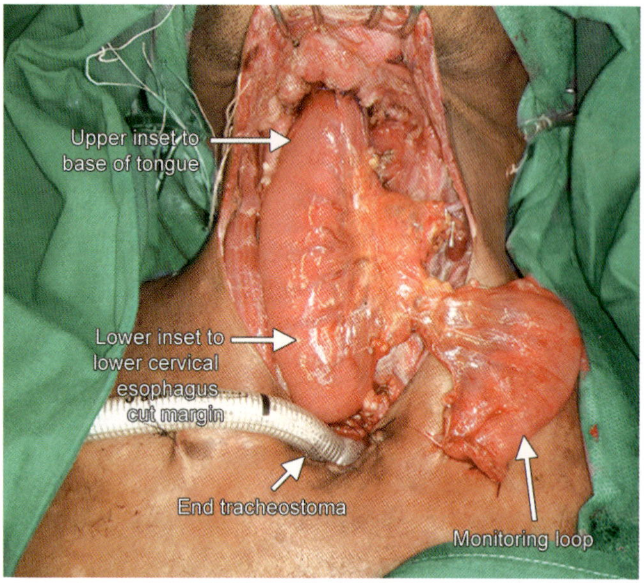

Fig. 11: Vascular and bowel anastomosis completed and monitoring loop exteriorized

- Proximal and distal luminal anastomosis is done end to end in single layer using extra mucosal sutures with 4-0 polydiaxonone suture.
- In the proximal end we mostly need to spatulate the antimesenteric border for luminal match along with the base of the tongue **(Fig. 10)**.
- Proximal luminal anastomosis done followed by the distal one.
- Posterior wall suturing is done at both ends after which Ryle's tube is passed and then anterior wall suturing is completed.
- The monitoring segment is representative of the vascular viability of the jejunal segment in the neck. It is not for the purpose of salvage but only for early intervention in case of any vascular thrombotic event before any infection develops **(Fig. 11)**.
- End tracheostoma suturing is done and the neck wound is closed primarily in most cases.
- If this is not possible a deltopectoral flap can be elevated and used for neck closure **(Figs. 12 to 14)**.

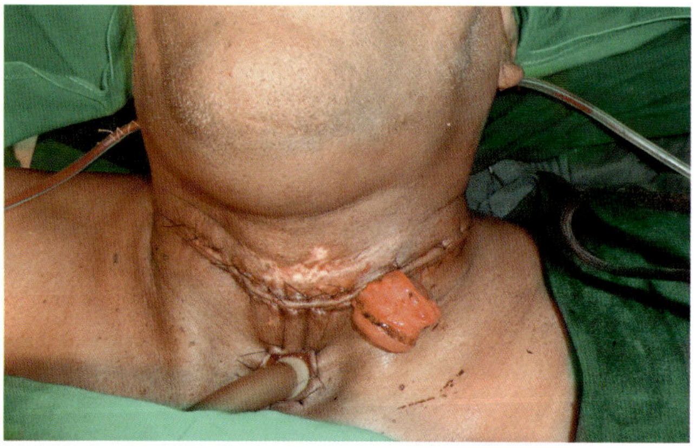

Fig. 12: Final appearance at skin closure

Donor Site Closure

- Done by second team
- Intestinal closure by hand sewn or stapler anastomosis.
- Mesenteric window closure
- Single layer mass closure of abdominal wall by No1 Loop nylon.
- Skin closure with stapler/suture technique
- No feeding gastrostomy or jejunostomy is required. A naso-jejunal tube is not required as Ryle's tube is sufficient.

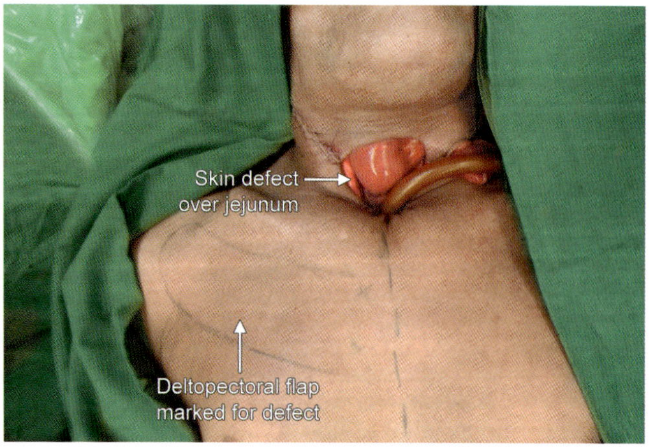

Fig. 13: Skin defect in the neck not amenable for primary closure

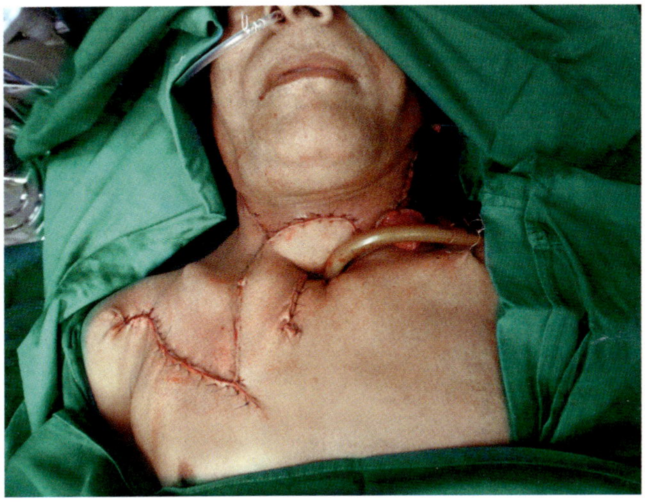

Fig. 14: Primary inset deltopectoral flap for neck skin defect

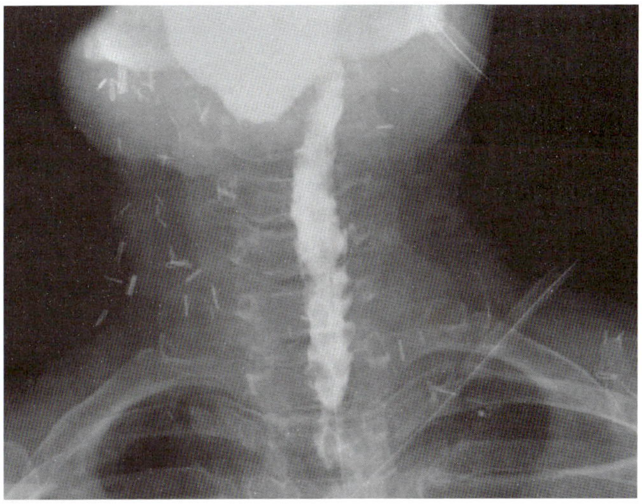

Fig. 15: Contrast X-ray image on POD10 showing no leak

POSTOPERATIVE CARE

- Patient is advised against excessive neck movements are restricted.
- Exteriorized segment to be kept covered by moist saline or paraffin *tulle* gauze and monitored as per protocol
- Restrict attempts at swallowing and speech to prevent movement of tongue so as to allow the upper anastomotic site to heal uneventfully.
- Ryle's tube feed to be started once peristalsis is confirmed by bowel sounds and patient nutrition parameters to be maintained as close to normal as possible.
- Abdomen to be checked routinely and managed as any case of intestinal bowel anastomosis .
- Monitoring segment is divided on 8th to 10th postoperative day in minor operation theatre and the neck wound closed under local anesthesia
- Contrast barium swallow is usually performed on 10th to 14th postoperative day **(Figs. 15 and 16)**.

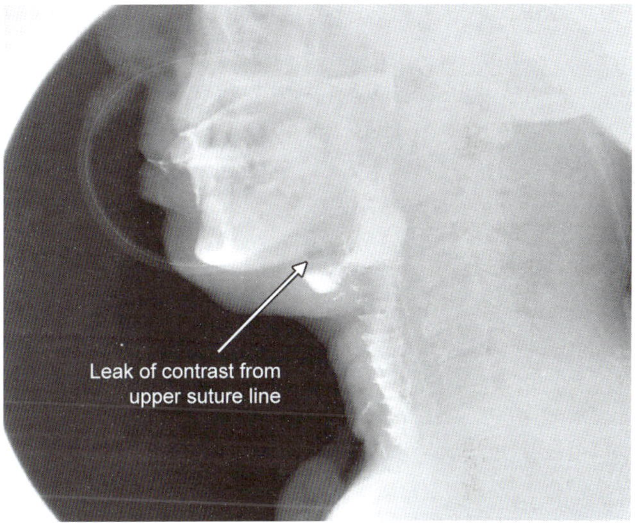

Fig. 16: Contrast X-ray image on POD10 showing minor leak at upper oropharynx to jejunal suture line

CONTRAINDICATIONS

Absolute

- Abdominal bowel pathology like tuberculosis.

Relative

- Previous abdominal surgery
- Intraperitoneal adhesions
- Poor general condition of patient

ADVANTAGES AND DRAWBACKS

- Tubular conduit and hence is best for circumferential defects.
- Most physiological reconstruction with diameter similar to pharynx and esophagus.
- Can cover defects up to 25 cm.
- Low postoperative fistula (most common at cervical anastomotic site) rates
- Faster postoperative rehabilitation with patient on oral diet.
- Short ischemia time
- Speech has a gurgling quality to it (has been describes as wet speech)

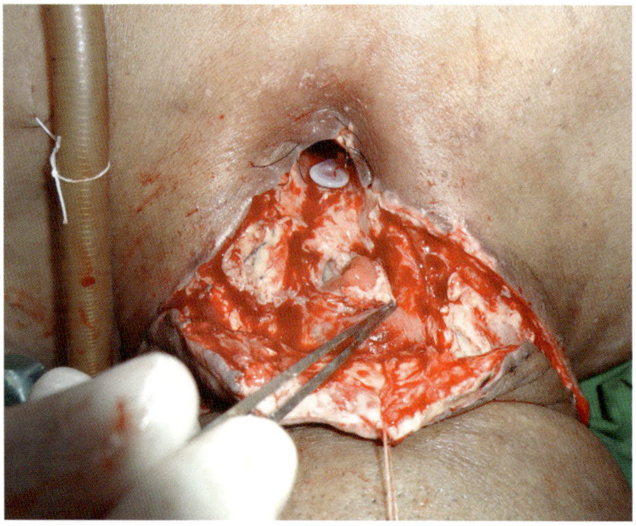

Fig. 17: Minimal leak at lower inset to cervical esophagus

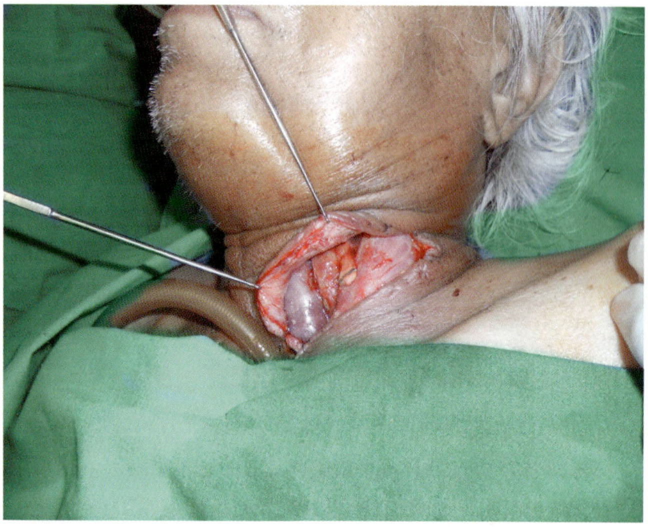

Fig. 18: Jejunum flap necrosed

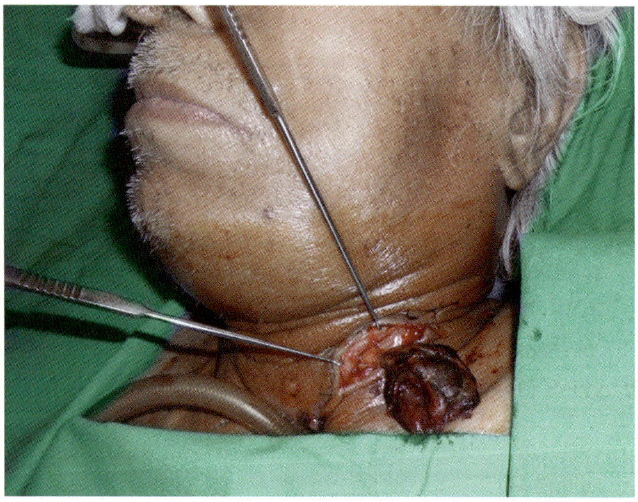

Fig. 19: Monitoring paddle discoloration indicating jejunal flap necrosis

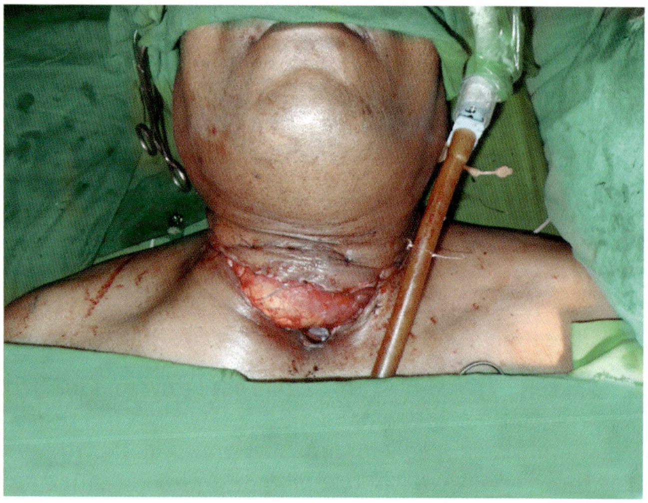

Fig. 20: PMMF inset for patching of the leak

MANAGING COMPLICATIONS

- Incase of flap loss, another free jejunum flap or a gastric pull-up **(Figs. 17 and 18)**.
- Minor leaks and orocutaneous fistulas are managed with a pectoralis major muscle flap **(Figs. 19 and 20)**.
- If overlying skin needs to be replaced due to necrosis or infection, deltopectoral flap is done.

CHAPTER 11

Medial Sural Artery Perforator Flap

Tanmay Mohan Joshi, Dushyant Jaiswal

INTRODUCTION

In 1975, Taylor and Daniel proposed the posterior calf as a versatile donor site for perforator-based flaps. Later Montegut, Allen and Hallock described technical refinements in harvest of perforator flaps of this region. The first clinical series of medial sural artery perforator flaps **(MSAP)** was done by **Cavadas** et al.

The medial sural artery originates from the popliteal vessels and enters medial gastrocnemius muscle and provides variable number of musculocutaneous perforators to the skin **(Figs. 1 and 2)**. They generally lie along an imaginary line joining the midpoint of popliteal fossa and center of medial malleolus. The perforators lie most commonly between 6 cm to 18 cm from the popliteal crease according to most studies **(Fig. 3)**.

The medial sural, median sural, and lateral sural are in a complimentary relationship in the calf and supply adjacent angiosomes.

What is the Need of this Perforator Flap?

The MSAP flap provides a flap of intermediate thickness between FRAFF and FALT with primary closure of donor site (~5–7 cm width).

Conventionally, the flap of choice for small to medium size defects in head and neck reconstruction has been Free Radial Artery Forearm Flap (FRAFF). The disadvantages of the FRAFF include

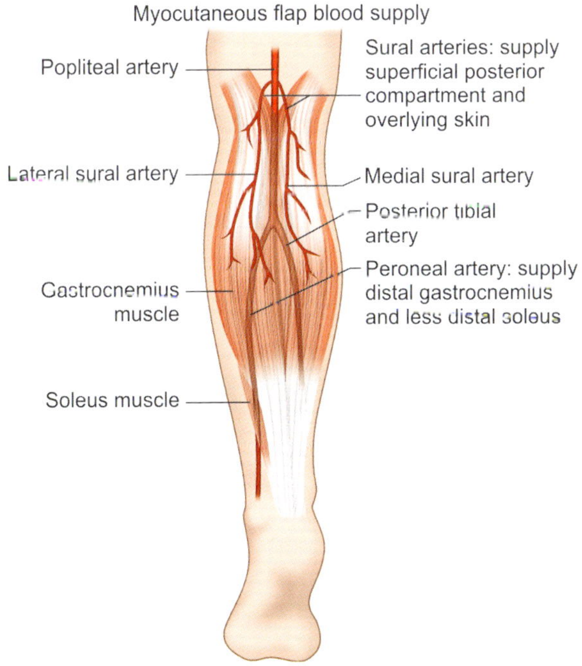

Fig. 1: The medial sural artery originating from the popliteal vessels, and entering medial belly of gastrocnemius

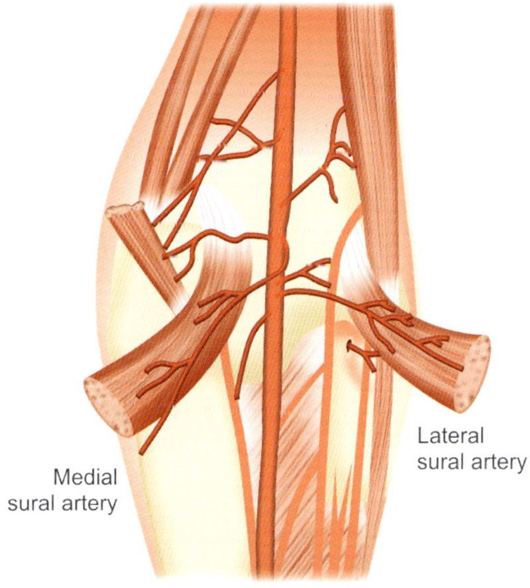

Fig. 2: The medial and lateral sural arteries and median sural are in complimentary relationship in calf

- Sacrifice of a major upper limb artery
- Conspicuous and cosmetically unfavorable STSG scar at donor site
- Contraindicated in patients with a positive modified Allen's test.

The free anterolateral thigh flap (FALT), another workhorse flap for head and neck reconstruction, used in moderate to large defects may not be a good choice in obese and/or hairy patients.

Advantages of MSAP Flap

1. Consistent presence of perforators
2. Long pedicle length
3. Can be harvested in supine position
4. Chimeric flaps including gastrocnemius muscle or another skin or adipofascial island can be harvested for complex soft tissue reconstruction.
5. Primary closure of the donor site is possible.

Harvesting the MSAP Flap

Use of Hand-held Doppler

We use the 8 MHz probe for marking the perforators. The surface marking includes the midpoint of the popliteal crease, medial malleolus and an imaginary line joining the two. The perforators lie along or beside this line, most commonly between 6 cm and 18 cm from popliteal crease. The side with the best audible perforator is chosen for flap.

CT angiography is used for perforator mapping for predictable harvest.

Patient Positioning

The patient lies in supine position with knee flexed and hip abducted and externally rotated. A split table with lithotomy has been described in literature for surgeon comfort.

Tourniquet

If a tourniquet is used, it should be used without exsanguination of the limb for better perforator visualization.

Marking and Incision

An elliptical skin paddle is marked centered on the perforator with the aim of primary closure **(Fig. 3)**. The medial incision is taken and subfascial dissection is continued by dissecting the epimysium of the deep fascia till a silhouette of perforator seen, followed by careful dissection to isolate the perforator with a bipolar cautery **(Fig. 4)**.

Dissecting the Perforators

All the perforators are dissected and the best perforator is chosen. Meticulous dissection is a crucial step in isolating the musculocutaneous perforators **(Fig. 5)**. When longer paddles are required, or if flap division is necessary, two perforators can be included. The skin paddle is modified so as to center the perforator and all incisions are committed **(Fig. 6)**.

MSAP can be harvested as a free style perforator flap.

Safeguarding the Nerve

The branches of the nerve to gastrocnemius are meticulously dissected away from the pedicle and preserved.

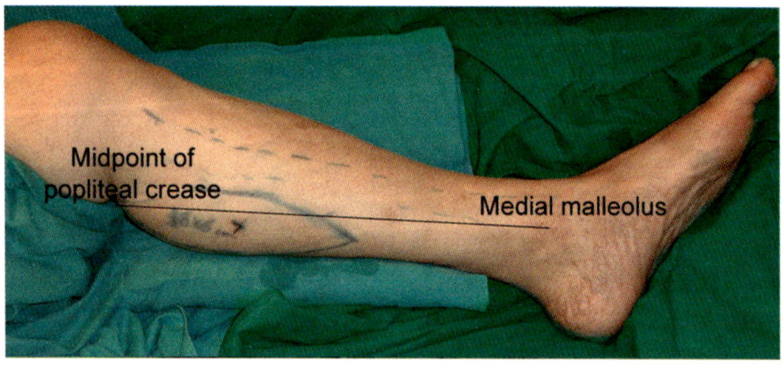

Fig. 3: A line joining the midpoint of popliteal fossa to medial malleolus is marked. The perforators generally lie along this line between 6 cm and 18 cm from popliteal crease

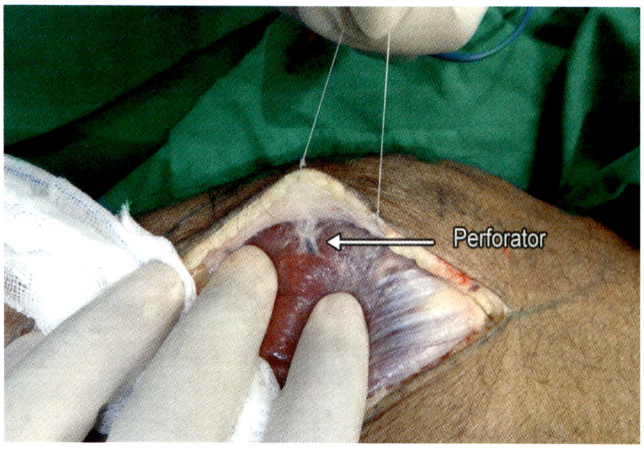

Fig. 4: A strong musculocutaneous perforator visualized

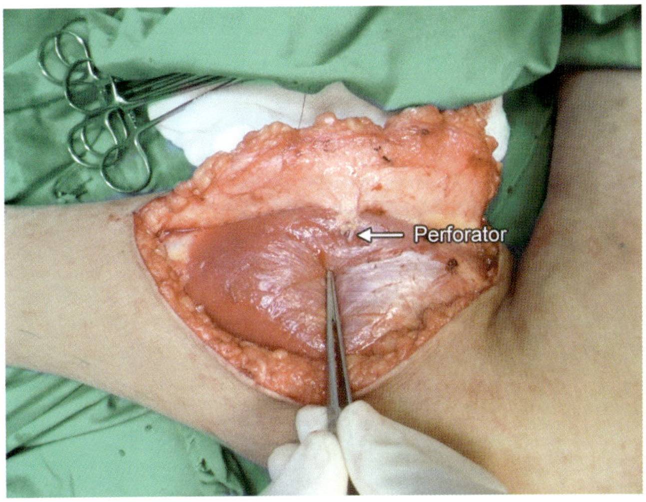

Fig. 5: Perforator visualized and intramuscular dissection commenced

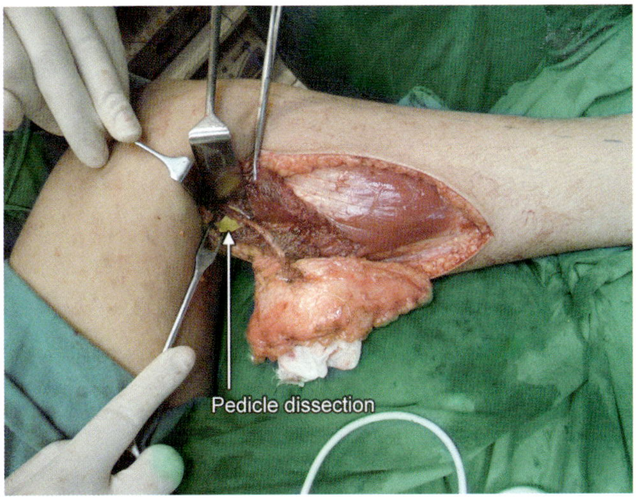

Fig. 6: Perforator dissection to source vessel

Pedicle Dissection

Pedicle dissection is continued toward the popliteal fossa till adequate vessel length or caliber is achieved. The short saphenous vein (SSV) and sural nerve are preserved.

The SSV can be harvested for augmenting venous drainage in case of a large flap **(Fig. 7)**.

Vascularity of the flap is confirmed and pedicle ligated **(Figs. 8 and 9)**.

Donor Closure

The donor site is closed in two layers with or without a suction drain **(Figs. 10 and 11)**.

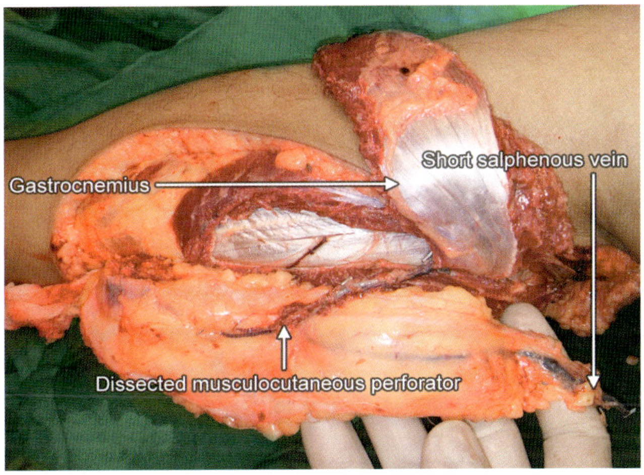

Fig. 7: Inclusion of SSV to augment venous drainage. Chimeric gastrocnemius has also been harvested

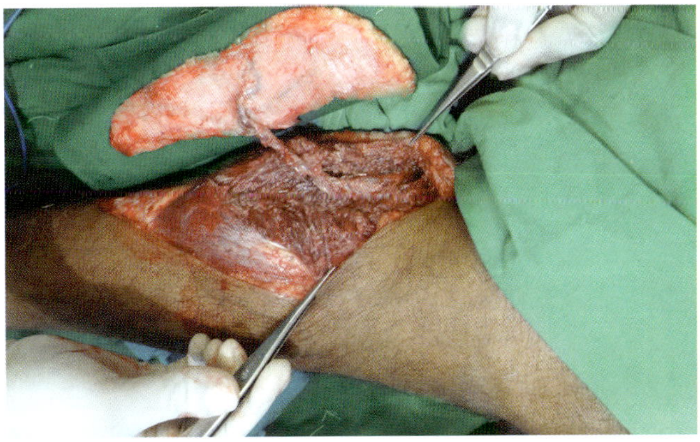

Fig. 8: Completed flap harvest ready for pedicle division

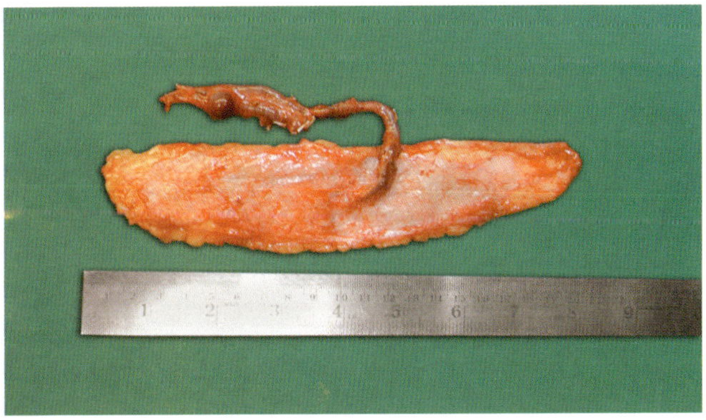

Fig. 9: Harvested MSAP flap harvested. A long intramuscular course provides a long pedicle

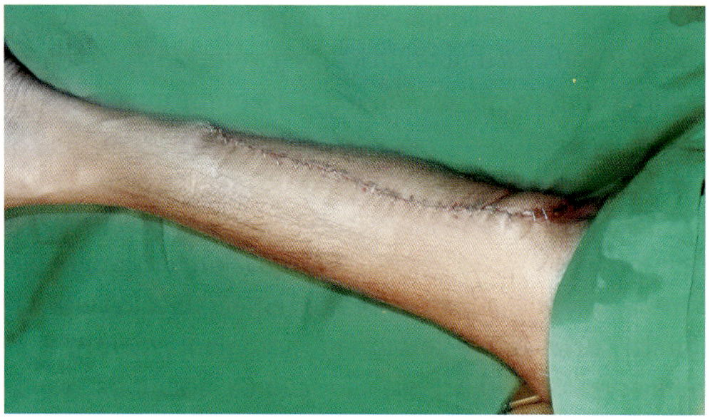

Fig. 10: Donor site closed in layers

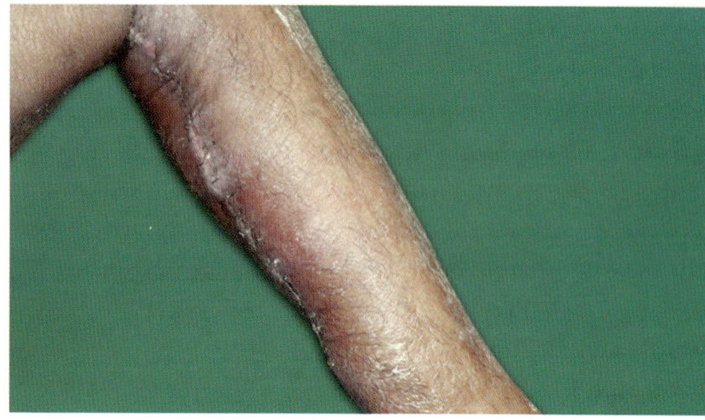

Fig. 11: Donor site scar

Disadvantages

- Steep learning curve associated with any free style perforator flap dissection
- A scar on the calf area may be undesirable in some patients.
- Not recommended in patients with varicose vein disease as flap venous drainage and wound healing may be compromised.

Uses

Free Flap

- For oral and oropharyngeal reconstruction.
  1. Buccal mucosa defect
  2. Composite buccal mucosa and skin defect **(Figs. 12A to D)**
  3. Tongue reconstruction, mainly hemiglossectomy, rarely total glossectomy **(Fig. 13)**.

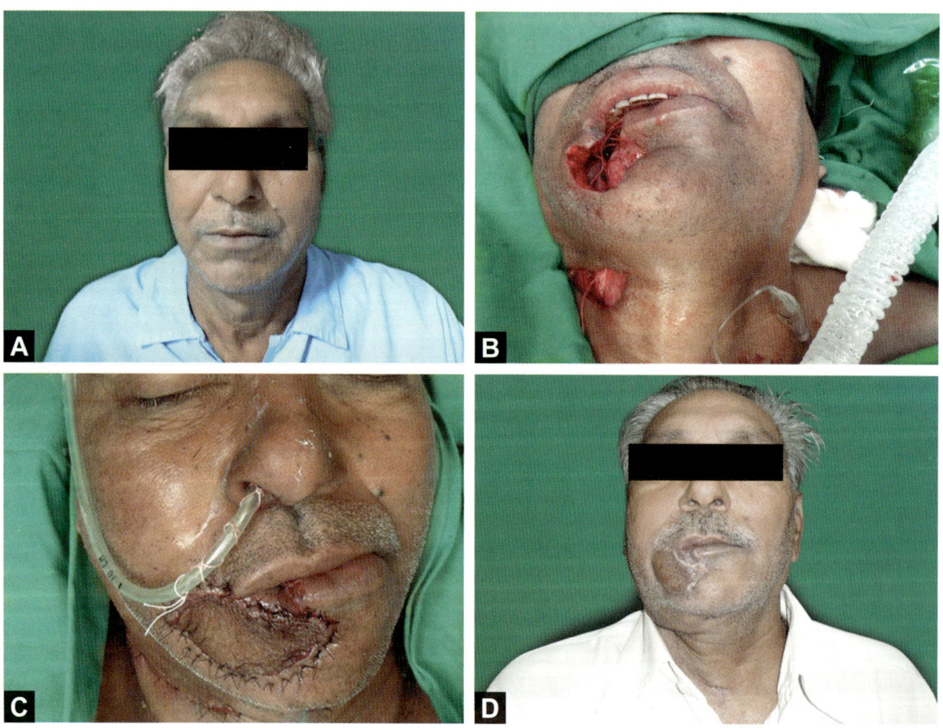

Figs. 12A to D: Clinical series of a patient with buccal mucosa with commisure and skin defect. (A) Preoperative view; (B) defect of buccal mucosa with commisure and skin defect; (C) reconstruction with MSAP; (D) postoperative view

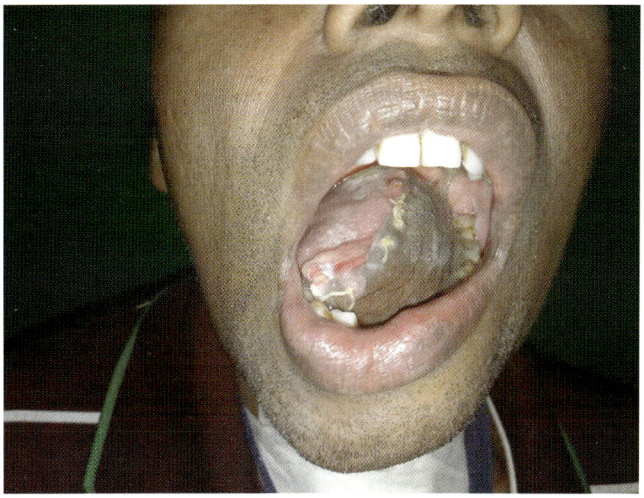

Fig. 13: Hemiglssectomy defect reconstructed with MSAP

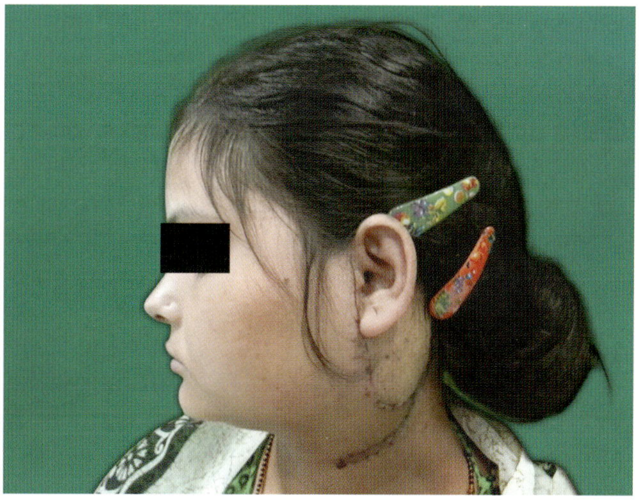

Fig. 14: Postoperative view of a post auricular defect covered with MSAP

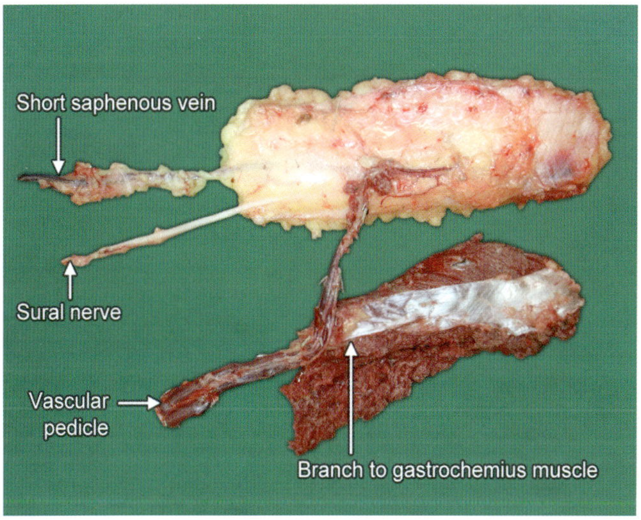

Fig. 15: MSAP with chimeric gastrocnemius muscle harvested. The SSV is included for added venous drainage

4. Palatal defects
5. Non circumferential pharyngeal defect reconstruction

- Soft tissue only defects of face and neck **(Fig. 14)**.
- Chimeric flaps with gastrocnemius muscle for use as filler or adjacent defect cover **(Fig. 15)**.

Pedicled Flap

This fasciocutaneous flap has a circular arc of rotation and the areas covered are

- Proximal third of the tibia (medial aspect and anterior crest)
- Anterior aspect of the knee till the lateral border of the patella
- Popliteal fossa.

We conclude that in our practice the MSAP can partly substitute a FRAFF/FALT when favorable donor characteristics exist. Thereby, increasing the armamentarium of a reconstructive surgeon.

Chapter 12

Free Latissimus Dorsi Flap

Amrita Rao, Vinay K Shankhdhar

INTRODUCTION

The latissimus dorsi flap was initially described by Iginio Tansini where he used it to close large post mastectomy wounds. Unfortunately, the knowledge was lost for the next 70 years until 1976 when Olivari in Cologne rediscovered it independently and used it for coverage of radiation-induced ulcers of the chest wall due to treatment of breast cancer. Then in 1978 three independent people used the flap in three unique ways. Bostwick modified Olivari's idea and used the islanded myocutaneous latissimus dorsi flap for breast reconstruction. Quillen first used pedicled latissimus dorsi flap for head and neck reconstruction. Finally Godina was the first to perform free transfer of the latissimus dorsi flap for coverage of extensive soft tissue defects in the leg.

Advantages of the Free Latissimus Dorsi Flap

- Large fan-shaped muscle which can cover extensive soft tissue defects
- Safe and reliable skin paddle which can be harvested along with muscle and donor area closed primarily
- Consistent anatomy and large caliber vessels with long pedicle length (2–5 mm caliber, 6–20 cm length if dissected upto the subscapular vessels)
- Possibility of harvesting chimeric flaps based on the subscapular vascular axis.
- Although a major muscle of shoulder joint is sacrificed , joint movement is not impaired if the rest of the shoulder girdle muscles are functional.

ANATOMY

The latissimus dorsi is a large fan-shaped muscle in the back. It takes aponeurotic origin from 9th to 12th ribs, lower five thoracic vertebral spinous processes, the lumbar and sacral vertebrae (via the thoracolumbar fascia), and the external lip of the posterior portion of iliac crest and the inferior angle of scapula. This large and triangular flat muscle belly converges to a flat broad tendon which is inserted on the lesser tubercle of the intertubercular groove of the humerus. The muscle is superficial to a large extent and covered only by the trapezius in the superomedial aspect. All muscle margins are clear and distinct except the superior where it may be fused with the teres major muscle and the lateral where it merges with the serratus anterior.

Vascular Supply

Latissimus dorsi is a type 5 muscle according to Mathes and Nahai classification system receiving dominant blood supply from the thoracodorsal artery and secondary blood supply from segmental perforating branches of the intercostal and lumbar arteries. All vessels enter through the deep surface of the muscle.

The subscapular artery originates from the third part of the axillary artery and divides into the circumflex scapular artery and the thoracodorsal artery which enters through the deep surface of the muscle about 6–9 cm from its origin. Usually the thoracodorsal artery also gives off a large branch to the serratus anterior muscle. This artery is accompanied by a large venae comitans. After entering the muscle the thoracodorsal artery divides into the transverse branch and the descending branch which independently give of cutaneous perforators **(Fig. 1)**.

On the basis of this vascular anatomy the free latissimus dorsi is amenable to a number of variations.

- Muscle only (whole or split muscle based on either the transverse or descending branch of thoracodorsal artery)
- Whole muscle with skin paddle
- Partial/split muscle with skin paddle (again based on either transverse or descending branch of the thoracodorsal artery)

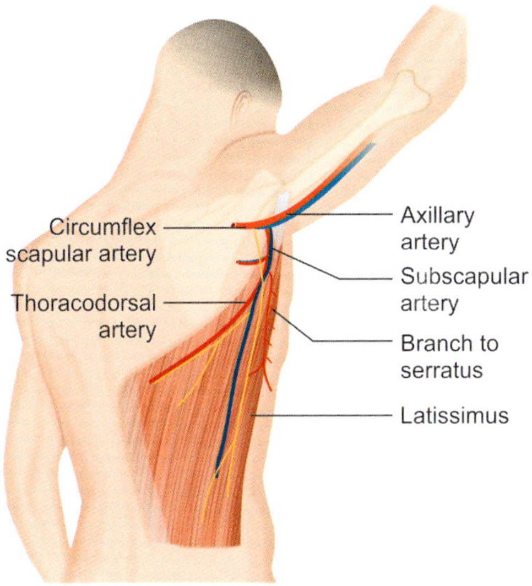

Fig. 1: Subscapular vascular axis

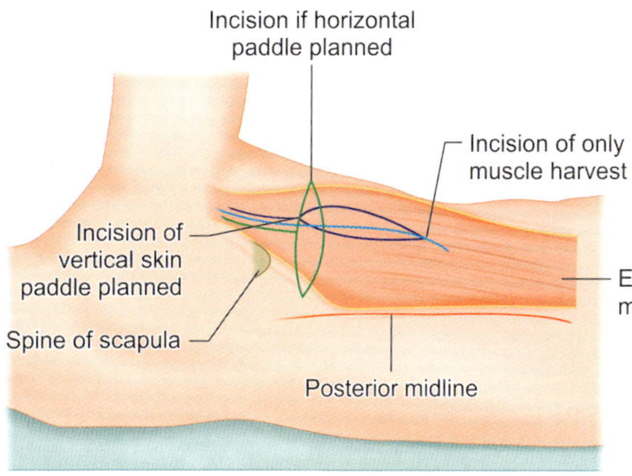

Fig. 2: Incisions for flap harvest

- Muscle sparing faciocutaneous flap—Thoracodorsal artery perforator flap (next chapter)
- Chimeric flap including the Serratus anterior muscle.

FLAP HARVEST

Patient Position and Draping

We prefer to harvest the flap in floppy lateral position and by open method. Draping is done keeping the arm free and sterile over an arm board so that it can be freely moved during the pedicle dissection toward axilla. Patient must be well-strapped to the table to allow for variable tilt of the table for convenience. Minimal access harvest with subcutaneous laparoscopic method is also possible.

Steps of the Surgery

- *The surface marking of the muscle and incision:* Mark the apex of the axilla and the posterior axillary line, the angle of the scapula and the posterior iliac crest. If only muscle is to be harvested, then a liberal incision along the posterior axillary line curving towards the surface of the muscle is made. The incision extends up to the axilla so to facilitate easy axillary dissection. If skin paddle is also to be harvested along with the flap, then it can be oriented either horizontally (so that the skin closure line is along the bra strap) or vertically (which is more reliable as maximum cutaneous perforators lie along the lateral margin of the muscle). The margins of the skin paddle then serve as the access incisions for the flap and an axillary extension can be added for ease of dissection **(Fig. 2)**.
- Monopolar cautery can be used for this part of the dissection. The supero-medial skin flap is raised first so as to identify the superior free border. Anterior margin of the muscle is delineated from the serratus anterior muscle. The LD is then dissected free from the trapezius muscle which is the only muscle which lies superficial to the latissimus dorsi. Inferiorly the muscle is dissected as far as required and divided from its origin from the thoracolumbar fascia the vertebral spines and the posterior border of the iliac crest.
- The muscle is then lifted off from its base starting from below upwards. Multiple lumbar and paraspinal perforators enter the muscle from its inferior aspect and these must be ligated or clipped securely. As we near the axilla the muscle must be separated off from the teres major by continuing dissection along the free border. Anteriorly the muscle most often mistaken for the latissimus dorsi is the serratus posterior inferior due to identical direction of fibers. This is avoided by continuing sharp dissection along the anterior border of latissimus dorsi after the serratus branch is seen arising from the thoracodorsal pedicle. It is advisable to change over to bipolar cautery at this juncture.
- The vascular pedicle is now visible entering the muscle from its inferior aspect. The thoracodorsal pedicle is detected up to its origin as per requirement of pedicle length and lumen. Additionally the serratus anterior muscle based on the serratus branch of the thoracodorsal can be harvested separately as a chimeric flap.

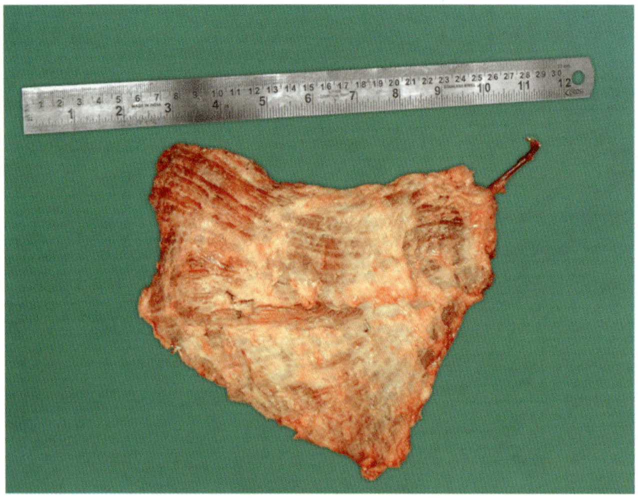

Fig. 3: Harvested muscle only flap with large surface area and pedicle length

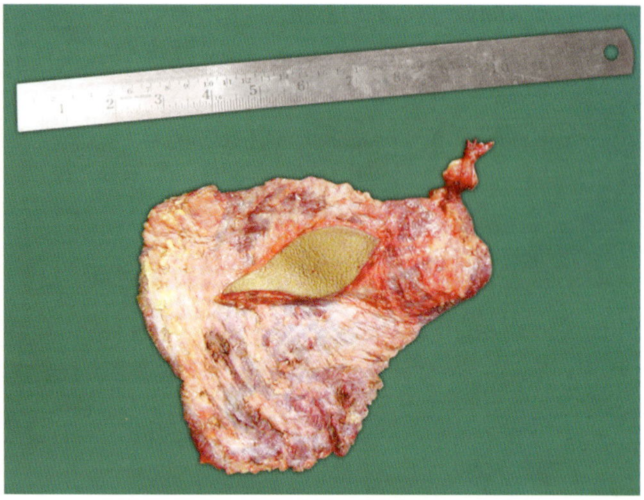

Fig. 4: Harvested flap with small skin island

- Another 4–5 cm of pedicle length can be obtained if the circumflex scapular artery is clipped and the subscapular artery harvested from its origin from the axillary artery whenever needed when used for scalp defects with anastomosis to neck vessels. The remaining muscles of the shoulder girdle will then derive blood supply from the anastomosis around the scapula.
- *Donor site*: It is closed after achieving adequate hemostasis and placement of suction drains **(Figs. 3 to 5)**.

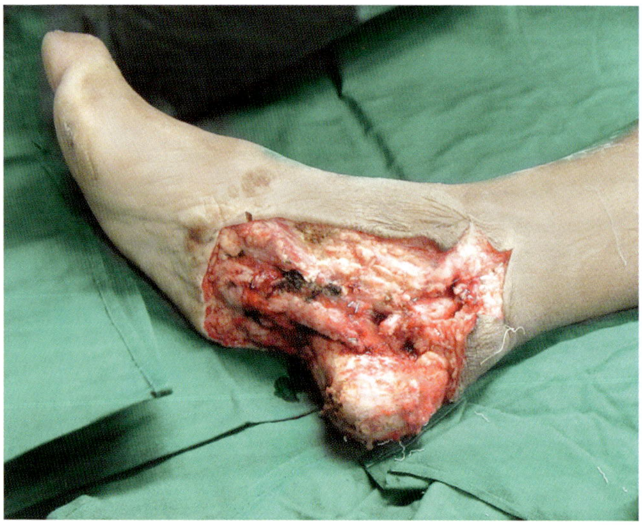

Fig. 5: Large soft tissue defect in the heel with exposed bone

Postoperative Management

- No restriction of shoulder movement and physiotherapy to be started on postoperative day 1
- Maintain suction drain for 10–14 days.

INDICATIONS

In head and neck reconstruction it is largely an alternative to anterolateral thigh flap where it is chosen due to its large surface area, volume and pedicle length.

- Soft tissue defects in the limbs secondary to sarcoma excision
- Cover of implant and nail cement spacer in lower limb
- Large irregular defects with multiple cavities after extensive maxilla and skull base resections.
- Large defects over scalp with exposed bone.

CONTRAINDICATIONS

- During previous neck dissection if the spinal accessory nerve is injured and the trapezius muscle paralyzed, the latissimus dorsi becomes an inexpendable muscle for movement of the shoulder joint
- If the patient is paraplegic/wheelchair bound/dependant on crutches.
- Patients indulging in extreme sporting activities like mountaineering and skiing.

In these cases, muscle sparing harvest of thoracodorsal artery perforator flap can be used.

- If the thoracodorsal artery has been ligated or clipped during previous axillary clearance, LD should not be harvested. In such cases, imaging to assess viability of pedicle can be done if no other expendable site is present.

Drawbacks

- Seroma over donor area requiring multiple aspirations.

Case Series 1 (Figs. 6 and 7)

Free Latissimus Dorsi Muscle with split thickness skin graft for heel defect.

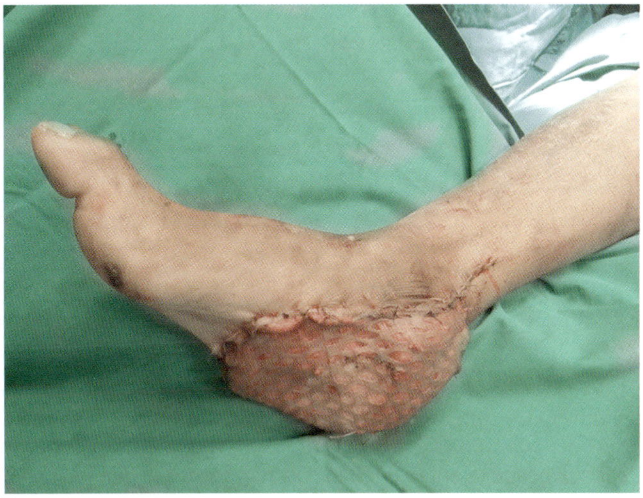

Fig. 6: Final flap inset with skin grafting of the exposed surface

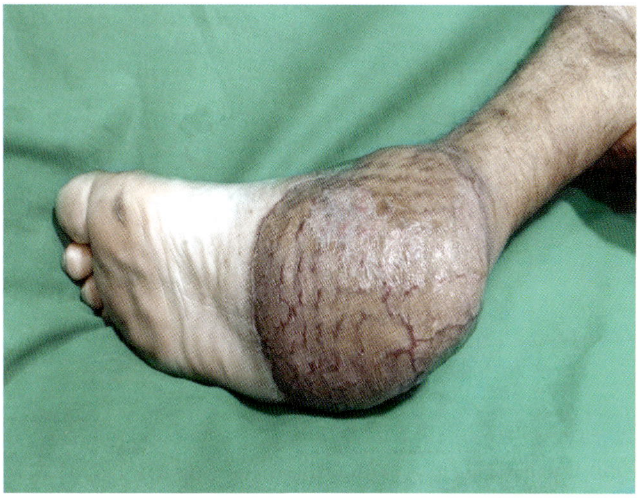

Fig. 7: After 2 months of surgery, well settled flap

Case Series 2 (Figs. 8 to 11)

Free Latissimus Dorsi Muscle flap for knee defect.

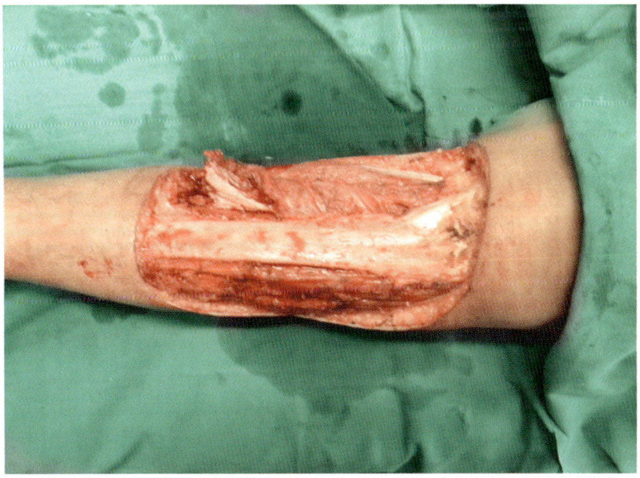

Fig. 8: Large defect over the knee with exposed bone

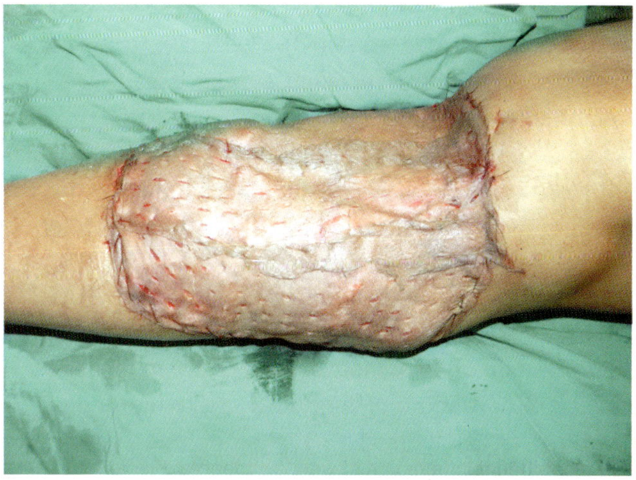

Fig. 9: Covered with free LD flap + STSG

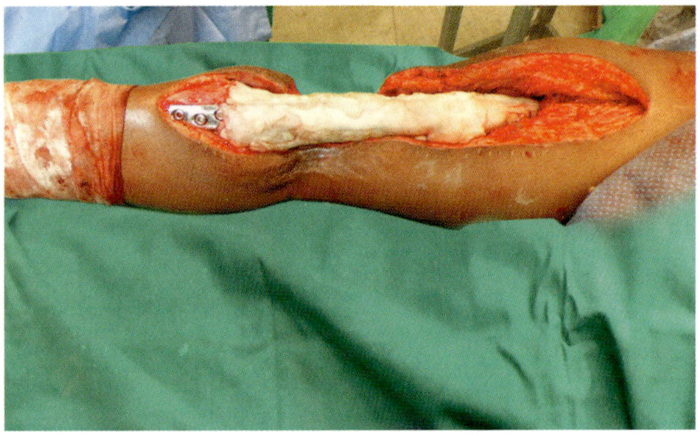

Fig. 10: Implant with nail cement spacer for right knee bony reconstruction

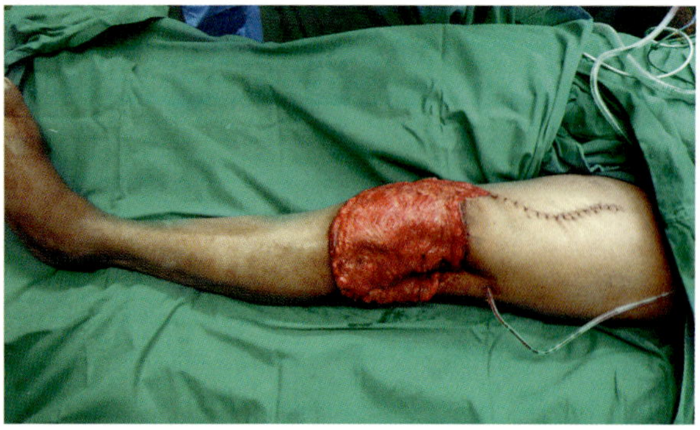

Fig. 11: Implant and bone covered with free LD flap

Case Series 3 (Figs. 12 to 18)

Chimeric Latissimus Dorsi myocutaneous with serratus muscle flap for complex maxillary defect.

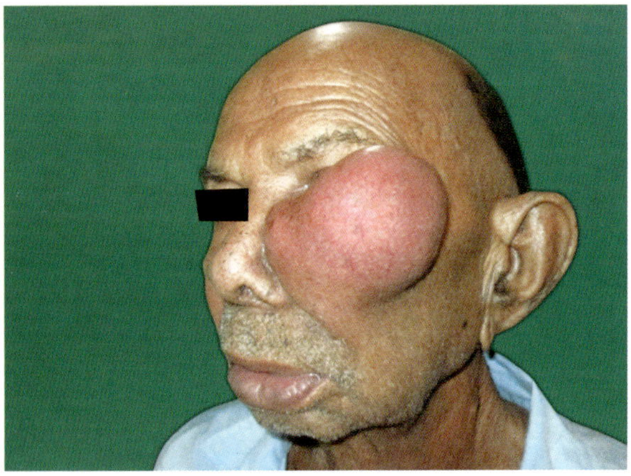

Fig. 12: Advanced carcinoma of left maxilla planned for total maxillectomy with orbital exentration

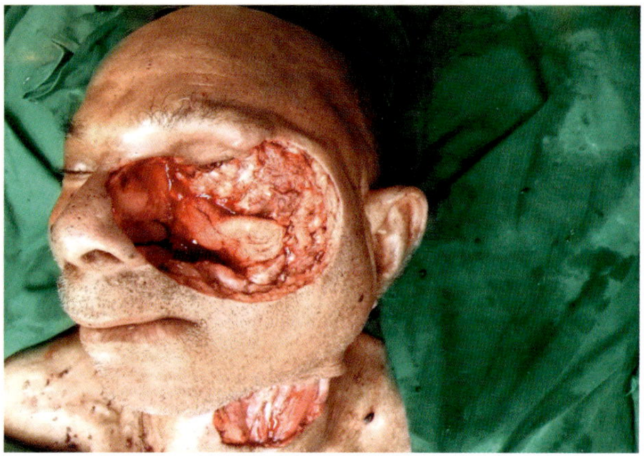

Fig. 13: Intraoperative defect with multiple large cavities (cavity looks smaller due to surgical mop in situ) and large skin defect

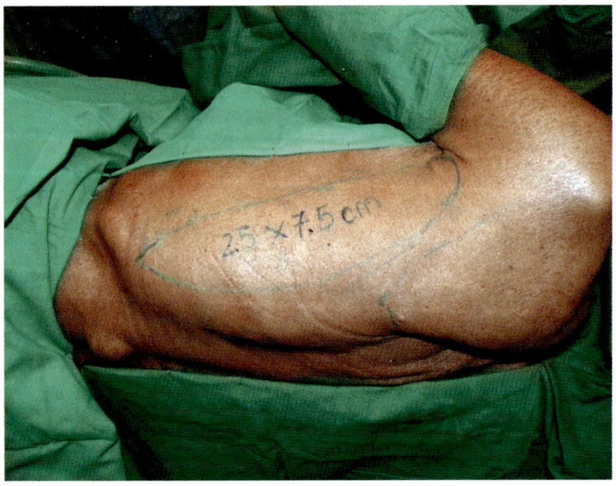

Fig. 14: Flap marking with skin island

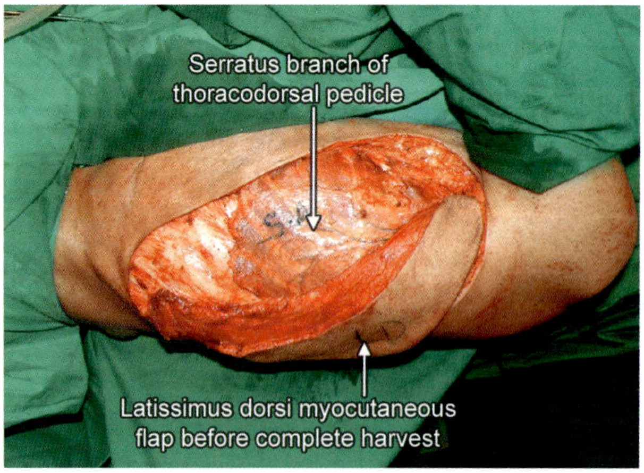

Fig. 15: Intraoperative photo showing large serratus branch

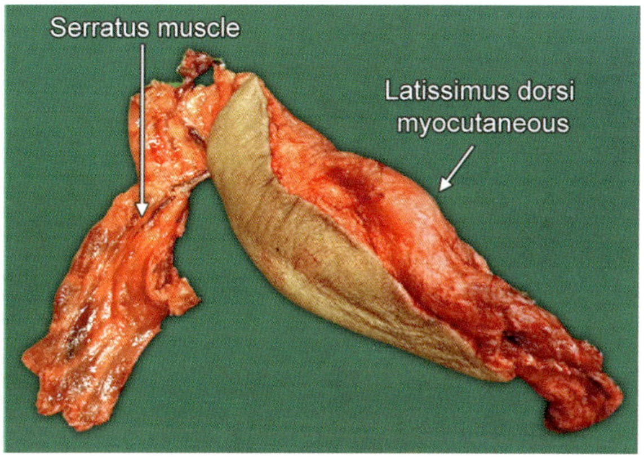

Fig. 16: Chimeric flap with serratus muscle and latissimus dorsi myocutaneous components

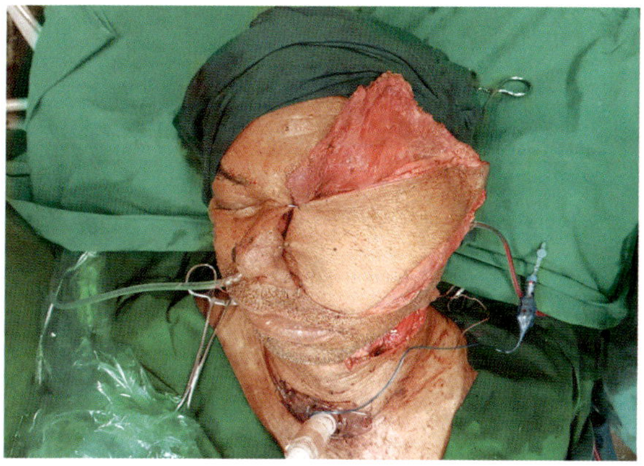

Fig. 17: Flap inset into defect with multiple cavities filled with muscular components and skin island for the cutaneous defect over left side of face

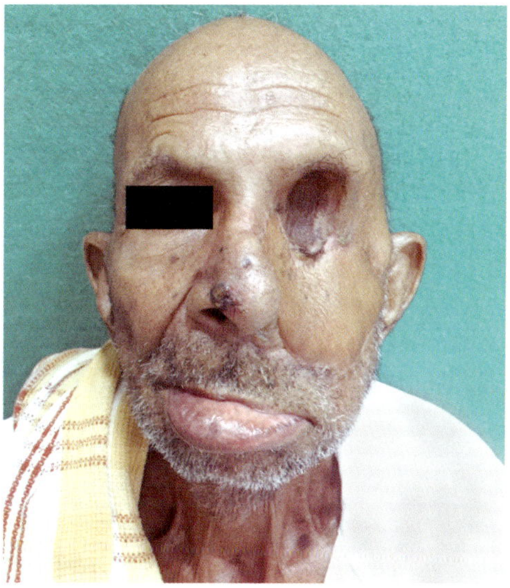

Fig. 18: Postoperative photograph (after completion of radiation) showing well-settled flap

Case Series 4 (Figs. 19 to 21)

Free Latissimus Dorsi muscle flap with split thickness skin graft for scalp defect.

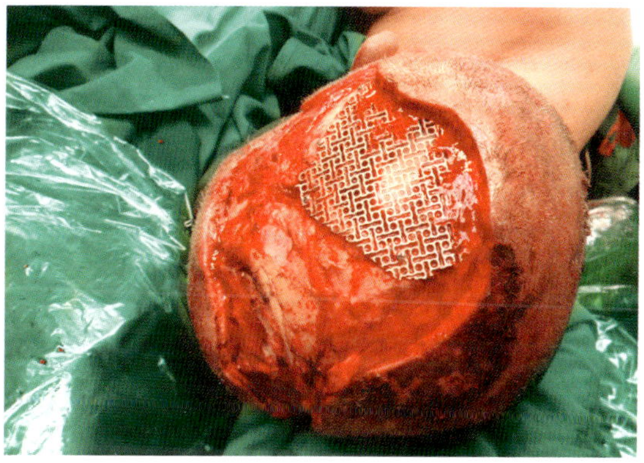

Fig. 19: Exposed cranial bone and implant

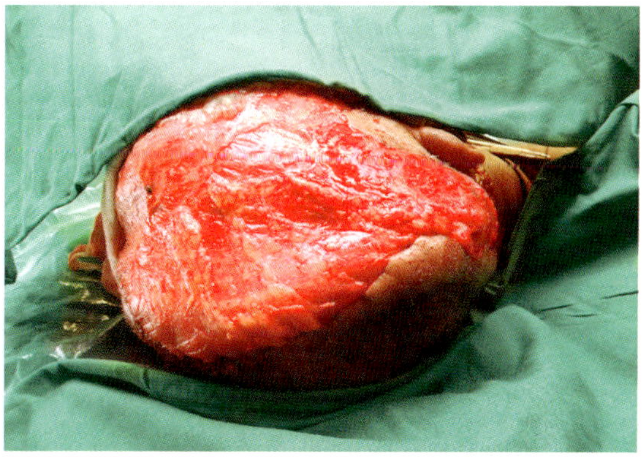

Fig. 20: After flap inset

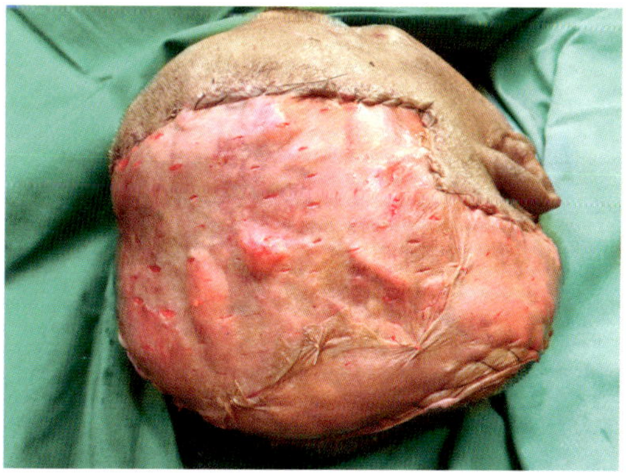

Fig. 21: Flap covered with STSG

CHAPTER 13

Thoracodorsal Artery Perforator Flap

Tanmay Mohan Joshi, Dushyant Jaiswal

INTRODUCTION

Thoracodorsal Artery Perforator Flap (TDAP), is a perforator-based flap first described by **Angrigiani et al. in 1995**. The adjacent angiosomes of the lateral chest are supplied by perforators arising from the lateral thoracic, serratus branch, thoracodorsal vessels and circumflex scapular vessels **(Fig. 1)**.

The TDAP flap is supplied most commonly by musculocutaneous and occasionally fasciocutaneous perforators that arise from either the lateral or the medial branch of the thoracodorsal artery **(Fig. 2)**.

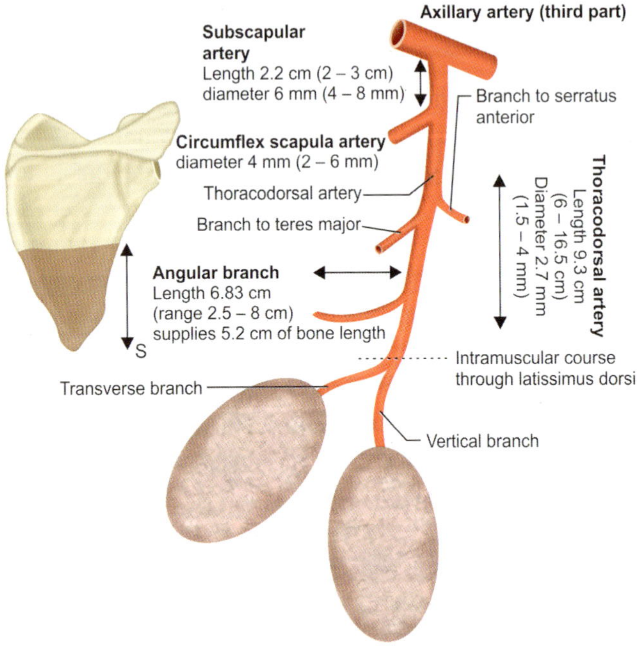

Fig. 1: Schematic showing the various branches of subscapular artery

Planning the Flap

Use of Hand-held Audio Doppler

We use the 8 MHz probe for marking the perforators. Preoperatively the patient is made to lie in lateral decubitus in a position similar to operative positioning. This is done to ensure minimum shift in location and direction of perforators with positioning. The surface marking includes the inferior angle of scapula, anterior free border of LD muscle and center of axillary fossa. The perforator usually runs posteriorly for a variable distance after exiting the muscle. Finding a perforator is a function of time and sufficient time is dedicated for the same to identify the strongest Doppler signal.

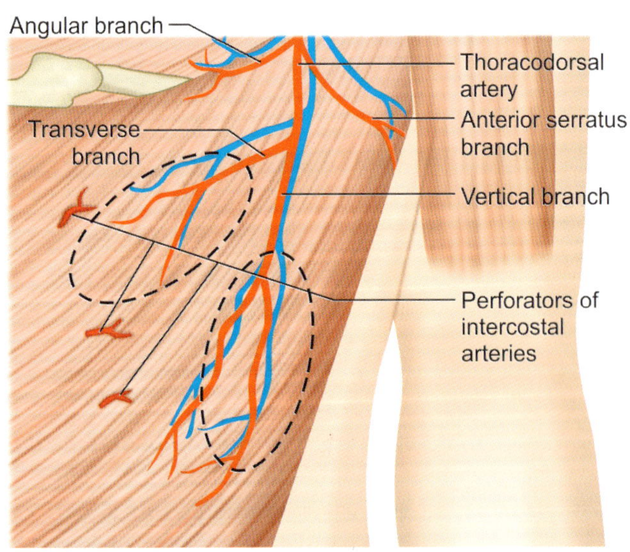

Fig. 2: The perforators from the medial and lateral branches of the thoracodorsal vessels can be used for designing various paddles

HARVESTING THE TDAP FLAP

Patient Positioning

We prefer to harvest TDAP flap in a lateral decubitus with arm kept free and entire hemi back exposed and prepared. It is possible to harvest smaller flaps in supine or semi recumbent position.

Marking: Flap Marking (Figs. 3 and 4)

The vertical skin paddle design is usually used as most perforators arise from the descending branch of Thoracodorsal artery. The disadvantage of a vertical paddle is that it is perpendicular to the relaxed skin tension lines, leading to stretching and widening of scars.

Horizontal paddle is designed in cases of pedicled flaps for breast.

When a horizontal paddle is used, retraction of skin flaps to dissect the pedicle is difficult and time consuming. Also converting into a parascapular flap or lateral thoracic flap not possible.

Incision

We prefer to place a linear vertical non-committal posterior incision. In case a TDAP perforator is not found or is injured, the same incision is useful to design a parascapular flap on circumflex vessels. We use the parascapular flap as a fall back rather than lateral thoracic perforator as it is more predictable. Parascapular flap is not our first choice due to short pedicle length and a scar over the scapula is not desired.

Dissecting the Perforators

Subfascial dissection is performed till a good perforator is seen. The perforators are usually musculo-cutaneous in origin **(Fig. 5)**. The perforator is dissected into the muscle cleavage plane. The muscle fibers are split along the length and fibers are retracted. Rarely septo-cutaneous perforators arise by curving around the anterior free border of the muscle. The muscle dissection is completely omitted in these cases **(Fig. 6)**. The anterior incision is committed and flap is elevated. Dissection continues till all perforators are visualized and the best perforator is selected. The perforator is carefully dissected and the distal end of thoracodorsal vessels is ligated **(Fig. 7)**.

Safeguarding the Nerve

The branches of the thoracodorsal nerve are meticulously dissected away from the pedicle. This is of prime importance as nerve damage defeats the purpose of muscle sparing harvest. Avoid any mechanical, thermal damage to the nerve during the dissection **(Fig. 8)**.

Pedicle Dissection

The serratus branch of vessel may be clipped. Pedicle dissection continues further towards the axillary vessels till adequate vessel length or caliber is achieved **(Figs. 9 and 10)**.

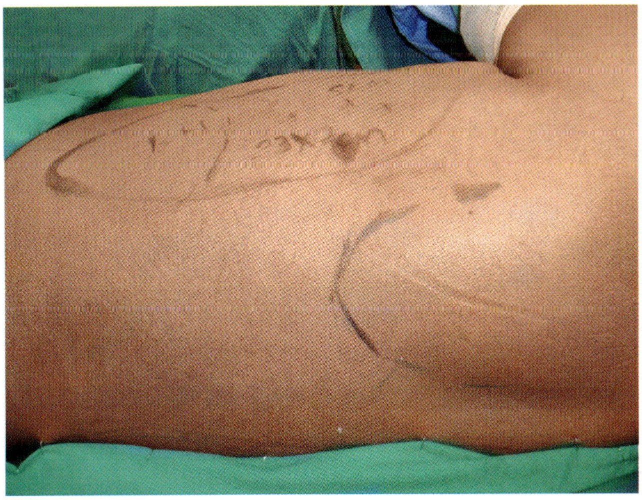

Fig. 3: Marking for vertical paddle TDAP

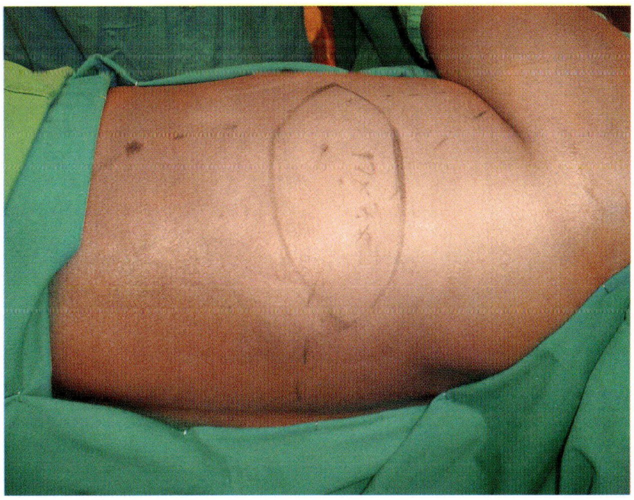

Fig. 4: Marking of horizontal paddle

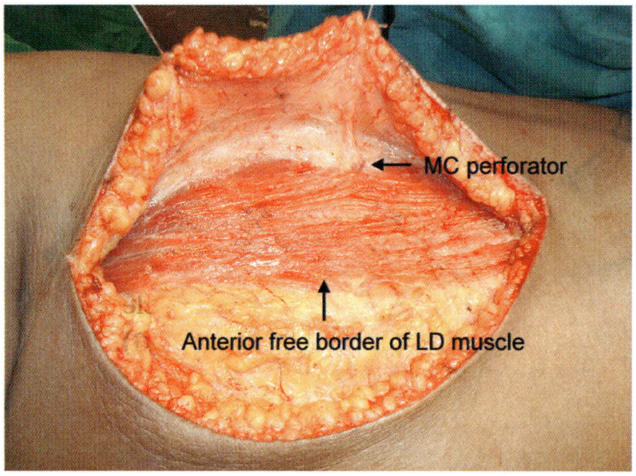

Fig. 5: A musculocutaneous perforator is seen

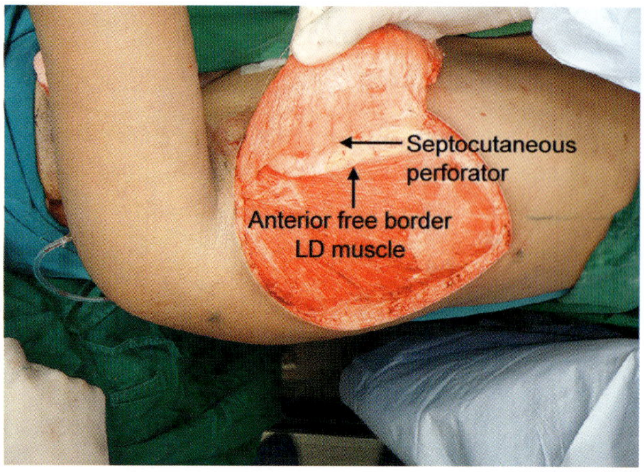

Fig. 6: Septocutaneous perforator arising anterior to free border of LD muscle

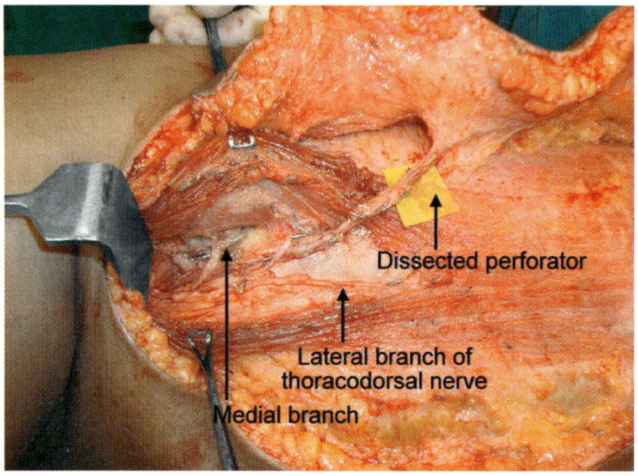

Fig. 7: Musculocutaneous perforator deroofed and dissected out

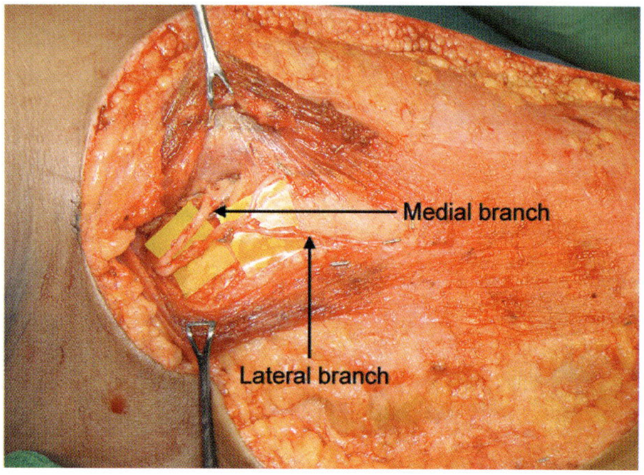

Fig. 8: The thoracodorsal nerve and its branches have been dissected and preserved

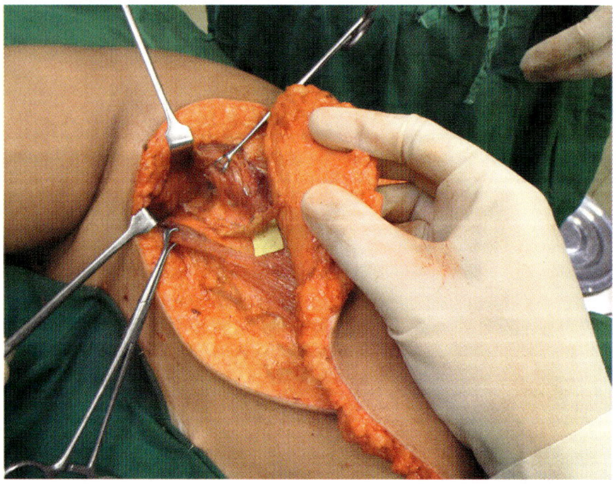

Fig. 9: Retraction and pedicle dissection to reach subscapular vessels

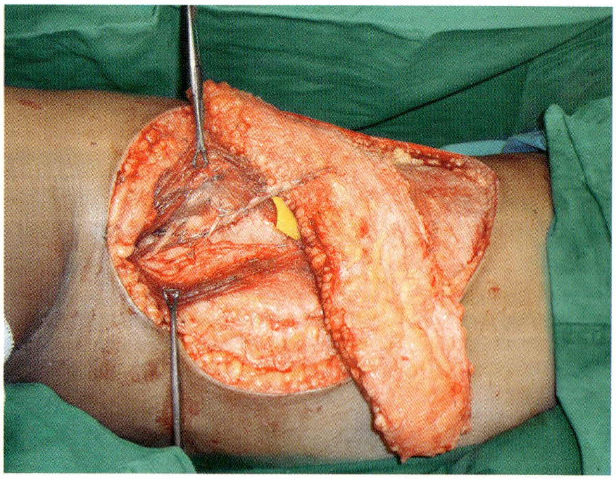

Fig. 10: Flap dissection complete and pedicle ready for ligation

Chimeric Flaps

The vascular network of the subscapular aretery gives several branches such as the circumflex scapular, thoracodorsal artery, angular artery to the tip of scapula and branch to serratus anterior.

- The skin paddle can be divided based on separate perforators.
- A part of the latissimus dorsi or serratus muscle can be harvested for use as a filler or commonly used for functional muscle transfer.
- Lateral border of scapula as vascularized bone flap.

The advantage of chimeric flaps is the comfort it offers in contouring according to the defect characteristics. This allows for a three dimensional reconstruction of irregular, multicomponent defects.

Donor Closure

The donor site is closed in two layers over a suction drain **(Fig. 11)**. The risk of seroma is lesser because of less muscle dissection. Larger flaps requiring skin grafts are not recommended as skin graft at this site is troublesome. **Figures 12 and 13** show stretched scars in late postoperative period.

Advantages

1. A thin pliable flap for contouring
2. Chimeras are possible on perforators of the subscapular arterial axis
3. Generally hairless skin beneficial for intra-oral reconstruction
4. Thinning of flap is possible **(Figs. 14 and 15)**
5. Intramuscular dissection allows long pedicle lengths 12–15 cm
6. No functional loss at donor site as innervated LD muscle is spared.
7. Reduction in donor site dead space seroma formation compared to muscle flaps
8. Scar is well-hidden in posterior axillary fold
9. Pliable skin at donor site enables easy primary closure.

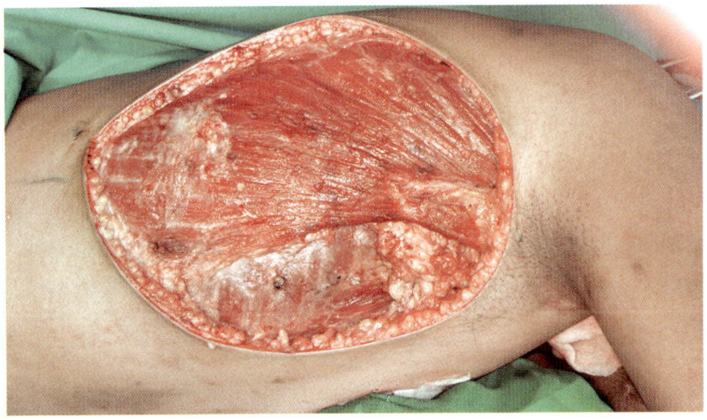

Fig. 11: Donor site after harvest

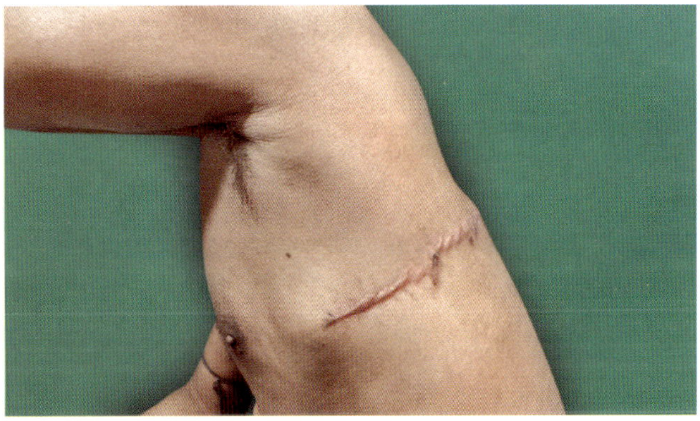

Fig. 12: Stretched healed scar of horizontal paddle

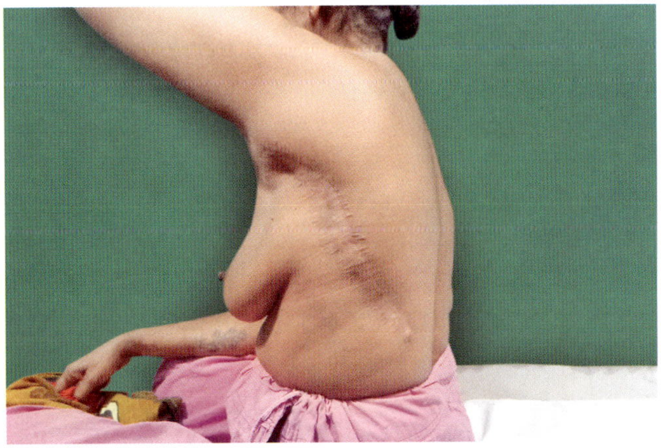

Fig. 13: Stretched healed scar of vertical paddle

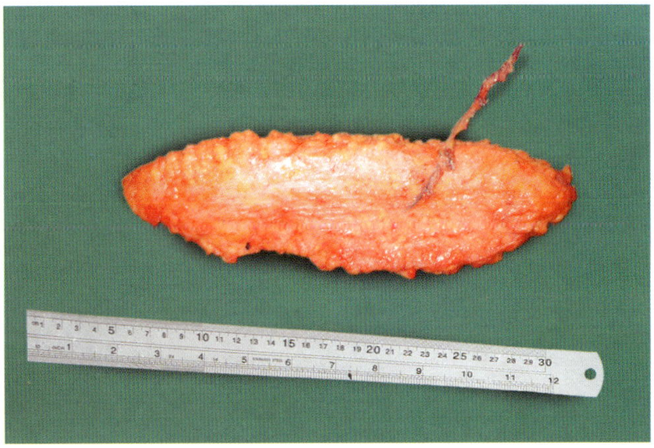

Fig. 14: Harvested flap

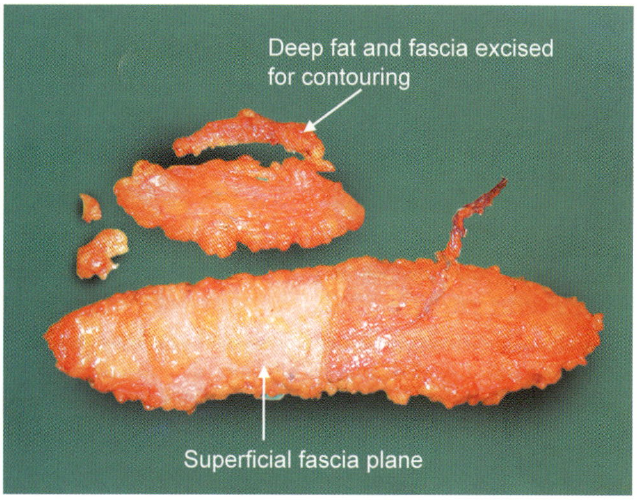

Fig. 15: Flap can be thinned in superficial fascia plane with magnification

Disadvantages

- Steep learning curve associated with any free style perforator flap dissection
- Lateral position precludes simultaneous harvest increasing operative time
- Flap size is usually limited by the pliability of the donor site, approximately 8–10 cms.
- Flaps may appear suffused in some cases due to stronger arterial inflow than venous outflow, giving a false impression of venous insufficiency. In our experience this problem settles due to auto regulation of blood flow in the postoperative period.

INDICATIONS

The TDAP flap provides a long large, relatively thin, hairless skin flap with a long pedicle length.

Free Tissue Transfer

The TDAP flap is a reliable alternative to the anterolateral thigh flap when the former site is excessively bulky, turgid, or hairy.

We have used the TDAP flap for reconstructing defects of:

Head and Neck Region

- Buccal mucosa composite defects **(Figs. 16A to F)**
- Buccal mucosa defects involving lip
- Buccal mucosa with marginal mandibulectomy **(Figs. 17A to C)**.

Limb Reconstruction

Cover defects post soft tissue sarcoma resection or bone/implant exposure where the thine, pliable flap allows for approximation of skin edges on convex surfaces **(Figs. 18A to C)**.

Pedicled Flap

Partial breast reconstruction after breast conservation surgery.

The arc of rotation of the flap allows its transfer to reconstruct defects of the shoulder, axilla, lower neck, arm, upper back, ipsilateral and lateral chest wall defects.

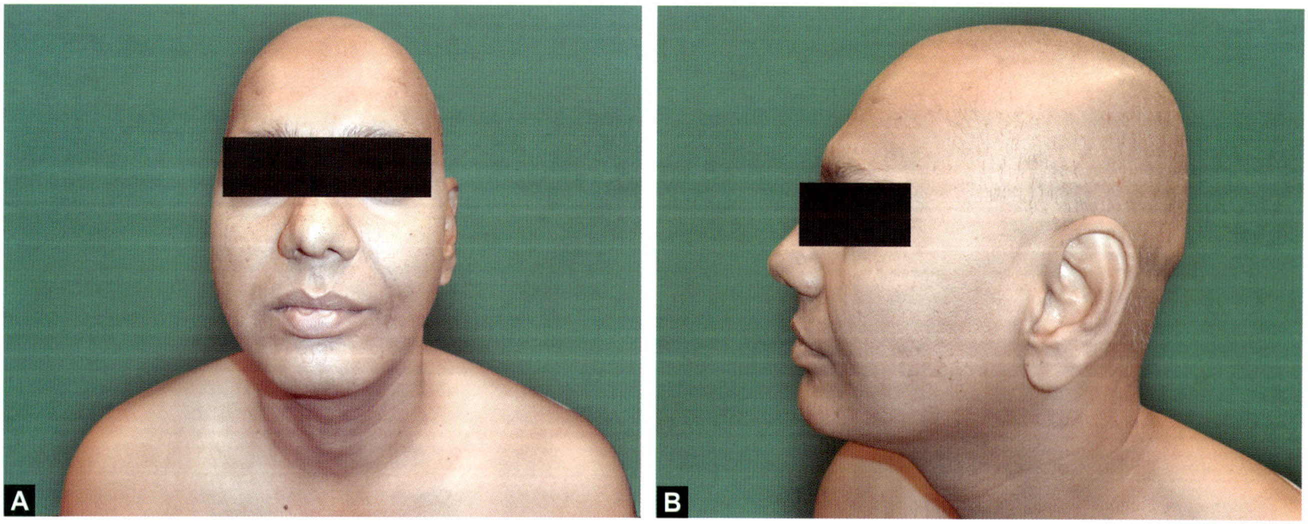

Figs. 16A and B

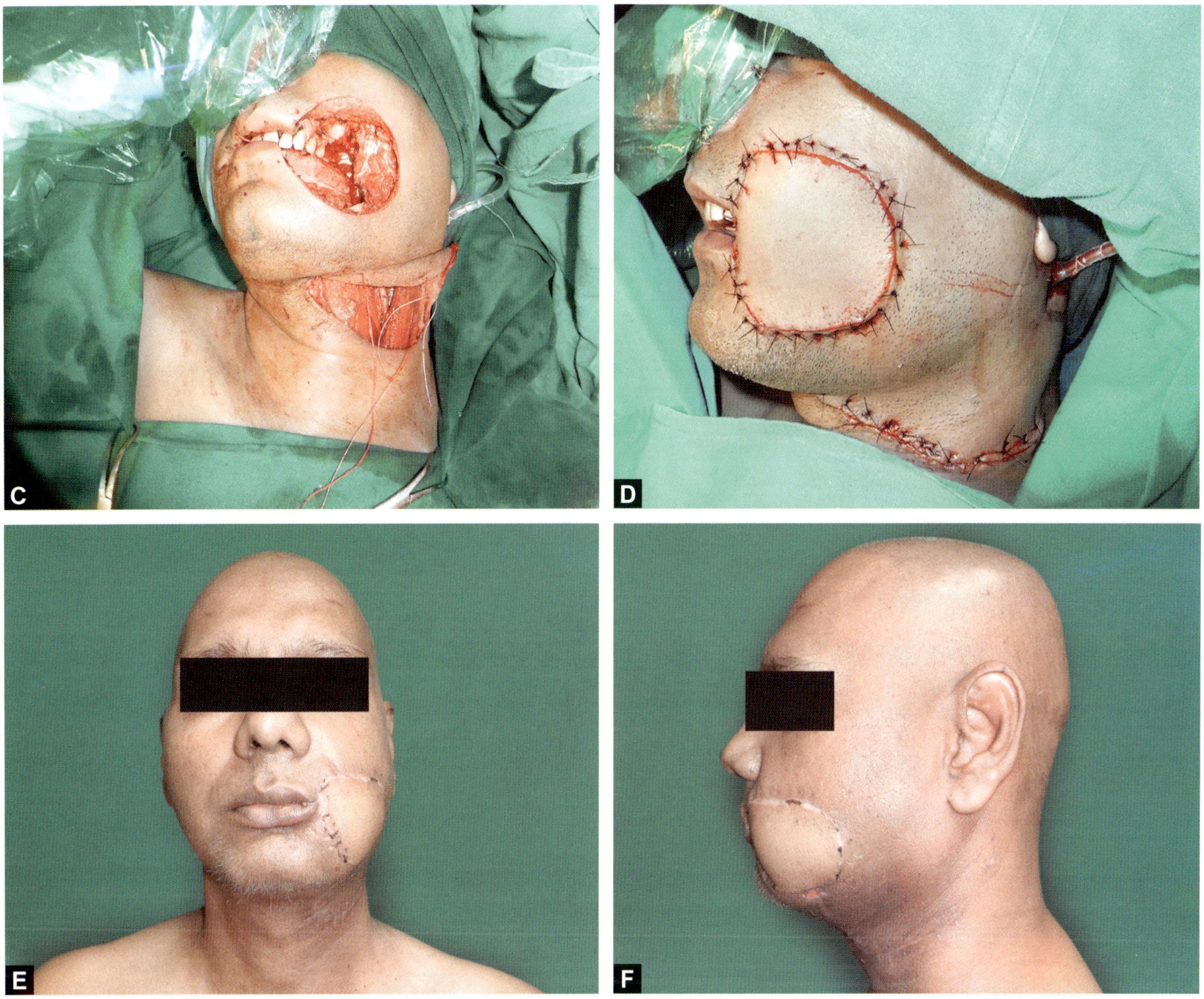

Figs. 16A to F: Preoperative, intraoperative and postoperative photos of a patient with reconstruction of a buccal mucosa + upper alveolectomy + marginal mandibulectomy defect

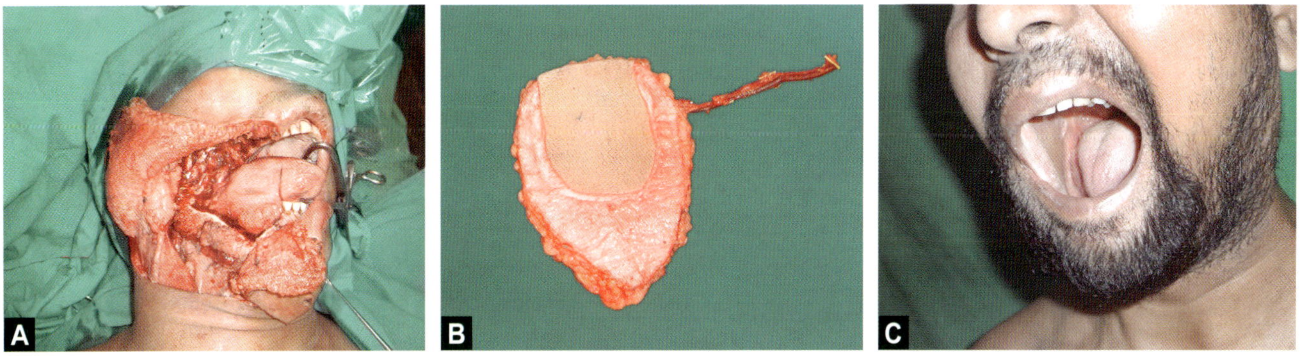

Figs. 17A to C: (A) Intraoperative defect, (B) a TDAP flap for buccal mucosa partially de-epithelized for fill, (C) postoperative

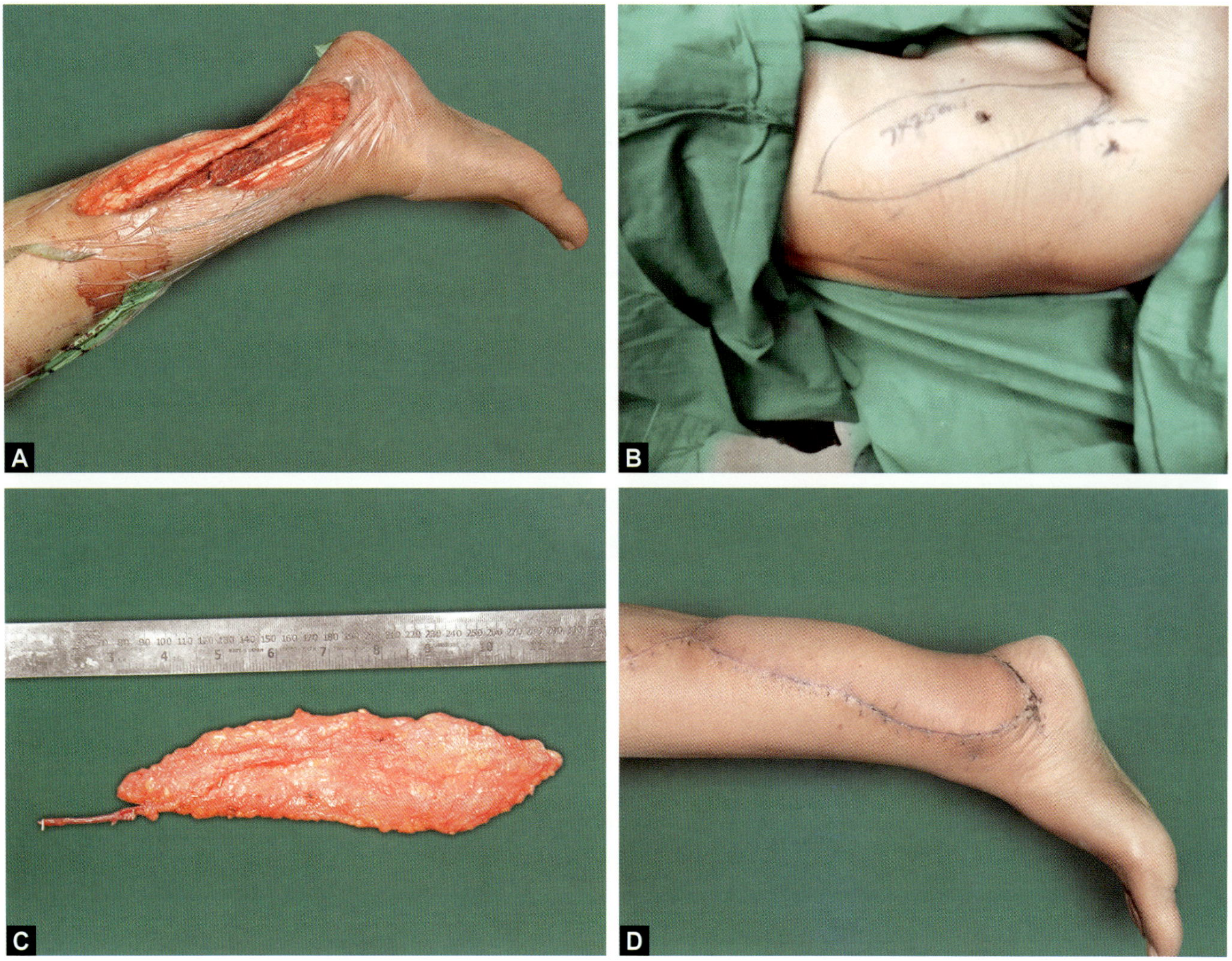

Figs. 18A to D: Reconstruction of leg defect with TDAP flap

CHAPTER 14

Gracilis Flap

Tanmay Mohan Joshi, Saumya Mathews, Prabha Yadav

ANATOMY

The gracilis muscle is a long slender muscle of the adductor compartment of the thigh. It originates from the inferior pubic ramus and is inserted on the medial surface and medial condyle of tibia **(Fig. 1)**. It is one of the five adductor muscles of the thigh. It has a Type 2 vascular pattern (Mathes and Nahai classification) of blood supply having dominant and minor vascular pedicles.

The dominant pedicle arises from the terminal branch of the medial circumflex femoral artery or sometimes from the Deep Femoral artery directly. Venous drainage is by two venae commitantes to the deep femoral vein. The nerve supply is from the anterior branch of the obturator nerve. The neurovascular pedicle is located about 8–12 cm inferior to the pubic tubercle **(Fig. 2)**.

The gracilis muscle or gracilis musculocutaneous flap is one of the most commonly utilised muscle flaps in microsurgery.

The salient features of this flap include:

1. Consistent anatomy
2. Perforators supplying the skin are concentrated in the upper two third of the thigh. The robust perforators are present in the upper one third.
3. Vertical (VUG) and transverse paddles (TUG) can be designed.
4. Superficial muscle that can be easily identified and dissected.
5. Neurotized free muscle flap is used for functional limb restoration and facial reanimation.

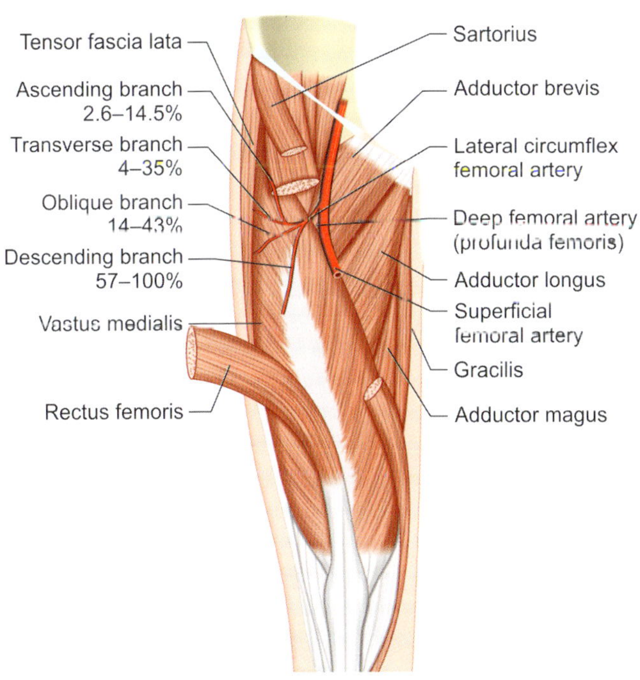

Fig. 1: Gracilis muscle in the adductor compartment

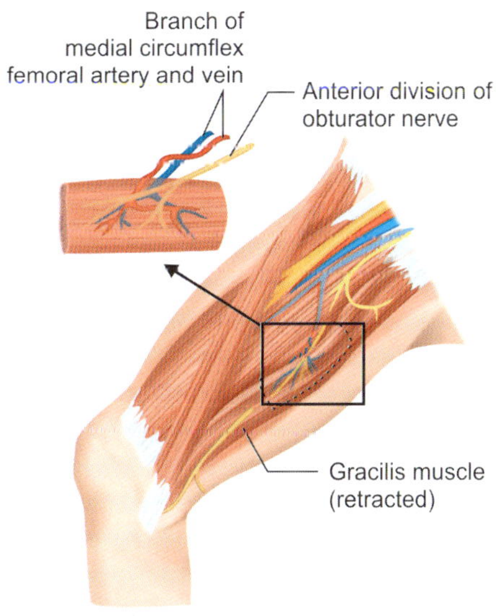

Fig. 2: Vascular pedicle from the medial circumflex femoral vessels and nerve from anterior division of obturator nerve

6. Donor area primary closure is possible
7. Expendable muscle with a minimum functional deficit
8. Two team approach is possible for upper limb or head and neck surgeries

It can be used as:

- Muscle flap
- Neurotised muscle flap
- Musculocutaneous flap
- Chimera including perforator-based skin island, or adductor longus muscle (same neurovascular pedicle).

FLAP PLANNING

Surface Landmarks

The patient is placed in supine position with hip joint in flexion and external rotation and knee in flexion. An imaginary line joining the pubic tubercle and the medial knee joint line is drawn to identify the position of the Gracilis. On forced adduction the tight adductor longus is palpable and is marked. The gracilis muscle is about 2.5 cm posterior to adductor muscle (*see* **Fig. 2**).

The skin island in a vertical paddle is designed in upper thigh centered over the gracilis with skin pinch used as marker for primary closure.

Similarly, the transverse paddle is designed as an ellipse centered over the vascular pedicle with limits being the posterior midline to anterior midline (**Fig. 4**).

FLAP HARVEST

Muscle Flap

The skin incision is placed directly on the gracilis muscle outlined. The great saphenous vein is preserved. The deep fascia is incised to visualize the gracilis muscle.

The gracilis muscle can be confused with the sartorius muscle in the proximal part of the thigh hence the incision is placed in the distal part of the thigh and Gracilis tendon is visualized and traction applied to identify the tendon. The muscle fibers of the Sartorius are obliquely oriented and bulkier than the Gracilis fibers. Then proceed proximally to dissect the gracilis from surrounding muscles and fascia till the pedicle is visualized. The adductor muscle is retracted and branches to adductor are ligated. Dissection continues till the origin of the Medial circumflex vessels from the Femoral Vessels. If the nerve is required it is dissected till its origin.

Musculocutaneous Flap

Skin Paddle Designs

- Vertical paddle design includes skin over the proximal 2/3 muscle. The distal skin is not reliable (**Figs. 5A to D**).
- Transverse upper gracilis (TUG)
- Trifoliate design for larger breasts

The skin paddle is marked. The anterior incision is committed till deep fascia and the fascia of the adductor is exposed. The epimysium over the adductor longus is

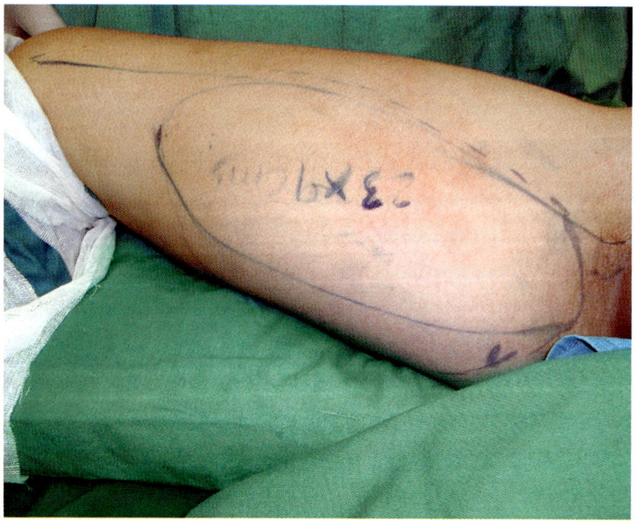

Fig. 3: Marking for vertical paddle upper gracilis

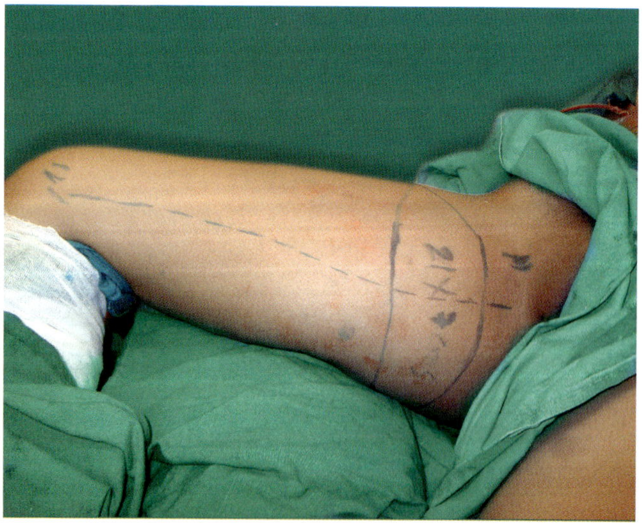

Fig. 4: Marking for a transverse paddle upper gracilis

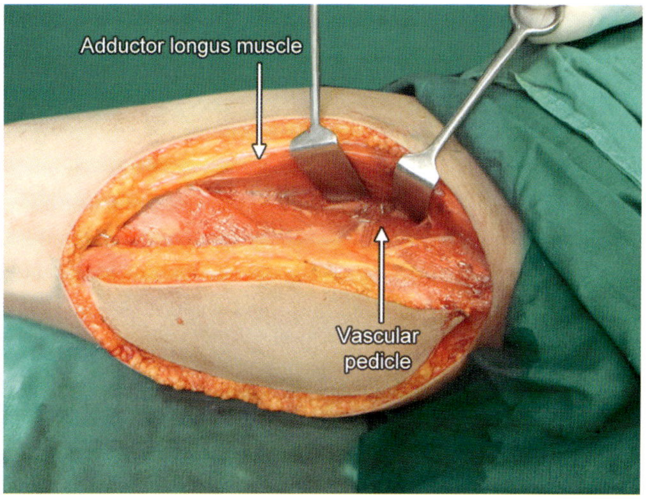

Fig. 5A: Adductor longus retracted to dissect pedicle

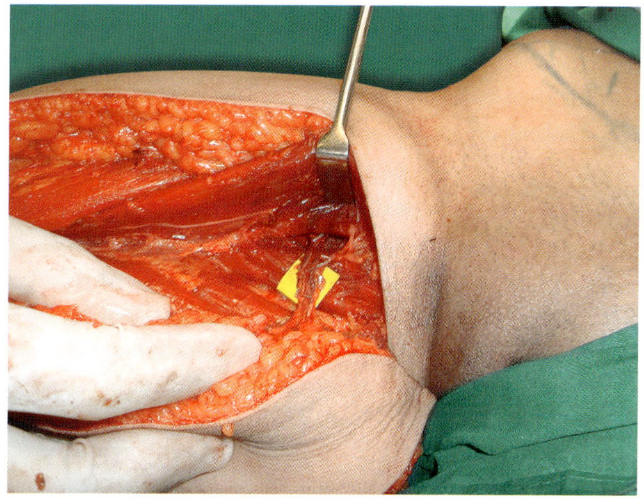

Fig. 5B: Pedicle dissection complete and ready for pedicle ligation

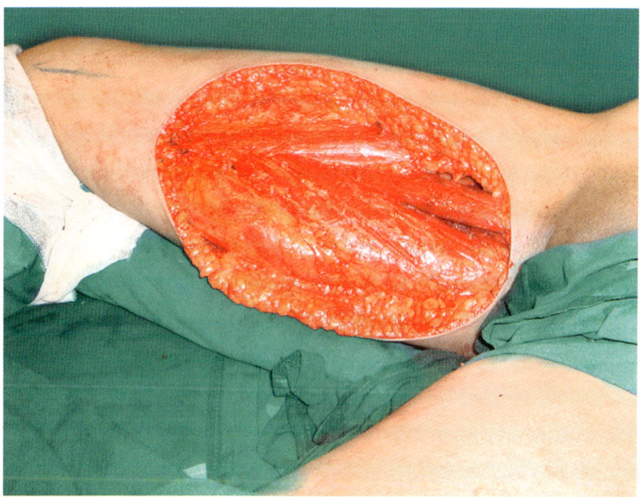

Fig. 5C: Donor site after flap harvest

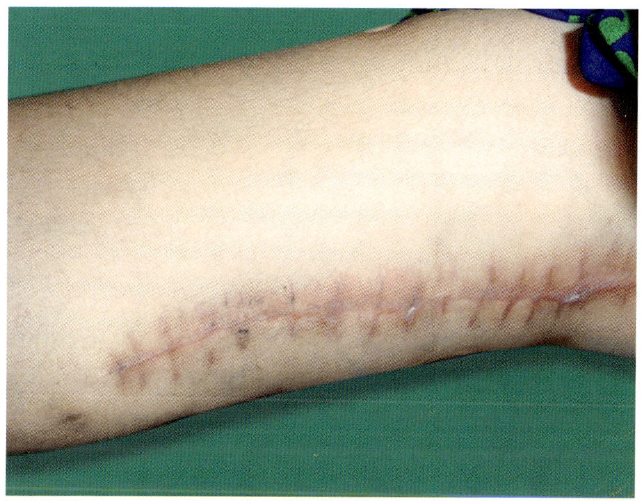

Fig. 5D: Donor site scar in patient of vertical paddle gracilis flap

incised vertically and muscle is retracted laterally. This ensures that the intermuscular septum and the septocutaneous perforators are included in the flap. Further pedicle dissection is same as that for the muscle flap.

Donor closure is done after achieving adequate hemostasis and placement of suction drains.

Donor Site Complications

- Stretched and hypertrophic scar
- Cosmetic contour deformity
- Lymphedema

Postoperative Course

- No restriction of movements required
- Physiotherapy and limb elevation at night
- TED stockings/pressure garments

Pointers to Reduce Lymphedema

- Safeguard the great saphenous vein
- Avoid over enthusiastic fat harvest
- Curtail skin paddle width according to exact requirements
- Judicious use of bilateral flaps when larger volume is required.

INDICATIONS FOR USE

Breast Reconstruction

In patients with a pear-shaped body habitus (Mesomorphic body type), there is inadequate fat in the abdomen (DIEP flap) but bulky lower body and thigh.

The texture is better in medial thigh than lateral.

We have used both the VUG and the TUG flap for breast reconstruction. The problems encountered include:

- Limited skin availability in short statured females
- Contour defect in thigh
- Lymphedema in patients with VUG flap with large skin paddles.
- Stretched sometimes hypertrophic scars

A result of vertical upper gracilis flap is shown in **Figures 6A to D**.

Clinical photos of transverse paddle upper gracilis flap is shown in **Figures 7A to D**.

A case of secondary reconstruction of the breast **(Figs. 8A to C)**.

Limb Reconstruction

We have used the gracilis flap for small to moderate size defects **(Figs. 9A to D)**.

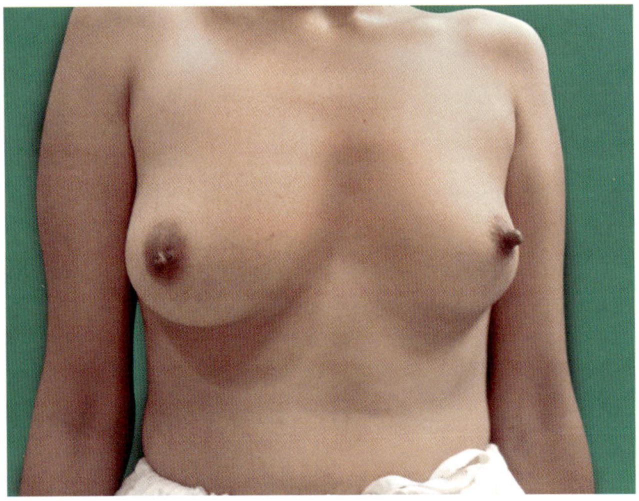

Fig. 6A: Preoperative photograph

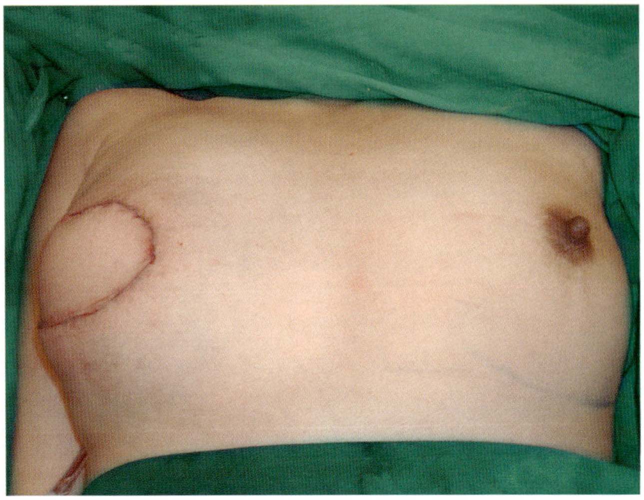

Fig. 6B: Intraoperative photo of right MRM reconstructed with VUG

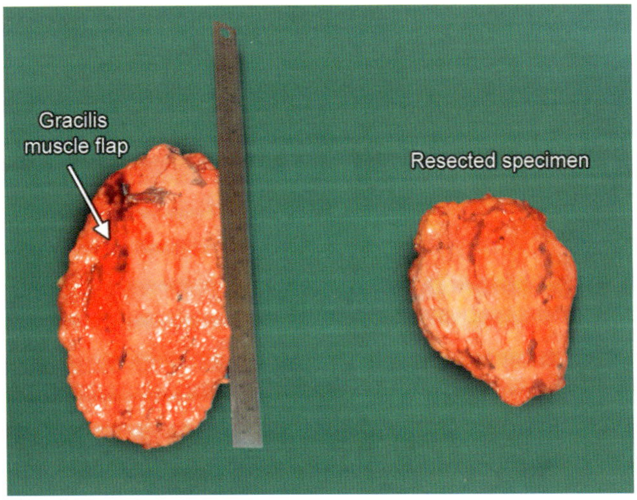

Fig. 6C: Harvested flap and specimen

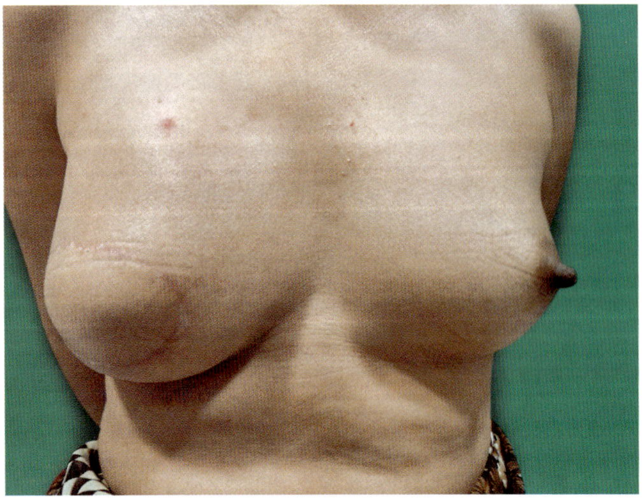

Fig. 6D: Late postoperative photo

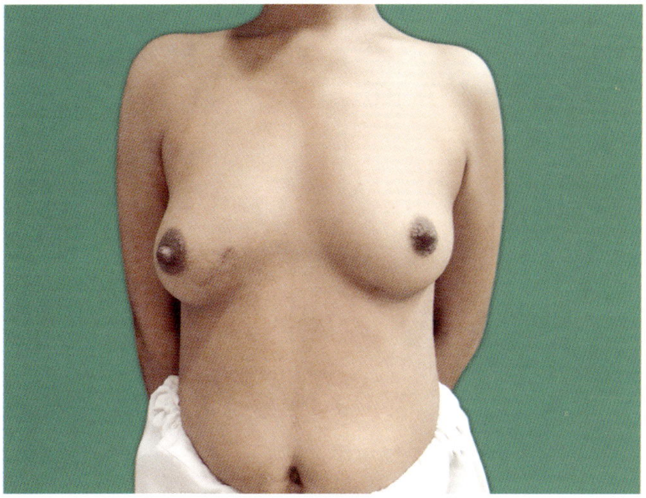

Fig. 7A: Preoperative photograph

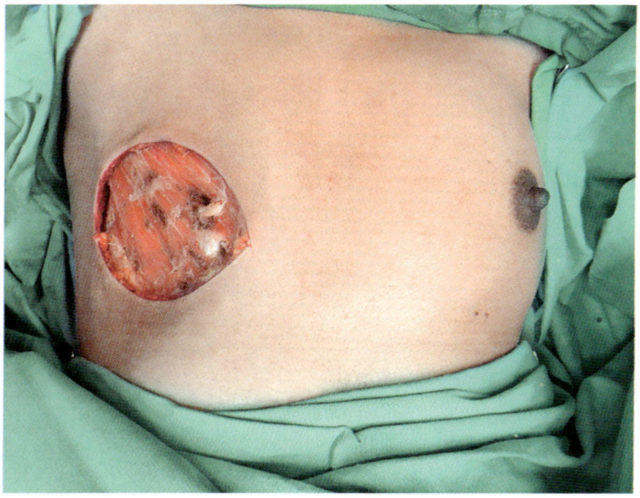

Fig. 7B: Right MRM defect

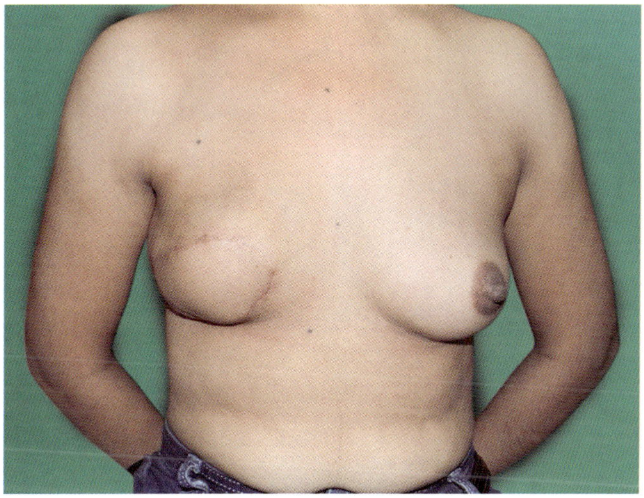

Fig. 7C: Late postoperative result of TUG flap

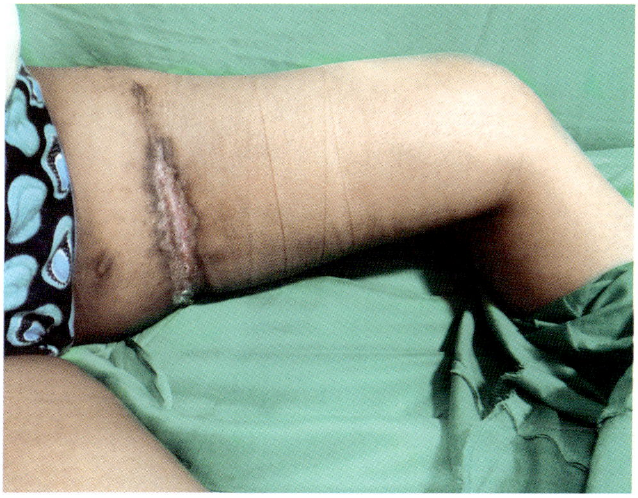

Fig. 7D: Old healed scar of TUG flap

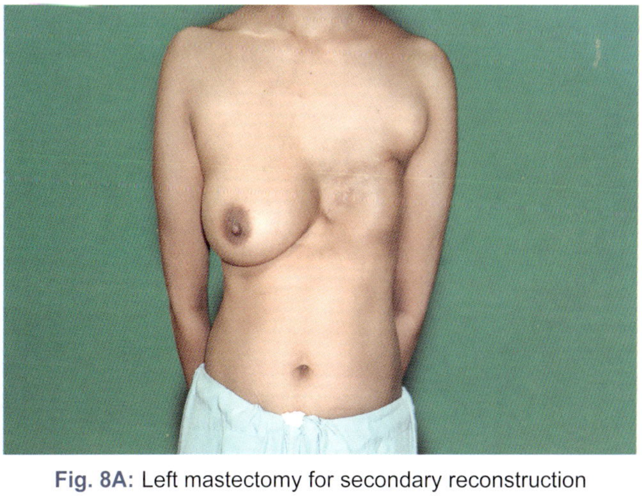

Fig. 8A: Left mastectomy for secondary reconstruction

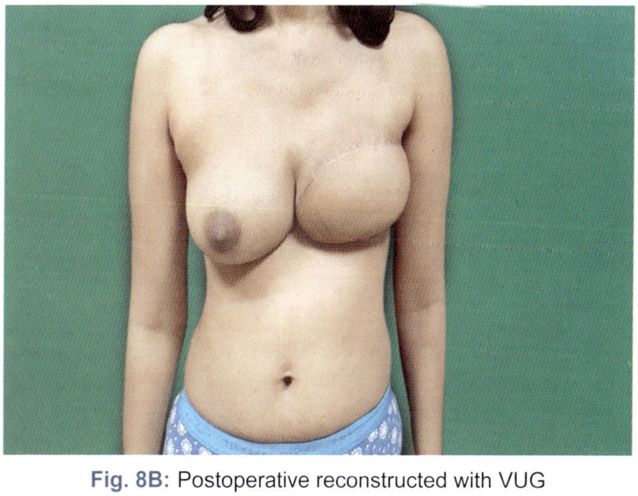

Fig. 8B: Postoperative reconstructed with VUG

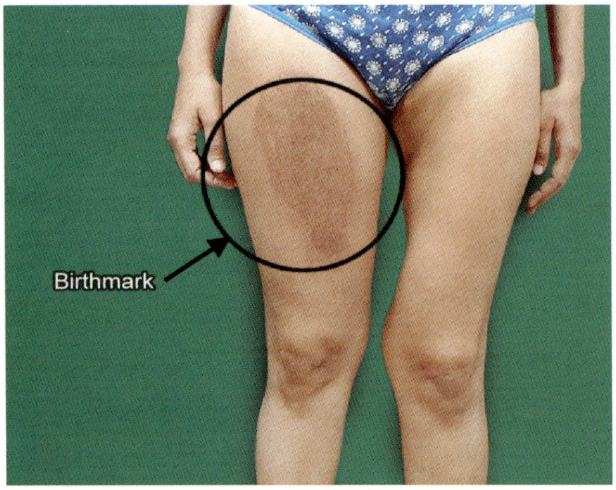

Fig. 8C: Shows the contour deformity of the left thigh

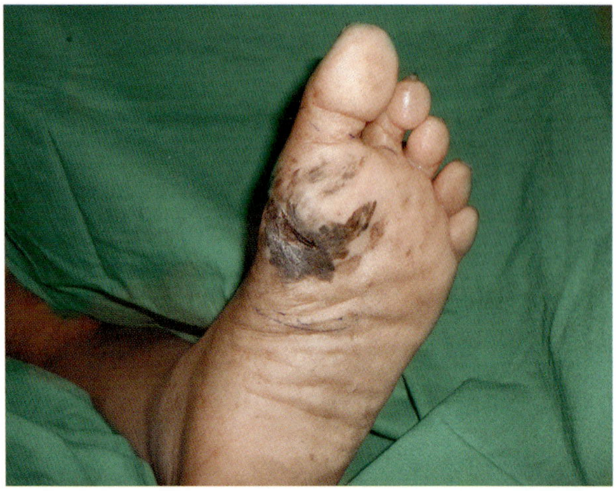

Fig. 9A: Melanoma of the left foot

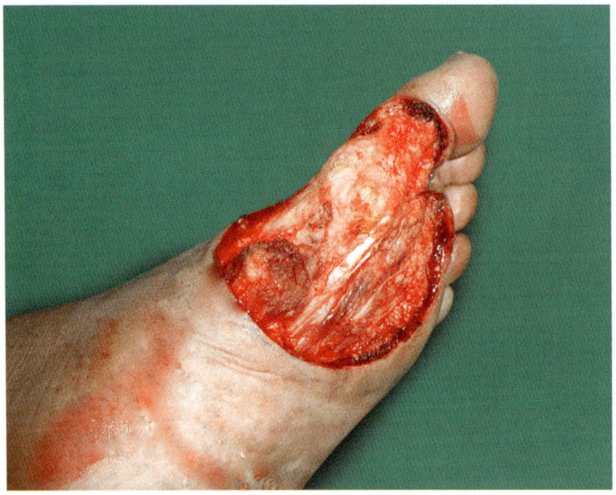

Fig. 9B: Defect over plantar aspect of foot

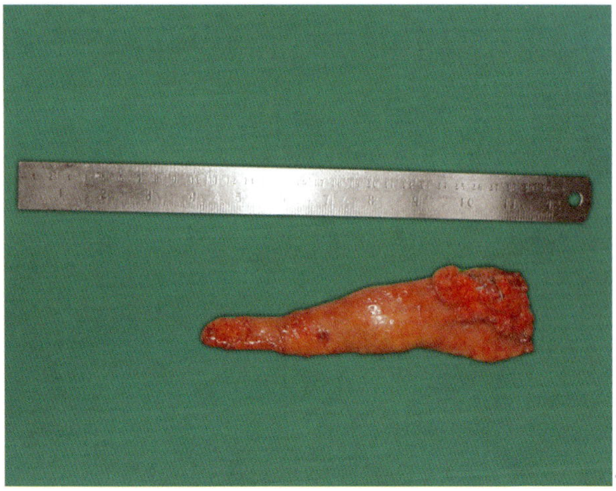

Fig. 9C: Harvested gracilis muscle flap

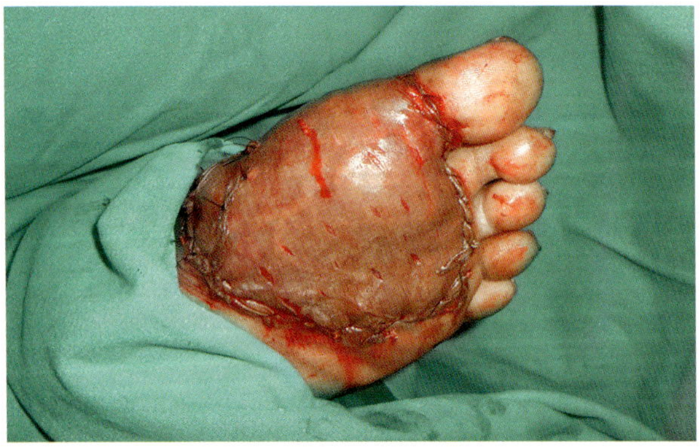

Fig. 9D: Reconstruction with gracilis muscle and STSG

Head and Neck

Tongue reconstruction with neurotised musculocutaneous flap.

Other Uses

- Facial reanimation
- Brachial plexus palsy, traumatic muscle loss (Forearm, Arm etc.)
- Anal sphincter reconstruction.

CHAPTER 15

Refinements in Free Flap Surgery

Dushyant Jaiswal, Chirag Bhansali

INTRODUCTION

We would talk about refinements in Microsurgery for Head Neck and Breast as they form the bulk of our workload and crux of most reconstruction solutions at Tata Memorial Centre.

The current state of microsurgery and free flaps for cancer reconstruction was not an overnight invention but a sequential evolution over last 4–5 decades. In terms of human medical history this could be called a very rapid revolution in a specialty, which existed only at a conceptual level till 1960's.

The Stage of Flap Survival

In the eighties flap survival was the prime aim of a free flap, generally refinements could wait for second stage.

The Stage of Standardization and Predictability

Nineties and early 21st century saw standardization in harvest methods and flap survivals improved consistently to above 95% at most centers. Simultaneously some new flap evolved. The ALT flap gained popularity as a panacea for all defects with some soft tissue element.

The Stage of Refinement and Surging Ahead

Current era presumes flap survival. Focus is on precise contouring ability for superior cosmetic outcomes, reducing donor morbidity, utilizing imaging for predictable outcomes, alternate donor sites, prefabrication, prelamination, perforators-based flaps and utilizing supercharging/turbocharging/multiplicity/chimerism of flaps for complex defects. Now a day has come where social media platforms and mobile mounted hand-held devices are also positively impacting decision-making and monitoring methods.

The below discussed concepts form the arsenal for 'Refinement'. It allows us to do more and better with the given flap.

THE PERFORATOR CONCEPT

It could be arguably said that the most significant and far reaching refinement in microsurgery in the last two decades is the establishment of the importance of the perforator concept **(Figs. 1A and B)**.

In the early days of microsurgery, latissimus dorsi muscle flap (LD) was the most commonly done flap. When skin was needed LD musculocutaneous was done. As the awareness dawned that underlying muscle is only incidental and the overlying skin is actually supplied by 'blood vessels traversing through muscle or in septum between muscles'—'The Perforator', had arrived. Musculocutaneous flap gave way to 'perforator flap of the source vessel', TRAM became DIEP, LDMC became TDAP **(Figs. 2 and 3)**.

Known axial pattern flaps became perforator based, groin flap became superficial circumflex iliac perforator flap (SCIP). The ALT perforator flap was a straight perforator flap entrant, it becoming a work horse really made the perforator concept popular.

So in summary, a skin element of a flap needs a perforator in it, not muscle below it. The skin flap is only as good as the perforator/s it has.

The fact that, the vascular source of the flap is visible so deep into the flap, is so small in proportion to the flap and could be multiple, opens up a whole new world of tricks for refinement in free flap surgery.

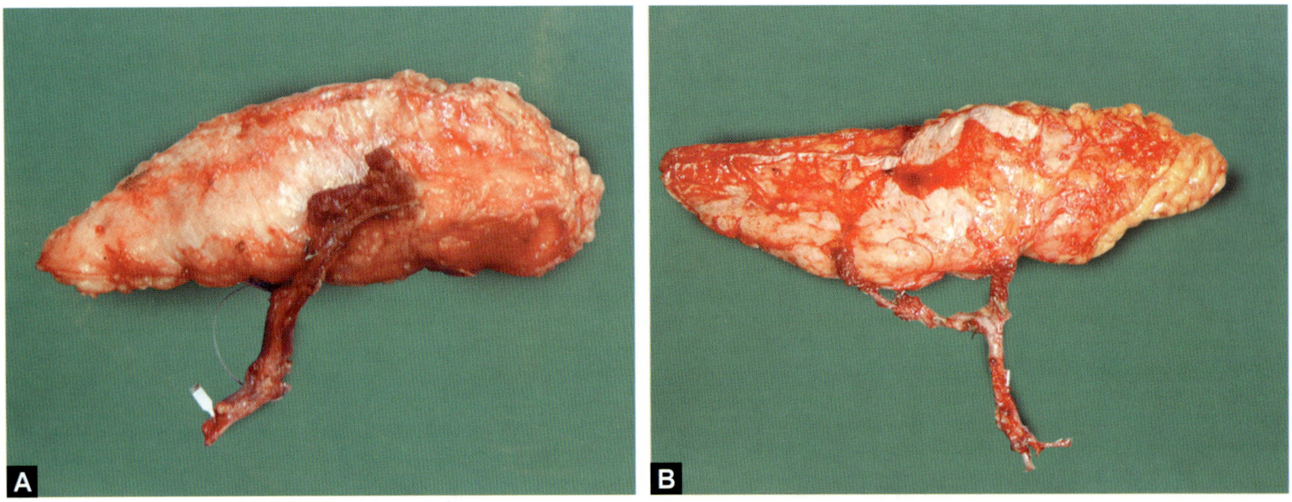

Figs. 1A and B: (A) Single perforator; (B) multiple perforators from same pedicle

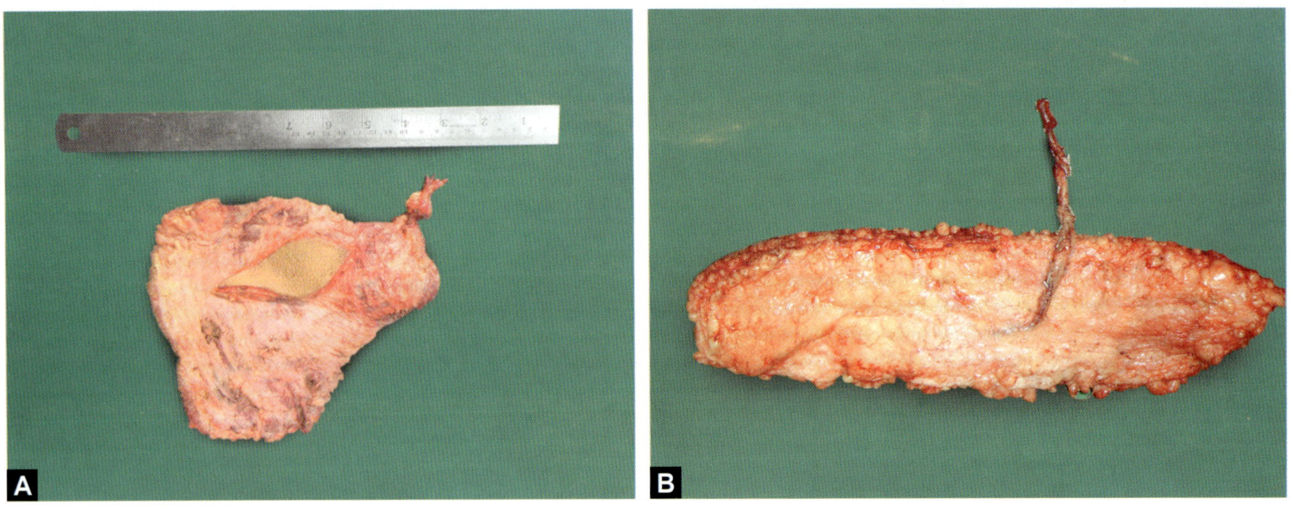

Figs. 2A and B: (A) Latissimus dorsi myocutaneous flap; (B) TDAP flap

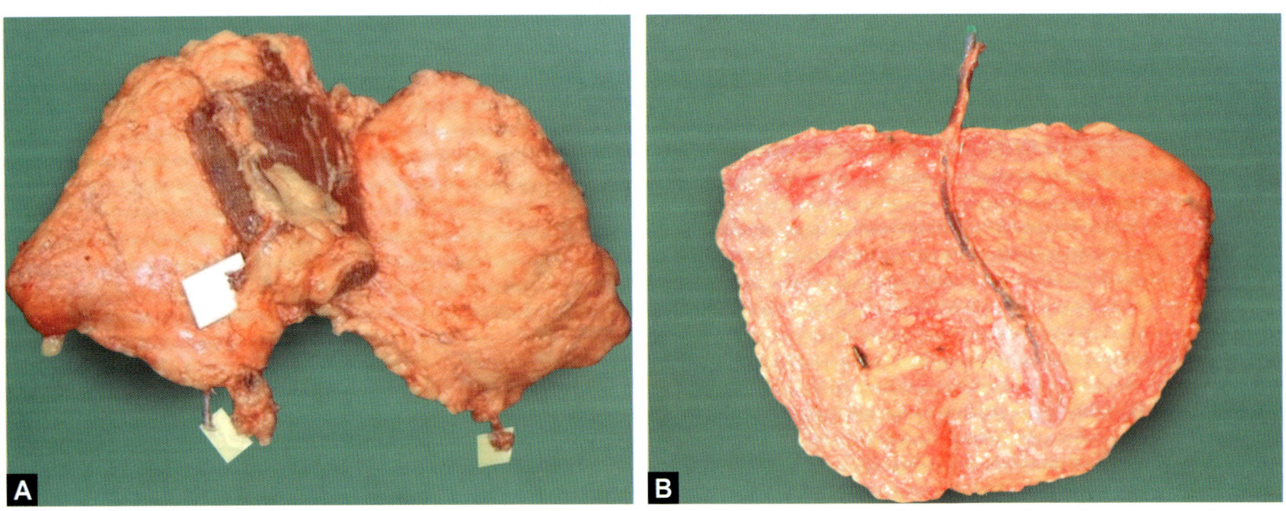

Figs. 3A and B: (A) Free TRAM flap; (B) DIEP flap

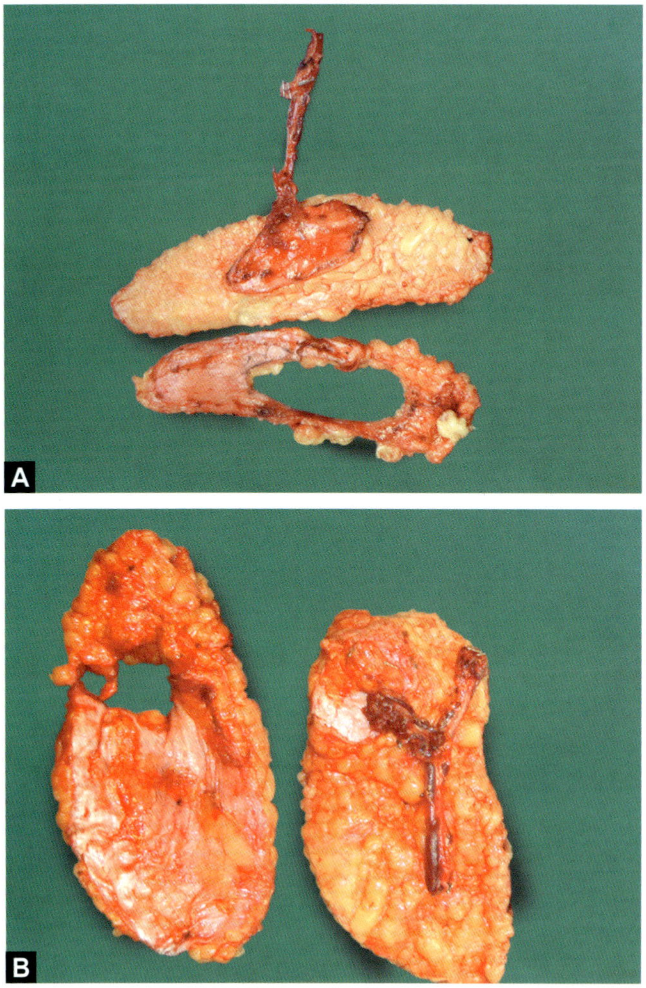

Figs. 4A and B: Thinned ALT flap

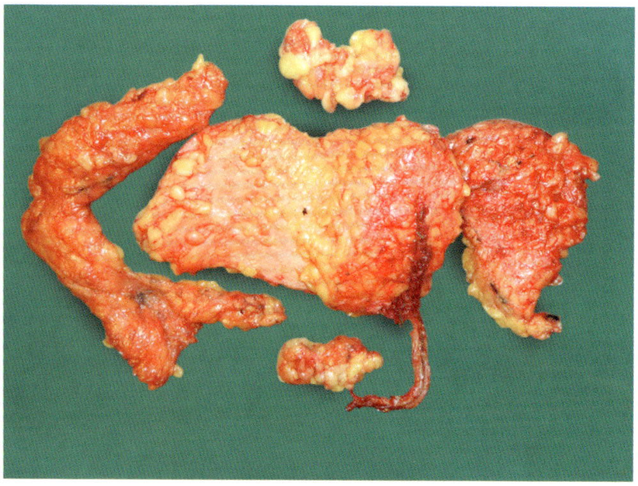

Fig. 5: Thinned DIEP flap

CONTROL ON THE THIRD DIMENSION/ VOLUME OF THE FLAP

Until the importance of perforators was realized the base or undersurface of the flap was sacrosanct. It was not to be touched or even better, protected by beveling to gather more subcutaneous tissue beyond its margins.

Often there is moderate to mild/subtle mismatch between the thickness of the flap to the thickness of the defect or the flap needed. Sometimes the thickness of the donor site can preclude its use at first glance.

Sometimes this discrepancy, in thickness of flap to the defect, is realized only while or after completion of the flap harvest. This situation may occur with simultaneous harvest of the flap as commonly with Head and Neck oncological resections. Sometimes the discrepancy is severe enough to cause problems with just putting the flap in place or good in setting of the flap, this might manifest as poor cosmetic outcomes or orocutaneous fistula related problems.

The ability to surgically reduce the volume of the flap, i.e. thin the flap, gives the surgeon ability to control the third dimension of the flap **(Figs. 4 and 5)**.

This in turn translates into the following:

Extended Indications for the Flap

The thinning changes the physical character of the flap. From a thick flap competing for indications with other thick flap, it can be converted to a thin flap competing for indications with thinner flaps, e.g. ALT remaining FRAFF, MSAP or Lateral arm.

Greater Contouring Potential

Control over the third dimension give the surgeon tremendous liberty to 'sculpt' the flap. This can translate into superior aesthetic results.

Better Pliability

The thinned flap has far superior pliability than the original flap. This makes it easier to turn the flap over itself, as in for a buccal mucosa and skin defect. It also makes 'twisting' the flap along its long axis too easier. This too gives better contouring potential in head and neck cases with complex defects.

Thinning can be safely done in the plane below superficial fascia, i.e. the deep fascia and the fat, between deep and superficial fascia, can be safely removed. A 1–2 cm radius, cuff of deep fascia and deep fat can be left around the perforator, this protects the perforator branches going to the dermis. It also captures the perforator arborization, if present, after piercing the deep fascia. If thinning is needed in this cuff too, it can be done under microscope, tracing the perforator to the dermis. Thinning to make the flap like a full thickness skin graft is rarely clinically needed. Monopolar and bipolar diathermy are used to do routine thinning.

CHIMERISM

Need for Chimeric Flaps

Head-neck cancer patients, in India, often present at an advanced local stage. Post-surgical resection this translates into defects which are:

1. Large (sometimes Extra-large, rarely OMG what is this!)
2. Multicomponent (buccal mucosa, skin, bone, soft tissue, tongue, palate etc.)
3. Multidimensional (length × breadth × variable thickness)
4. Irregularly shaped (odd shaped defects, due to lesions in continuity).

A single paddle of skin, has its limitations, when you need to move it in different directions. The thickness of flap, pliability of skin and singularity of the perforators might result in very restricted maneuvering liberty of the flap.

Chimeric flaps give you that liberty.

Chimera is a Greek mythological creature. It has the head of a lion, body of a goat and tail of a serpent. Though some lot other animals and their parts are described, this is the most common description. The basic idea is a common soul (vascular basis) with different attached bodies (similar or disparate tissue components with no morphological continuity, except for the vascular axes) **(Figs. 6 to 11)**.

Chimeric flaps find utility in HN reconstruction due to the nature of complex, multidimensional defects.

With a chimera, complex defects can be managed satisfactorily with a single set of microvascular anastomoses (MVA), a lot of times. In cases where the different vascular axes don not meet, 2 separate set of MVA can be done. This would take some more time, but there would be no compromise in the result as all 'morphological needs' of the defect would be met.

So, an attempt at chimerism almost always works!

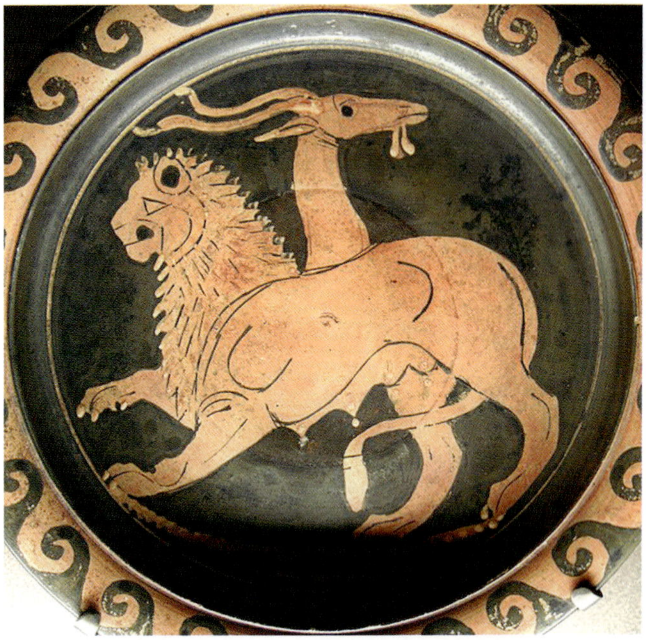

Fig. 6: Chimera—Greeek mythological creature

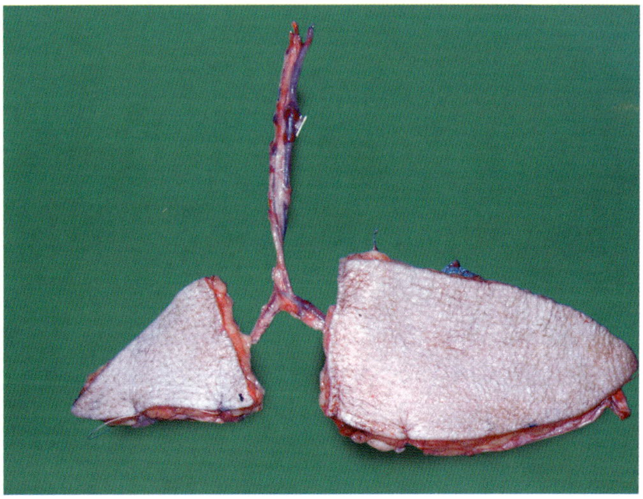

Fig. 7: Chimeric ALT flap based on 2 perforators of a single source pedicle

TURBOCHARGING AND SUPERCHARGING

When large size flaps are harvested or an attempt at chimerism is made, following possibilities exist:

1. Single large perforator perfusing the entire flap
2. Two or three perforators, having the same source of pedicle origin.

In both these situations the question of supercharging or harvesting muscle for vascularity sake does not arise.

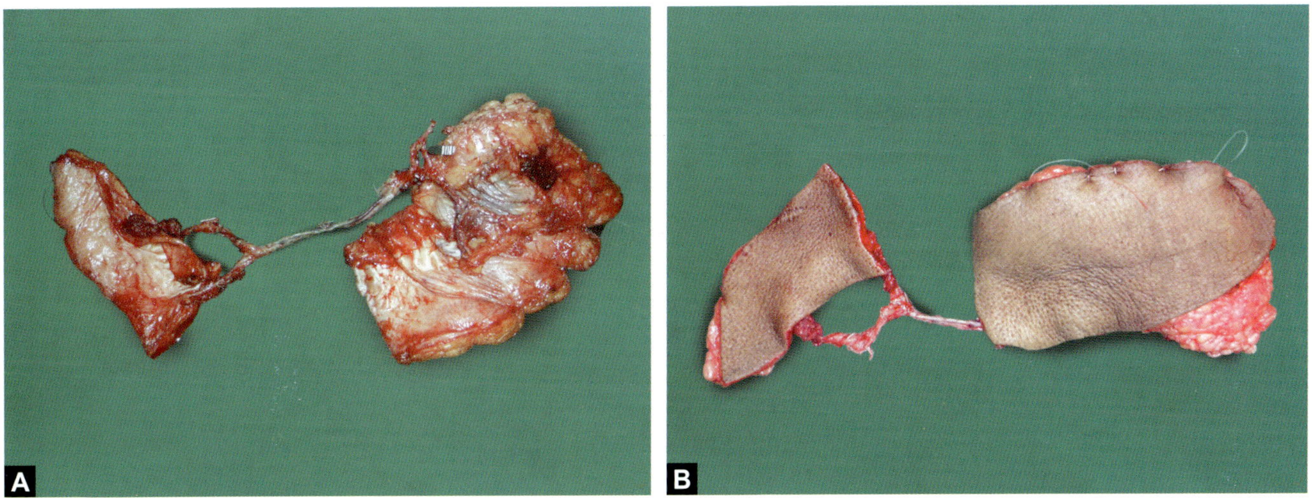

Figs. 8A and B: (A) Chimeric ALT on descending and oblique branch; (B) chimeric ALT on descending and oblique branch

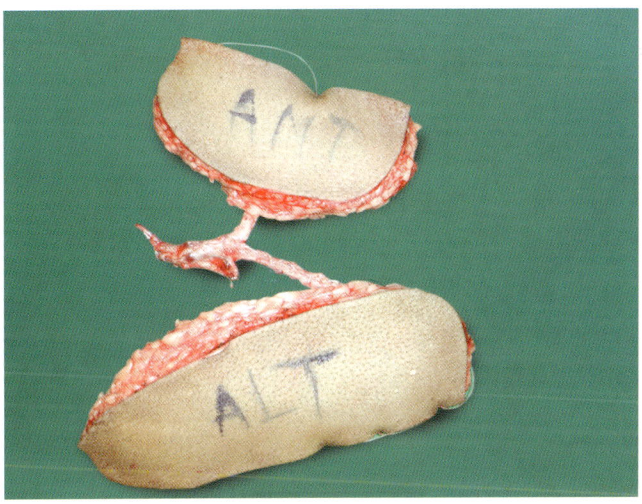

Fig. 9: Chimeric ALT plus AMT

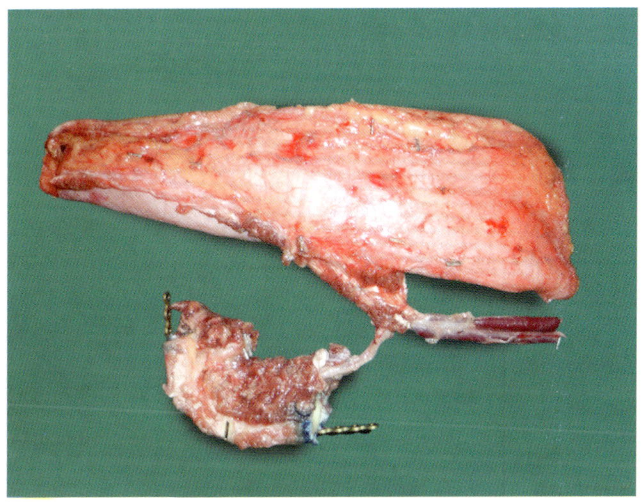

Fig. 10: Chimeric fibula flap

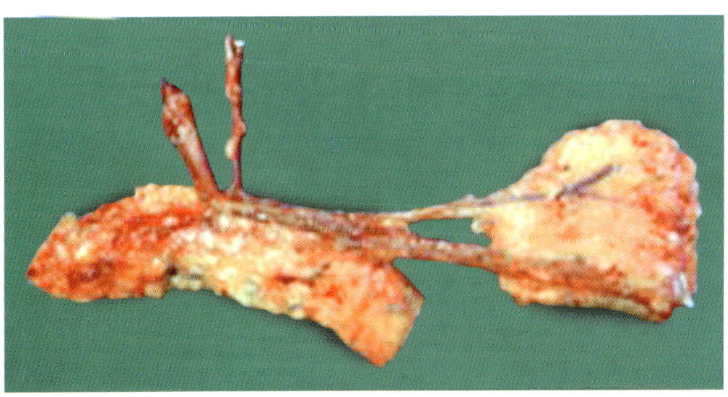

Fig. 11: Chimeric radial artery forearm flap

3. Two or more perforators arising from 2 different pedicles
4. Two or more perforators arising from 2 different pedicles, joining each other close to source vessel and with a lot of intermingled nerves, such that harvest of the pedicle after joining would entail severe nerve damage.

In the latter 2 scenarios, common sense would dictate restoring blood supply to both the sources. It would be the safer option to pursue and be respecting the native anatomy of the flap.

In these situation, it is preferable to augment the vascularity especially if:

1. Clearly inadequate or any doubt of perfusion on one pedicle
2. Flap needs to be surgically thinned
3. Lots of maneuvers (deepithelization, turning or folding on itself etc.) to contour the flap is needed, as these would cause some ischemic insult to the flap.

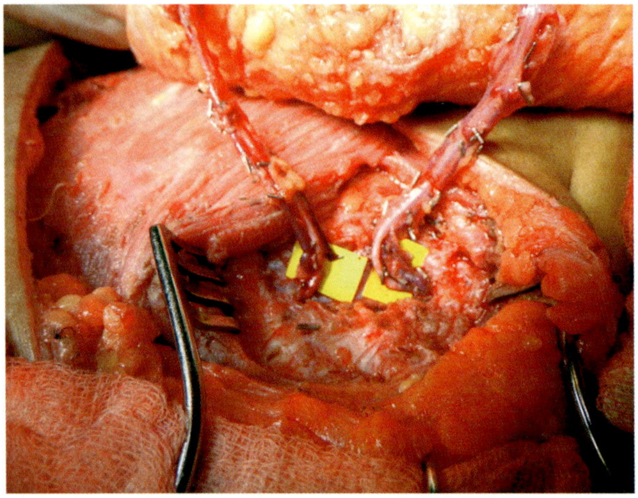

Fig. 12: Supercharging, use of both ends of IMA

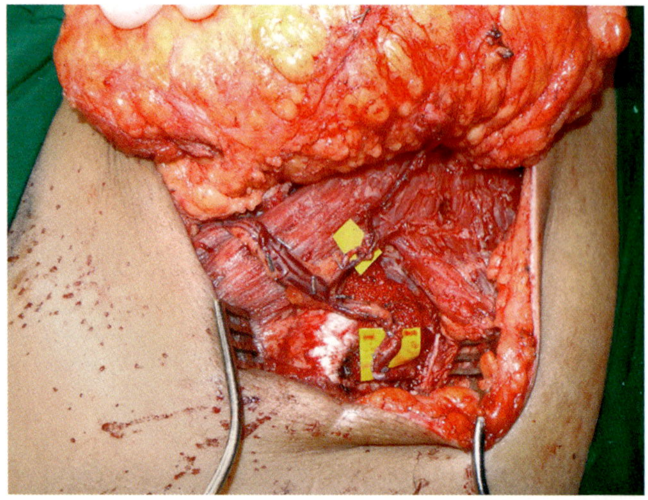

Fig. 13: Turbocharging to side branch of DIEA/V

4. Chimerism is needed for a complex multicomponent, multidimensional defect, this could convert a single free flap into two free flaps.

Supercharging: Adding an additional vascular source by anastomosing the second pedicle to a different artery and vein **(Fig. 12)**.

Turbocharging **(Fig. 13)**: The second pedicle is anastomosed to the distal runoff or a side branch of the first pedicle. The first pedicle artery and vein are anastomosed to donor vessels.

We prefer supercharging, when technically feasible without vein grafts. The two sets of microvascular anastomoses are independent of each other, thrombosis of one does not affect the other.

Turbocharging can be resorted to when supercharging not feasible (vessel depleted neck) or would necessitate vein grafts.

MULTIPLE FREE FLAPS

Now that the survival rates of free flaps are 95% upwards, using two of them in one go, is logical when needed.

Multiplicity is often the easiest way to counter skin/soft tissue deficiency and defect complexity. This situation often arises in Head-neck cancer patients presenting late with advanced local disease, combined with deficient donor sites due to a frail body habitus.

Multiple free flaps are needed mostly for severe mismatch of skin surface area and soft tissue volume between the defect and donor site. Sometimes it could be employed in a complex defect to modulate an attempt at chimerism or to enable better contouring ability. Rarely it could be forced due to the available perforator and pedicle anatomy of the donor site or be electively used to reduce the potential donor site morbidity.

Most common use of multiple free flaps in our center is for segmental mandible defects with large skin excision, when the skin paddle with fibula is insufficient. Free fibula with ALT is the most common **(Figs. 14 to 16)**.

Fibula with FRAFF, ALT with TFL and 2 ALT on separate perforator and pedicles from the same thigh, are the other combinations we have used.

When judiciously employed an extra set of microvascular anastomosis can make a relatively complex and tricky defect easy to manage, at the cost or rather investment of some extra time.

THE IMPORTANCE OF DONOR SITE

The decision of reconstruction cannot be done seeing the defect alone. The donor site parameters are equally important; thickness, pliability, color, amenability to primary closure, perforator characteristics, pedicle size and length. A match of defect and donor on all these points is the easiest path to a good outcome. Any reconstructive decision should be done with assessment and matching of the defect and donor areas.

In the current era of reconstructive microsurgery, the outcome of donor site is as vital as the defect reconstruction. Primary closure of the flap donor site is desirable as a skin graft creates another wound which heals with secondary intention. In Indians skin graft donor sites often heal

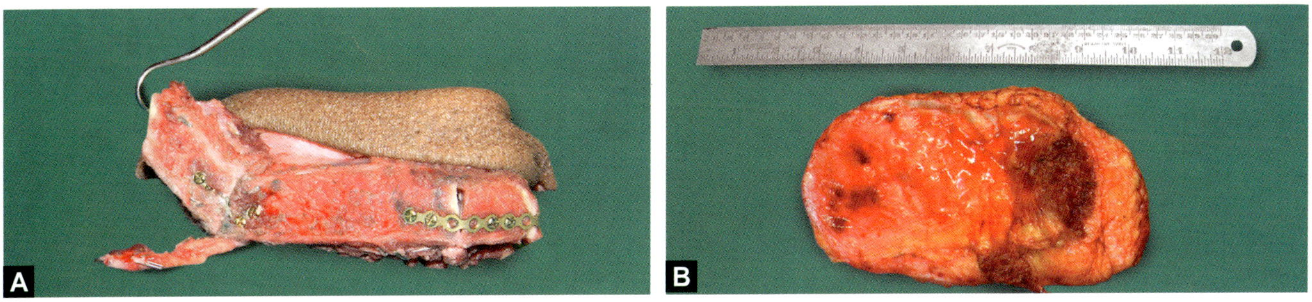

Figs. 14A and B: Double free flap, fibual osteocutaneous + ALT

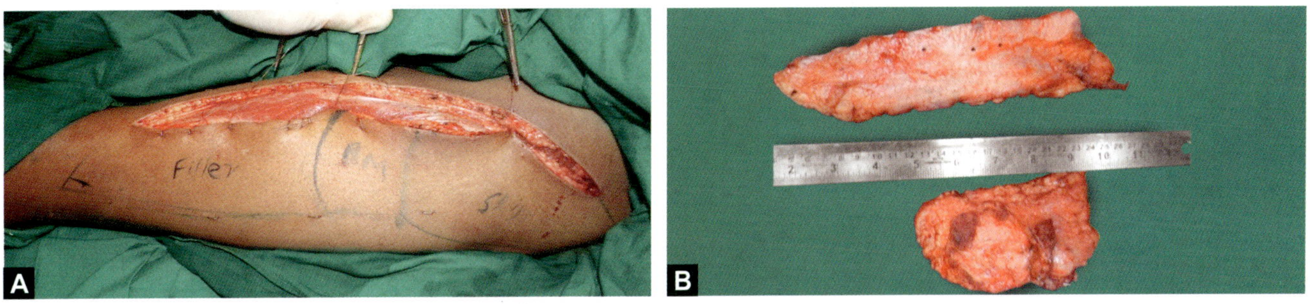

Figs. 15A and B: ALT and TFL from same thigh

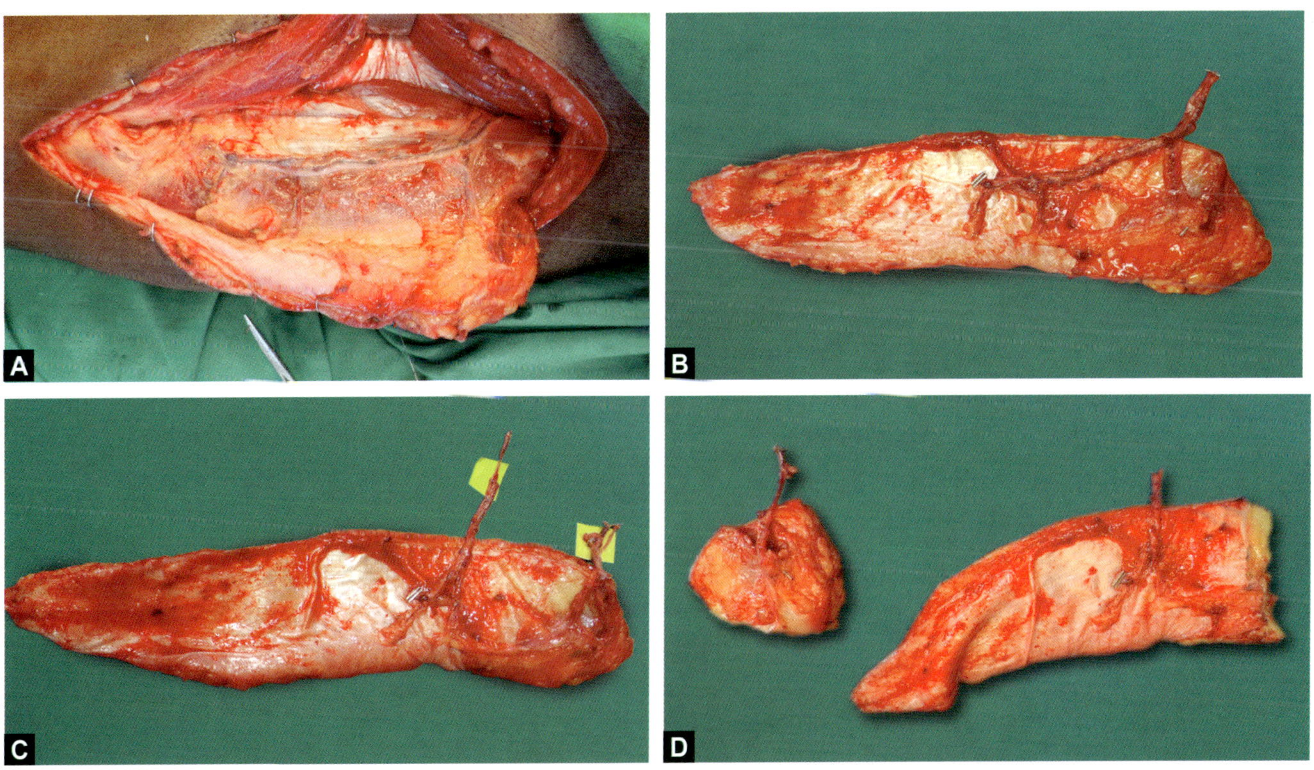

Figs. 16A to D: (A) ALT pedicle with 3 septocutaneous perforators; (B) harvested ALT flap with 3 perforators from same pedicle; (C) 2 pedicles carved, 1 perforator on proximal, 2 perforators on distal; (D) one ALT flap split into two

with a lot of hypertrophy, hyperpigmentation and itching, this often being the only complaint in late follow-up patients at TMH.

ALTERNATE FREE FLAPS FOR A LARGER ARMAMENTARIUM

Most Head and Neck defects can be managed with the safe and standard 3 free flaps. Radial for thin, ALT for thick and Fibula for bone.

Alternatives to fibula are scapula and the iliac crest (DCIA), at TMH we have literally never used them in all these years, fibula has been our default choice whenever bone is needed. World over Scapula bone flap, based on the subscapular system is used when an associated large skin and soft tissue defect is also present. DCIA is used for small bone defects where a superior bone quality is desired for osteointegration.

Alternative soft tissue flaps find indications more often. When the defect and flap thickness are too disparate either for RAFF or ALT alternatives can be used. Sometimes they can be employed for a better outcome of the donor site or in presence of an unfavorable donor site like, morbid obese thighs, forearms with chemotherapy to veins and previously exhausted sites donor sites. At TMH we sparingly use TDAP, MSAP, DIEP and scapular/parascapular flaps. Ultimately a surgeon should be comfortable with using any possible flap in the body **(Figs. 17 to 20)**.

Sometimes a given defect can be reconstructed equally well, harvesting tissues from one of many donor sites. With a larger armamentarium the patient can be given a choice of the donor site! This might sound superfluous for HN cancer reconstruction but is a routine practice in breast reconstruction in the best centers.

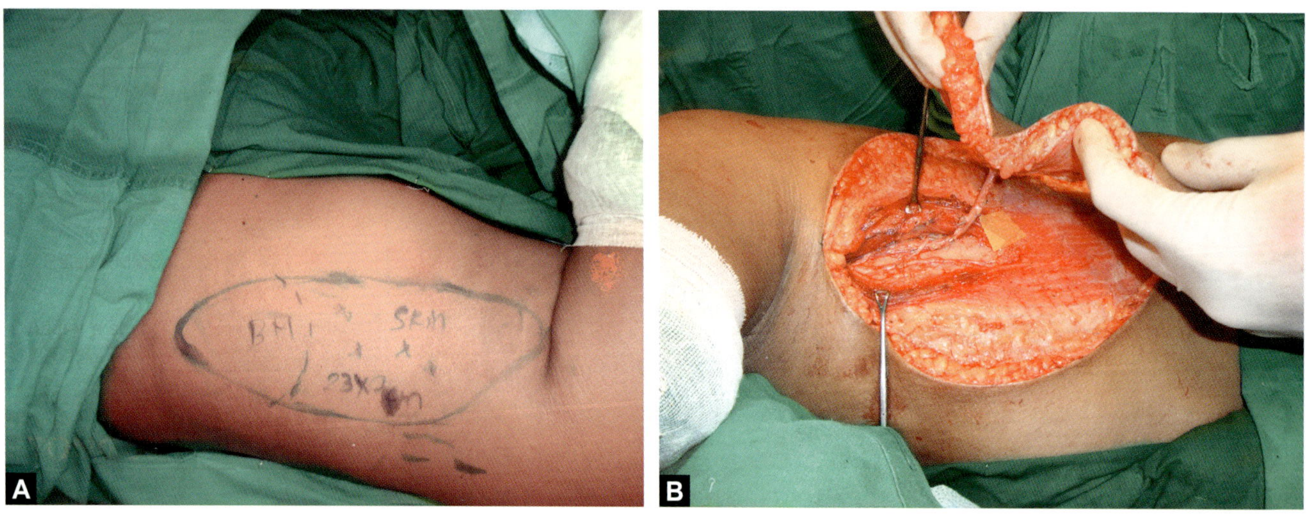

Figs. 17A and B: (A) TDAP flap-marking; (b) TDAP, perforator dissected and nerve preserved

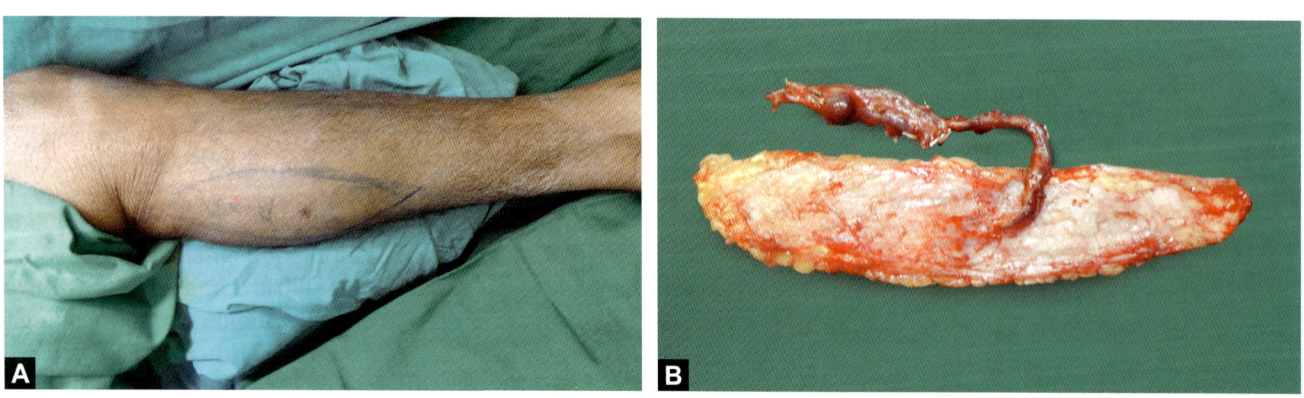

Figs. 18A and B: (A) MSAP flap planning and marking; (B) MSAP flap harvested on perforator with pedicle

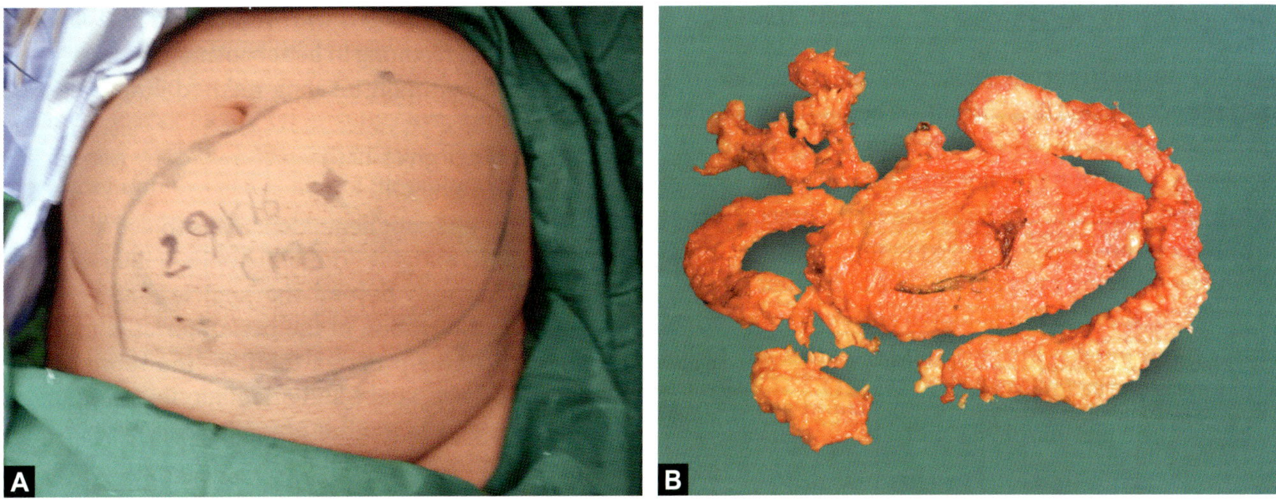

Figs. 19A and B: (A) DIEP flap for thigh defect 29 × 16 cm; (B) DIEP flap harvested and thinned for contouring

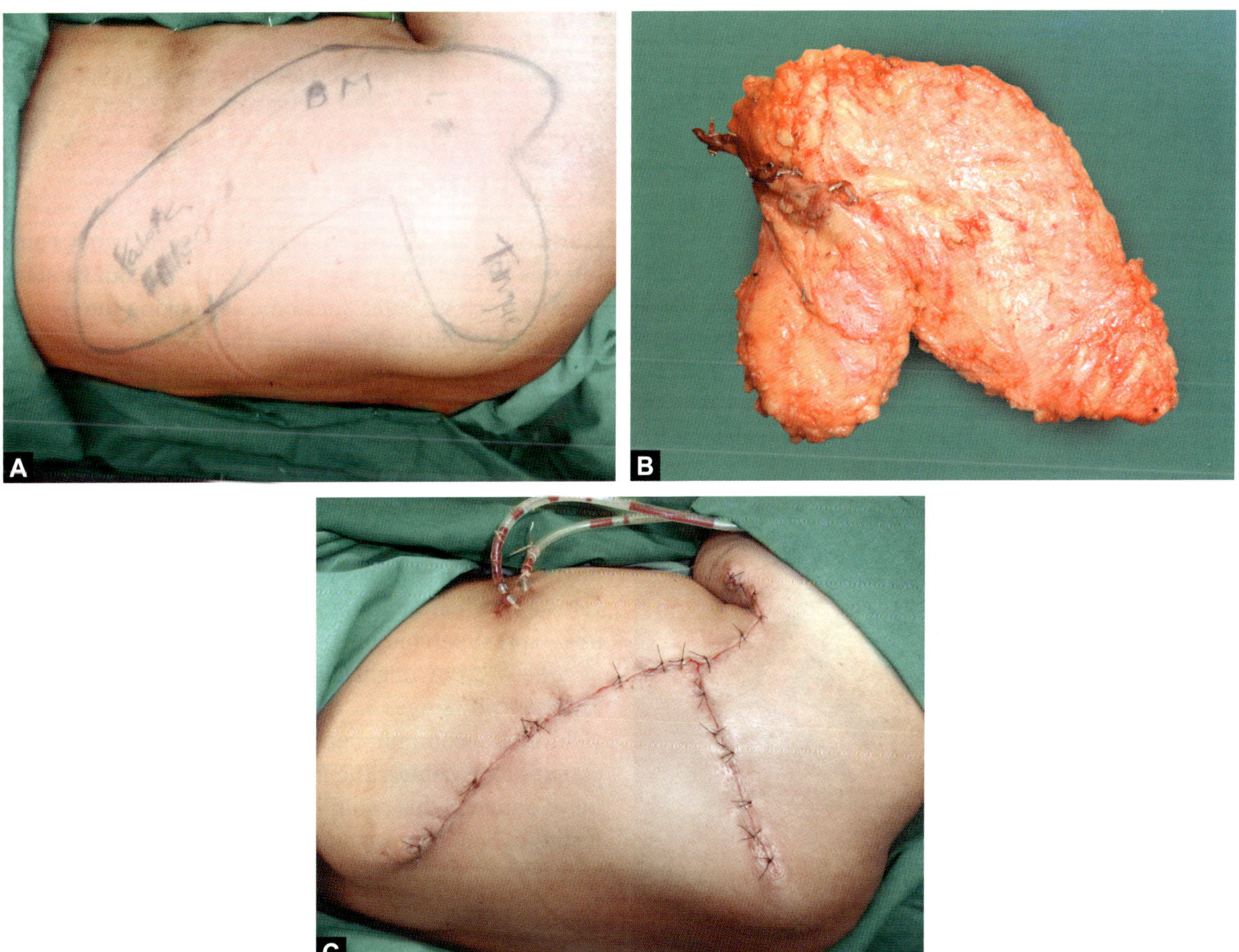

Figs. 20A to C: (A) Scapular-parascapular conjoint flap, marking; (B) Harvested flap; (C) Primary closure of the donor site

CHAPTER 16

Prosthetic Rehabilitation and Reconstruction

Kanchan Dholam, Sandeep Vivek Gurav

INTRODUCTION

The Dental Services at TMH work in close coordination with the Head Neck DMG and Plastic & Reconstructive Services. Their services significantly contribute to improving QoL (Quality of Life) issues in patients. They provide whole range of dental rehabilitation from dentures to permanent osseointegrated implants and varied external prosthesis as needed. They are an important complimentary and completing element in our 'Adding life to years' philosophy of reconstruction.

INTRAORAL PROSTHETIC REHABILITATION

Intraoral prosthetic rehabilitation following reconstruction can be done either by:

1. Tissue supported prosthesis
2. Osseointegrated implant supported prosthesis.

Tissue Supported Prosthesis

These type of prostheses are fabricated by conventional method of denture fabrication. The prosthesis is always removable and takes support from contralateral (nonreconstructed) side alveolus and teeth. These prostheses are not possible in cases where complete arch reconstruction is done. However in segmental reconstruction, these prosthesis are boon to the patients.

Advantages

- Less time consuming
- No additional surgeries required
- Less post prosthetic complications and are economical
- These prostheses are also favored in pediatric patients whose jaw growth is not completed, and diameter of free fibular graft does not allow placement of implants. **(Figs. 1A to C)**.

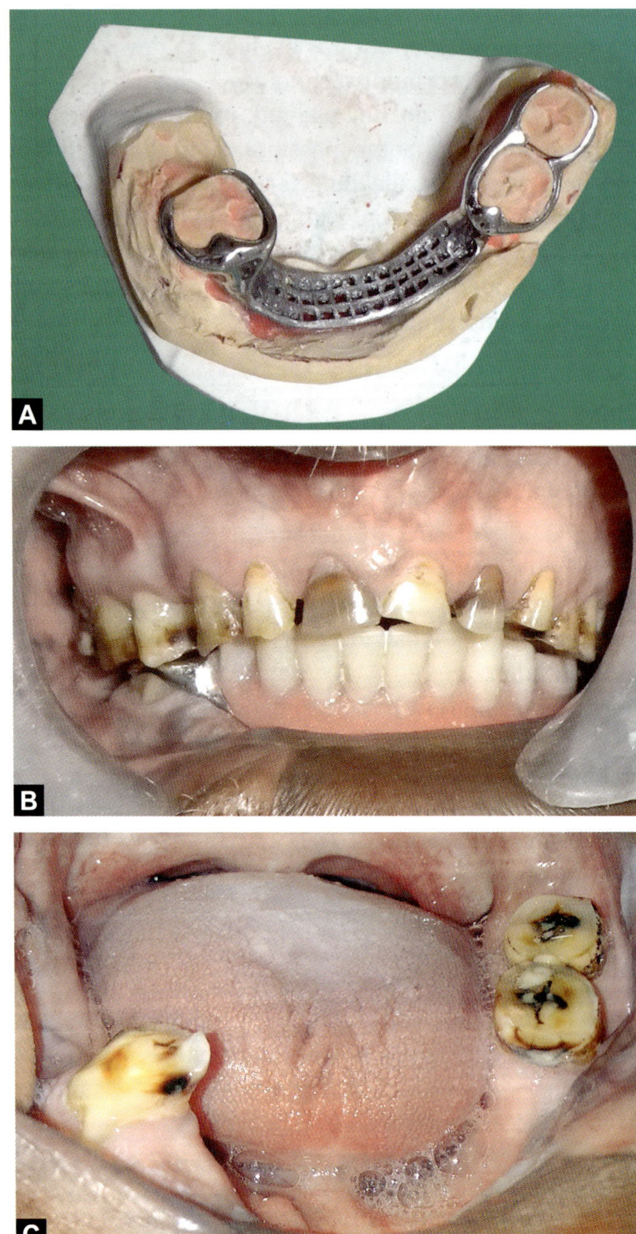

Figs. 1A to C: Tissue supported prosthesis on fibula

Disadvantages

- They are always removable so patients acceptance rate is low
- Sometimes prosthesis may not be stable and retentive, due to lack of firm base and teeth support causing problems in mastication.

Osseointegrated Implants Supported Prosthesis

Osseointegrated implants, can play a pivotal role in the rehabilitation process by augmenting the available retentive base or replacing critical missing teeth. Osseointegrated implants rehabilitation has huge potential for rehabilitation of reconstructed jaws. Free fibular flaps are more favored for implant supported prosthesis because of availability of sufficient bone and flexibility of its use in reconstruction.

Factors to be Considered before the Osseointegrated Implants

Number of Implants

Number of implant per arch is dependent on various factors. Minimum of two, optimum of four and maximum of one implant per tooth is required for rehabilitation. However, taking into consideration effects of radiation, low integration rate, increased complication rate in reconstructed jaws, over treatment by placing more number of implants per arch is recommended.[1] Though there is no significant difference in QoL outcomes in patients with two- or four-implant supported removable prostheses,[2] there is increased marginal bone loss when over denture is retained on two implants as compare to four implant supported over denture.[3]

Choice of Prosthesis

Two types of prosthesis are possible on reconstructed jaws.
1. Fixed prosthesis
2. Removable prosthesis.

Fixed prosthesis generally requires more number of implants (ideally one per tooth) as compare to removable prosthesis where even two implants can retain prosthesis. Overall removable prosthesis has lesser soft tissue complication rate as compared to fixed prosthesis and effectively manageable **(Figs. 2 to 4)**.

Unilateral fibular reconstruction where continuity of the mandible is missing, the jaw deviates to resected side. Guidance prosthesis are utilized on an interim basis until acceptable occlusal relationships and proper proprioception are reestablished.

Single barrel and double barrel fibular reconstruction and dental implant placement: In most of the cases, jaw reconstruction can be satisfactorily done with single barrel technique. However in indicated case, double barrel is advantageous as it decreases vertical discrepancy between alveolar bone and free flap thus giving better esthetic results with acceptable occlusal plane **(Figs. 5A to H)**.

Timing of Implant Placement

Implant rehabilitation can be done either

a. At the time of reconstruction (Primary implant placement) or
b. After completion of sufficient time of successful reconstruction (Secondary implant placement) (6 months in non-irradiated and 1 year in radiated patients).[1]

Primary implant placement: It is favored in non-malignant cases or early malignant stages as chances of radiation are less. Radiation might affect the osseointegration of titanium implants if given during integration phase. However, after integration phase there is no influence of

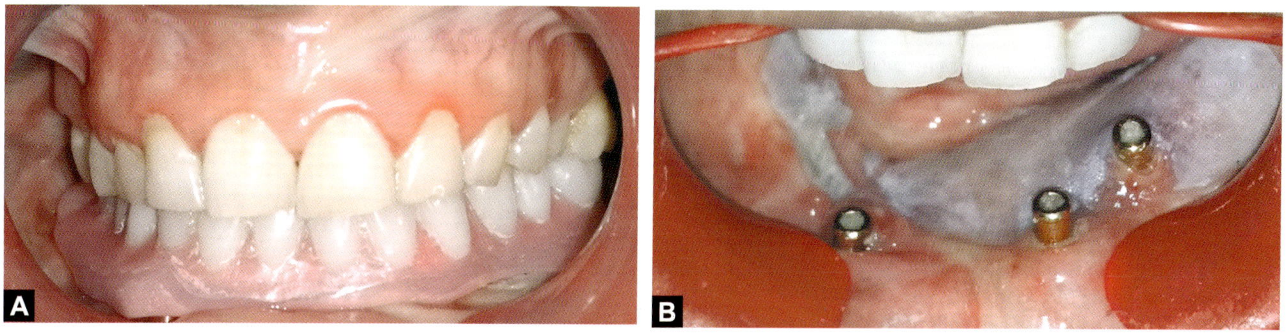

Figs. 2A and B: Implant retained removable over denture

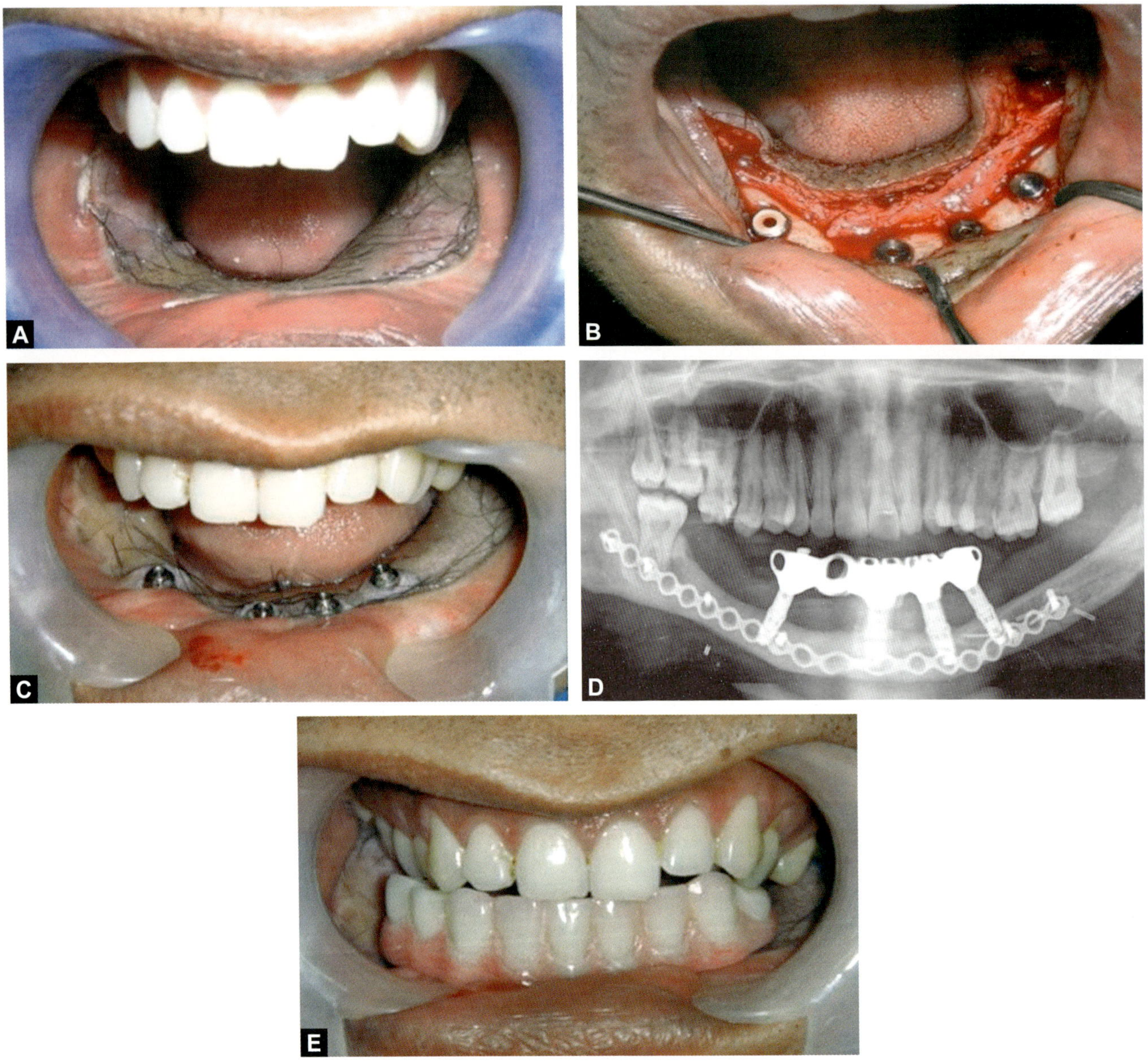

Figs. 3A to E: Implant retained fixed prosthesis

radiotherapy of implants. Advantages include early rehabilitation even in cases requiring radiotherapy where integration gets completed before deleterious effects of radiotherapy. However, it requires meticulous planning of reconstruction as well as implant positioning. Osseointegration rate of primary implants is similar to native bone implants, however, prosthetic success rate is much lower (75%)[4] **(Figs. 6A to E)**.

- **Secondary implants placement in free fibula**: Implant insertion done after completion of cancer treatment. Advantage is that it allows for more comprehensive assessment of disease status, oral function, and patient motivation, as well as more precise prosthetic planning. But disadvantages are that lack of interest or motivation shown by the patient for an additional dental procedure after completion of cancer treatment resulting in postponement or even cancellation of prosthetic rehabilitation. Vascularization and regenerative ability of the irradiated tissues can decrease, which may lessen the prospect of successful osseointegration of the dental implants. Apart from radiotherapy many other factors influence implant rehabilitations in free fibular reconstruction.

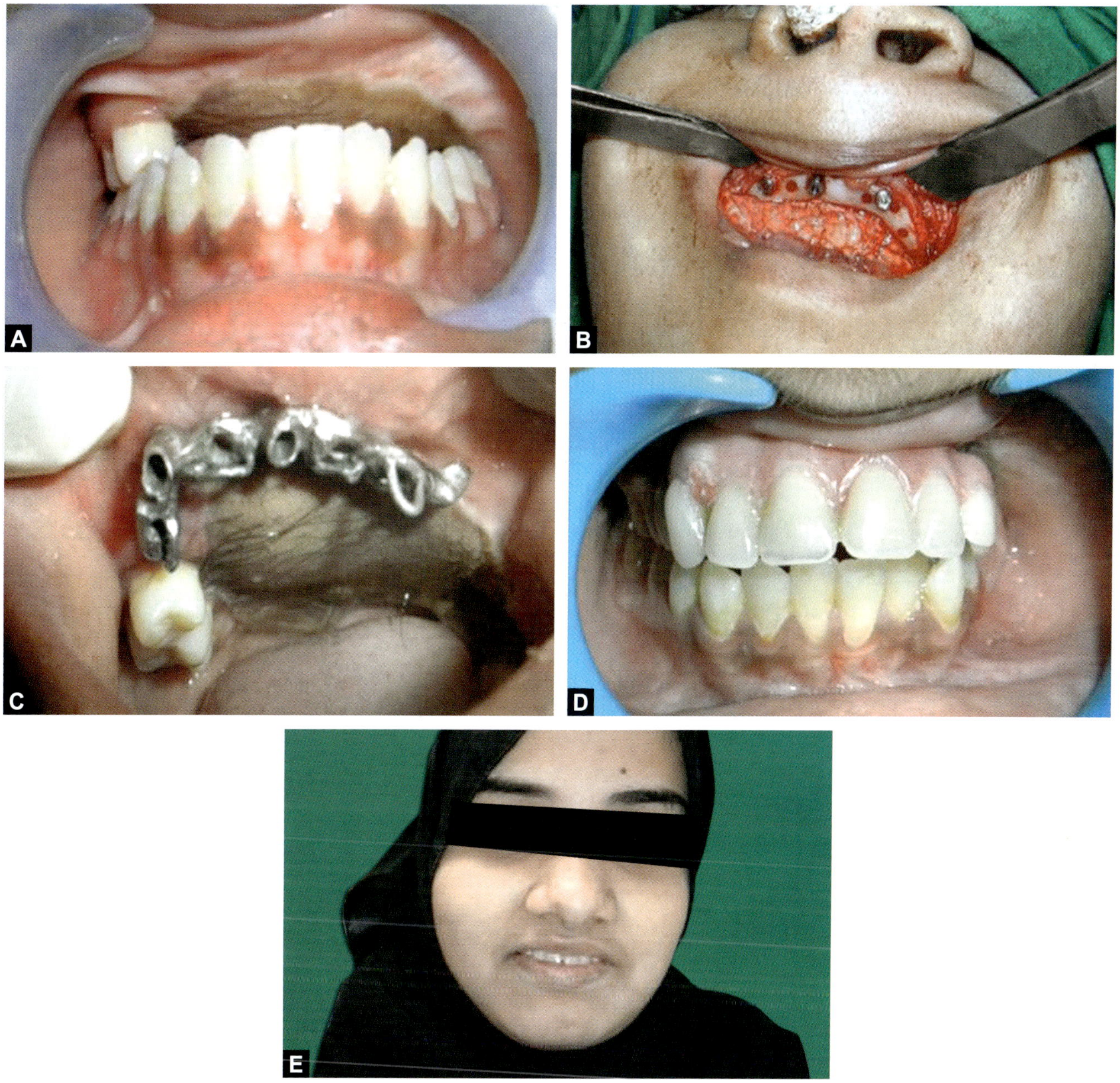

Figs. 4A to E: Implant retained fixed prosthesis in maxillary arch

FACTORS INFLUENCING DENTAL IMPLANT REHABILITATION IN FREE FIBULAR RECONSTRUCTION: TMH EXPERIENCE

A study was conducted on 138 patients in Tata Memorial Hospital (TMH) to study the factors affecting dental rehabilitation following jaw reconstruction with free-fibular graft in head and neck cancer patients. All the possible relevant factors which could influence dental rehabilitation were noted and subdivided into four groups psycho-social and patient-related factors, disease-related factors, surgical resection and free fibula reconstruction-related factors, existing anatomic factors hindering prosthetic rehabilitation.

In this study it was found that 60% patients could not undergo dental rehabilitation with osseointegrated implant supported prosthesis, 26% patients were rehabilitated right away, 4% patients were not willing for the rehabilitation

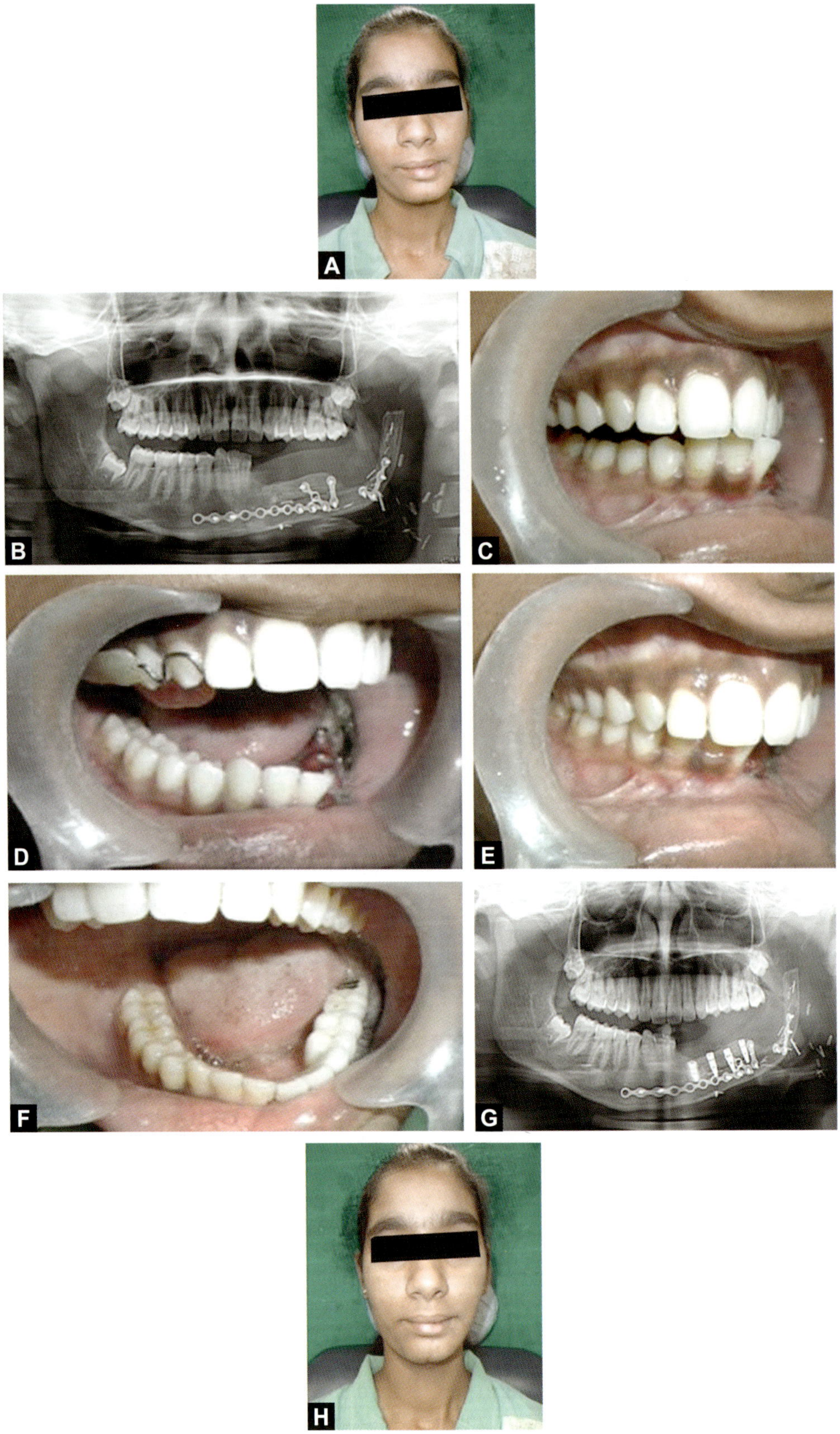

Figs. 5A to H: Implant retained fixed prosthesis after correction of deviation in double barrel free fibular graft

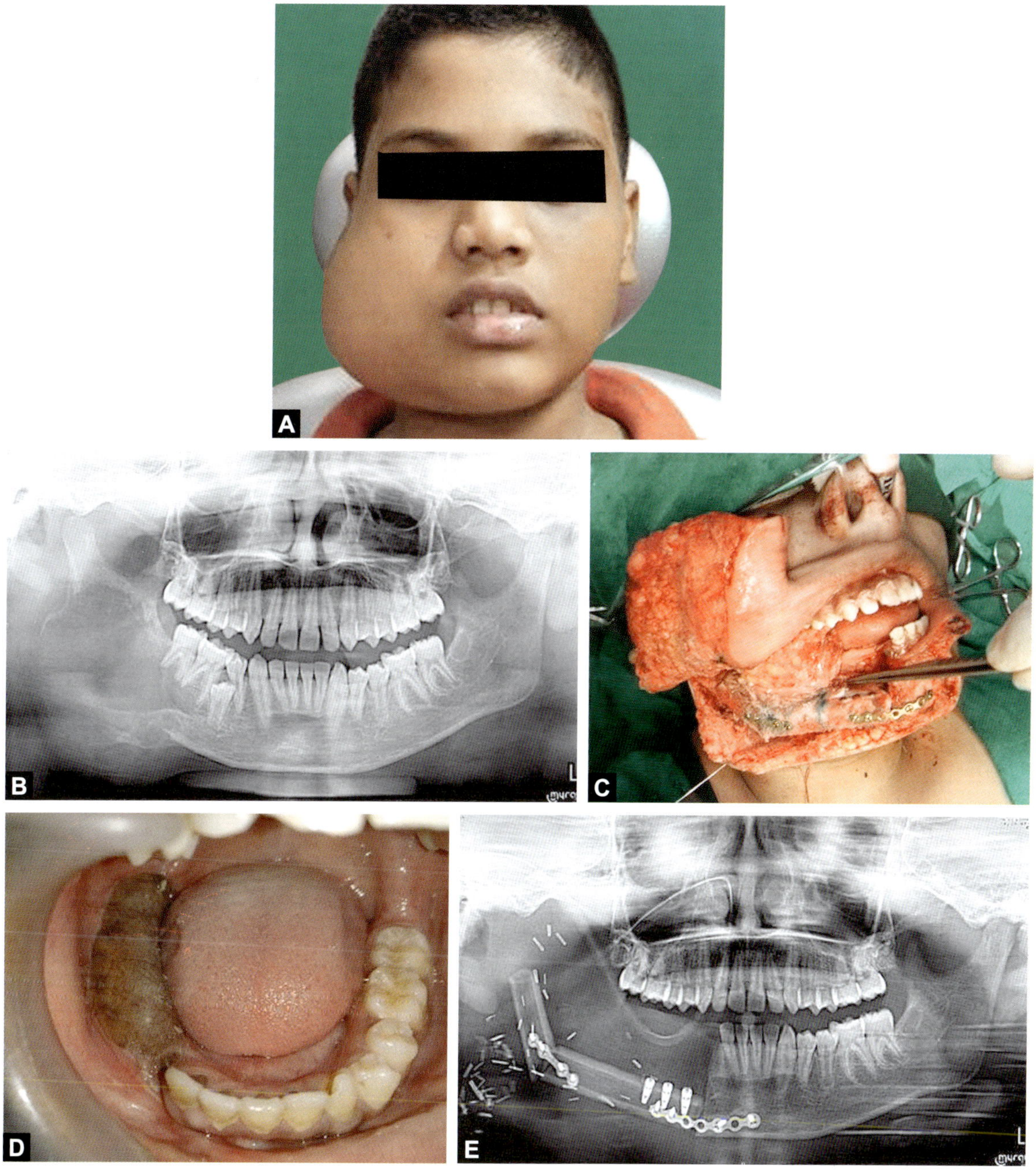

Figs. 6A to E: Primary implant placement

while in 10% patients implants could be placed by additional surgical intervention such as vestibuloplasty.

Multivariate analysis showed 3 factors showed a statistically significant association with the main outcome measure. Interference to placement of implants by reconstruction plates and screws, unfavorable diagnostic maxilla-mandibular relationship and obliterated vestibule were statistically established ($p < 0.05$) as the most significant reasons for not carrying out dental rehabilitation in patients who had undergone free-fibular graft reconstruction.

Also there is the issue of additional financial burden which such implant-based treatment entails; which assumes even greater significance in a developing resource-limited country like ours. However, financial incapability of the patients was not included as factor in this study.

COMPLICATIONS AND FAILURE IN IMPLANTS

Soft Tissue Complication

Peri-implant inflammation is most common complication in implant supported rehabilitation in reconstructed jaw bones.

It was noted that peri-implant soft tissue inflammation (peri implantitis) was one of the deterrent factors for the success of implant-retained prosthetic rehabilitation in reconstructed mandible **(Figs. 7A and B)**.[5] The rate of peri-implantitis was considerably higher in implants in skin grafted mucosa than in implants inserted in native bone with normal oral mucosa. Thick soft tissue coverage that is more mobile than attached gingival of the oral mucosa leads to pseudo pockets. Altered implant environment due to radiation induced xerostomia lead to peri-implant inflammatory process.[6]

This lead to implant failure and at times needed surgical removal.[7] Failure to maintain optimum oral hygiene lead to the failure of implants after prosthetic loading. Peri-implantitis can be minimized to some extent by de-epithlization and de-bulking of the flap. A recently developed protocol by Kumar VV et al.[8] has shown significant reduction in occurrence of peri-implantitis **(Figs. 8A to D)**.

- Unnatural loading by connecting implant with natural tooth for a fixed prosthesis leads to failure of implant and sometimes even fracture of free fibular graft **(Fig. 9)**.

Retrospective study by Dholam et al[9] showed five year rate of osseointegration and overall success rate was 88% and 77% respectively. Rate of osseointegration was 93% for grafted, 85% for native, 83% for irradiated and 100% for non-irradiated jaws. Overall success rate was 73% for grafted, 80% for native, 71% for irradiated and 89% for non-irradiated jaws.

EXTRAORAL PROSTHESIS

Maxillofacial prosthetic repair is indicated when anatomic parts of head and neck are not replaceable with living tissue. Reconstructive surgical procedures can reduce the extent of the bone and soft tissue defects, but in many patients persisting deficits remain, leading to severe functional disability and obvious cosmetic deformity. In these cases, the use of tissue integrated prosthesis in oral and maxillofacial reconstruction is indicated.

Material for extraoral facial prosthesis is room temperature vulcanizing silicone. Extraoral prosthesis needs to be retained with anatomic retention, and or with external source such as adhesives, mechanical retention using eye glasses, embedding magnets in nasal, or orbital prosthesis to assist in securing to maxillary obturator.

Types of extraoral prosthesis

Rehabilitation of Ocular Defects

Immediate rehabilitation of ocular defects is done by inserting conformer at the time of enucleation. These conformers are either pre-fabricated or custom made and made up of either acrylic resin or heat vulcanizing silicone. The conformer prevents collapse and shrinkage of soft tissue maintains space for future final ocular prosthesis **(Figs. 10A and B)**.

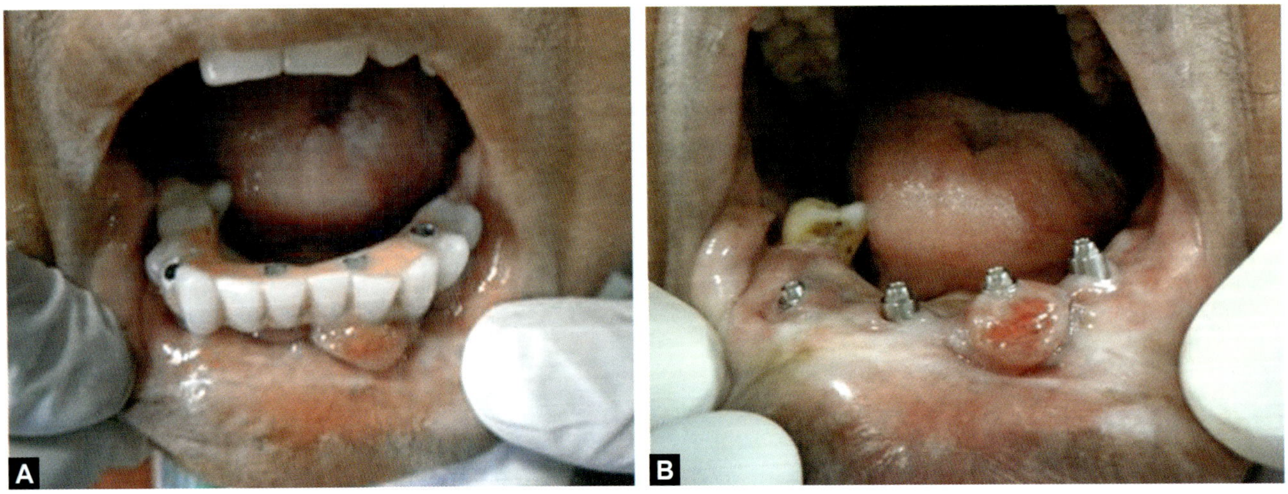

Figs. 7A and B: Peri-implantitis

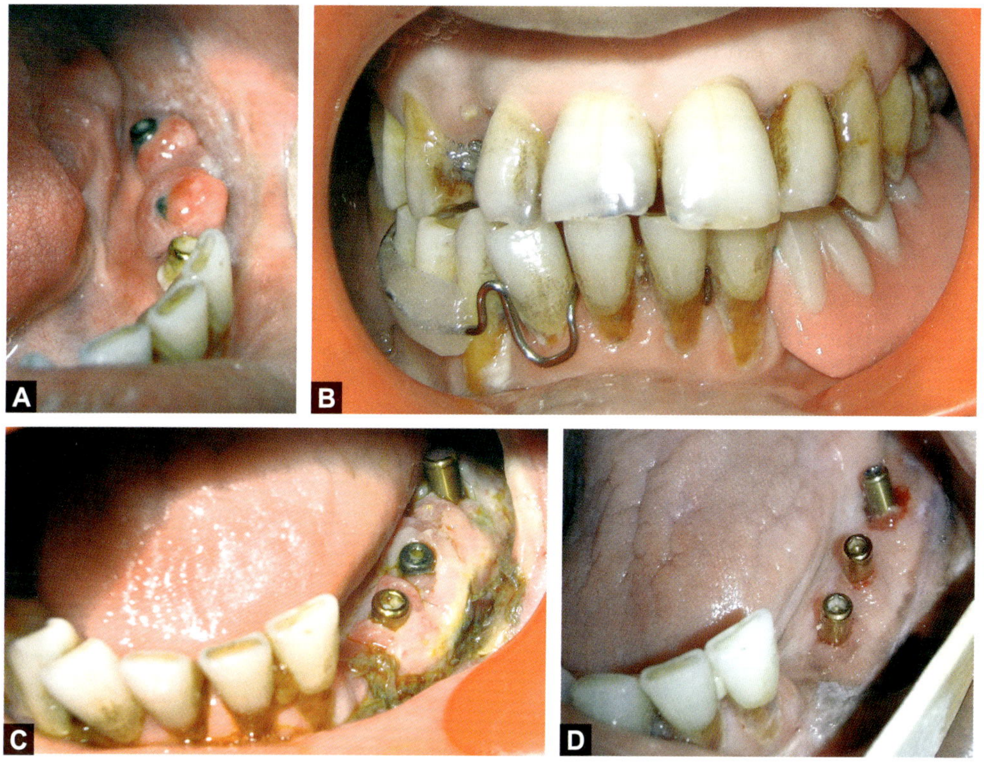

Figs. 8A to D: Subperiosteal dissection with denture-guided epithelial regeneration

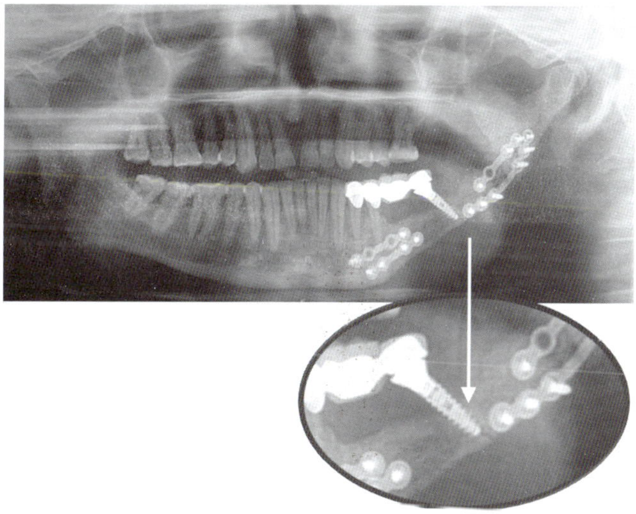

Fig. 9: Fracture fibula due to unnatural loading

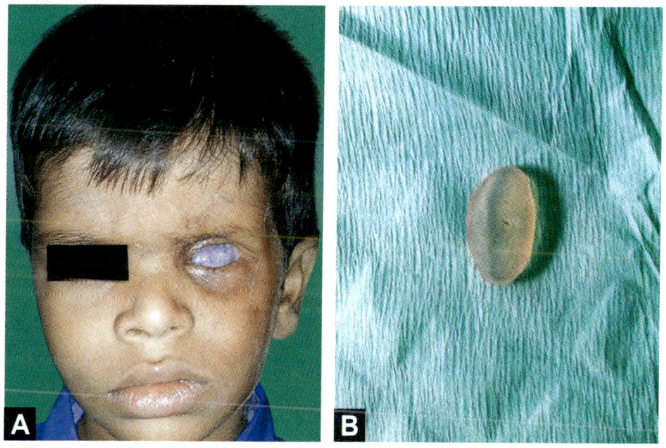

Figs. 10A and B: Insertion of conformer after enucleation

Ocular Prosthesis

Made up of acrylic resin with either stock or custom made iris matching contralateral iris. If eyelids and extrinsic muscle bed is well-preserved, ocular prosthesis gives excellent esthetics and sometimes even reproduce movements of contralateral eye ball **(Figs. 11A and B)**.

Orbital Prosthesis

Indicated in exenteration where all the contents of orbital cavity along with eyelid are resected and lined either with skin or free muscle flap. The eyeball part is made up of acrylic and surrounding skin is made with silicone prosthesis for life-like appearance. It can be retained with ana-

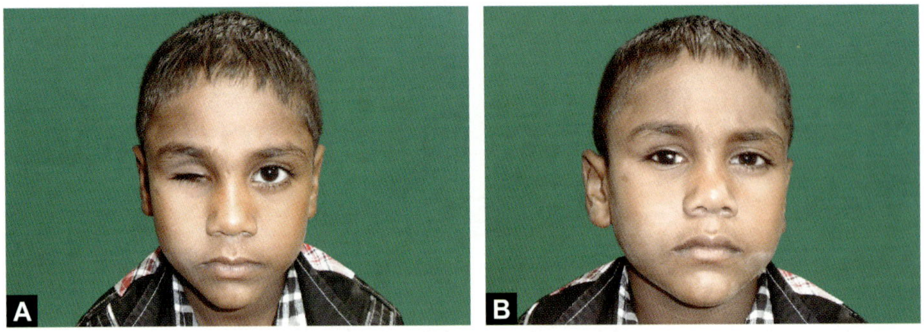

Figs. 11A and B: Ocular prosthesis

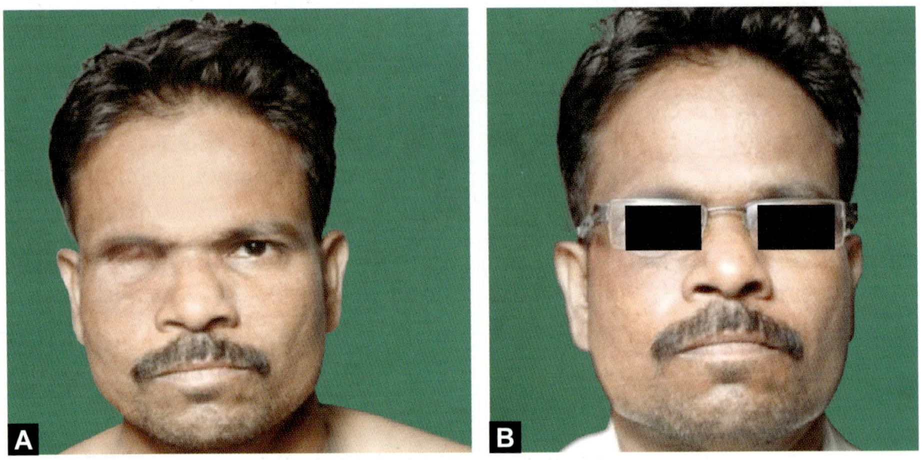

Figs. 12A and B: Orbital prosthesis—adhesive retained

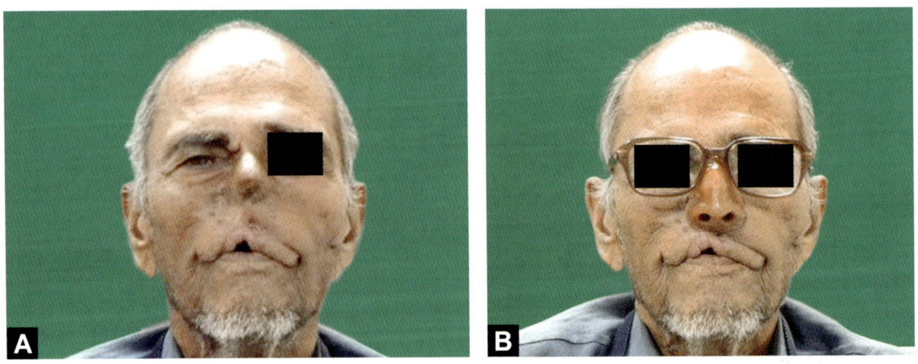

Figs. 13A and B: Acrylic nasal prosthesis retained with spectacles

tomical undercut, with adhesives, spectacle mounted or with the help of osseointegrated implants **(Figs. 12A and B)**.

Nasal and Auricular Prosthesis

These prostheses replace missing facial parts with either acrylic or Room Temperature Vulcanizing (RTV) silicone. Retention can be achieved with adhesives, eye glasses or implants **(Figs. 13 to 15)**.

Patch Prosthesis

These skin colored patch prosthesis covers and obliterates extra oral fistulas. Extra oral fistulas occur when vascularization of free or pedical flap fails during radiotherapy. In radiated patients, resurgery to achieve acceptable plastic closure may become problematic hence patch prostheses are recommended **(Figs. 16 and 17)**.

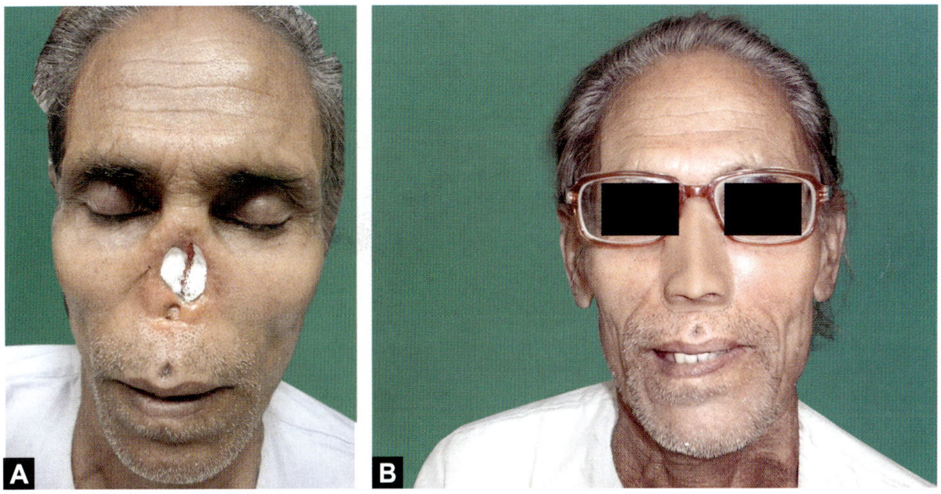

Figs. 14A and B: Adhesive retained nasal prosthesis (RTV silicone)

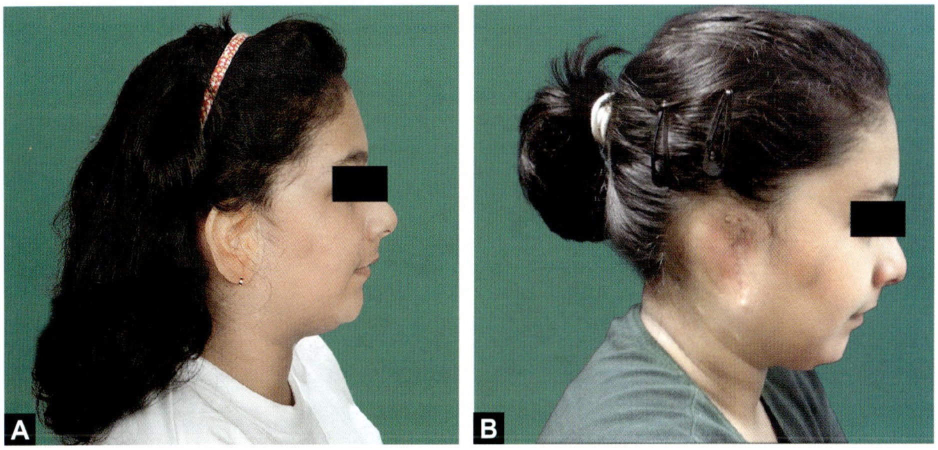

Figs. 15A and B: Silicone ear prosthesis

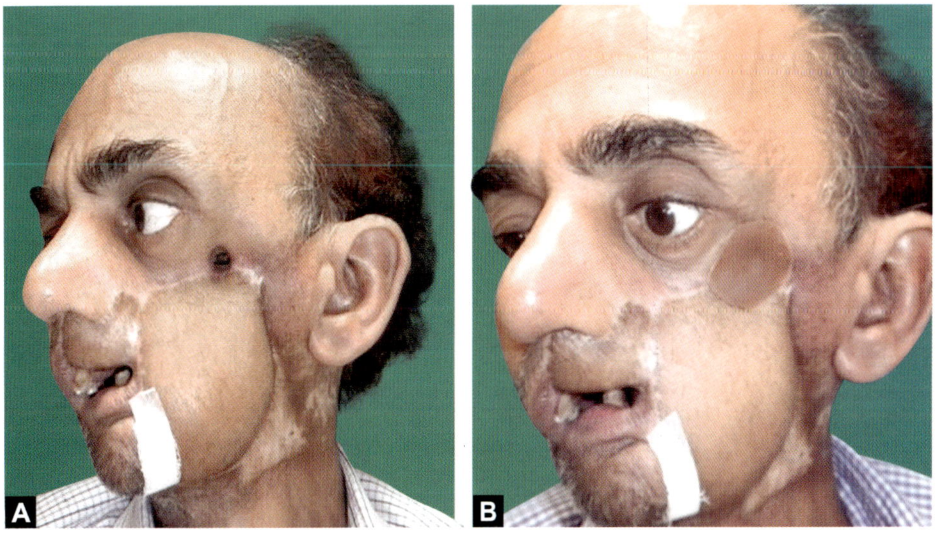

Figs. 16A and B: Closure of orocutaneous fistulas

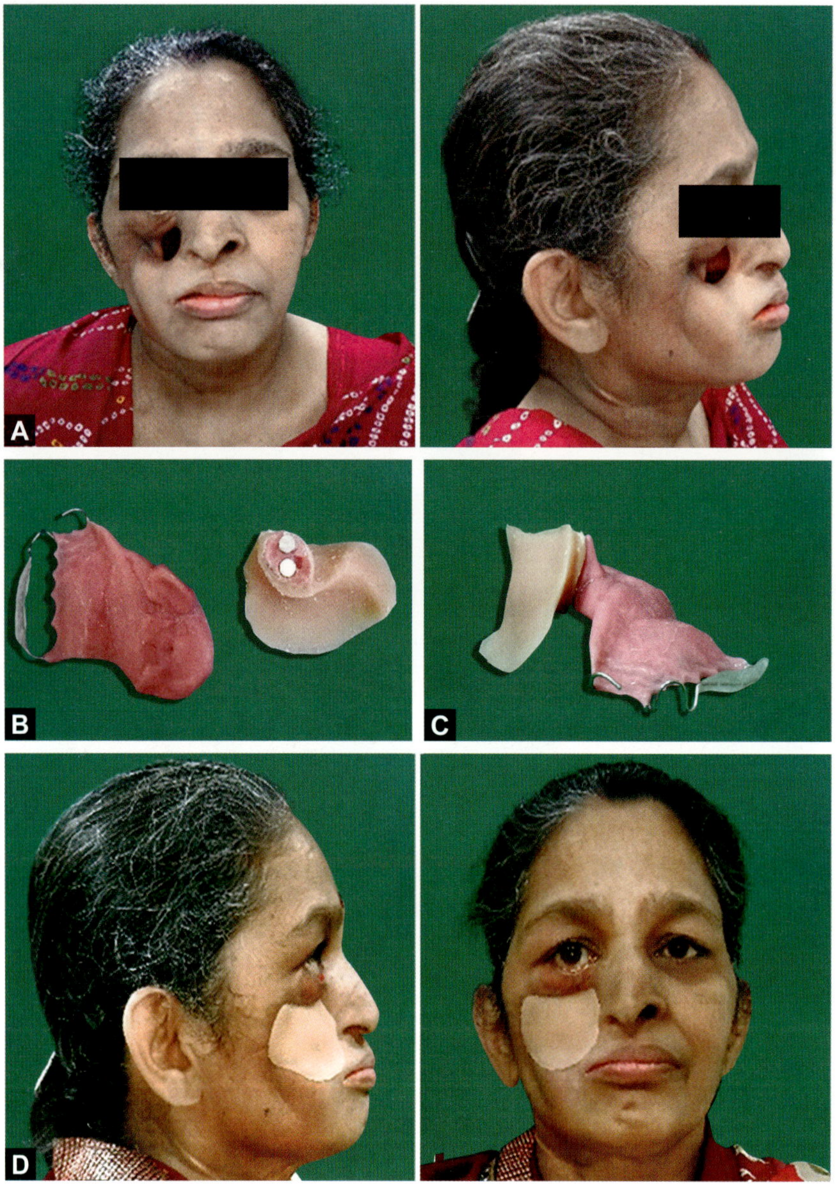

Figs. 17A to D: Magnet retained fistula closure

OSSEOINTEGRATION AND EXTRAORAL PROSTHESIS

Conventionally, the silicone prosthesis is used for this purpose and an adhesive is used for fixing it to the surrounding skin. Unfortunately, this adherence is often not satisfactory and the prosthesis can detach, leading to an embarrassing situation to the patient in the society and cause a negative impact for the suffering patient. Use of adhesive is controversial due to its unpredictable performance, difficulty of manipulation, decreased durability of the prosthesis and its application to compromised tissue surface. With the introduction of osseointegrated implant biotechnology to the facial prosthesis there is opportunity to provide secure retention of prosthesis without jeopardizing the integrity of the skin and underlying tissue or prosthesis when inherent retention with in defect is absent or external forms of retention are unacceptable to the patient. The osseointegrated implants offer a rigid fixation which will not allow the prosthesis to slip away and also conceals the deformity satisfactorily.[10] This improves the patients confidence enormously, and he/she can function normally and makes them socially acceptable **(Figs. 18 and 19)**.

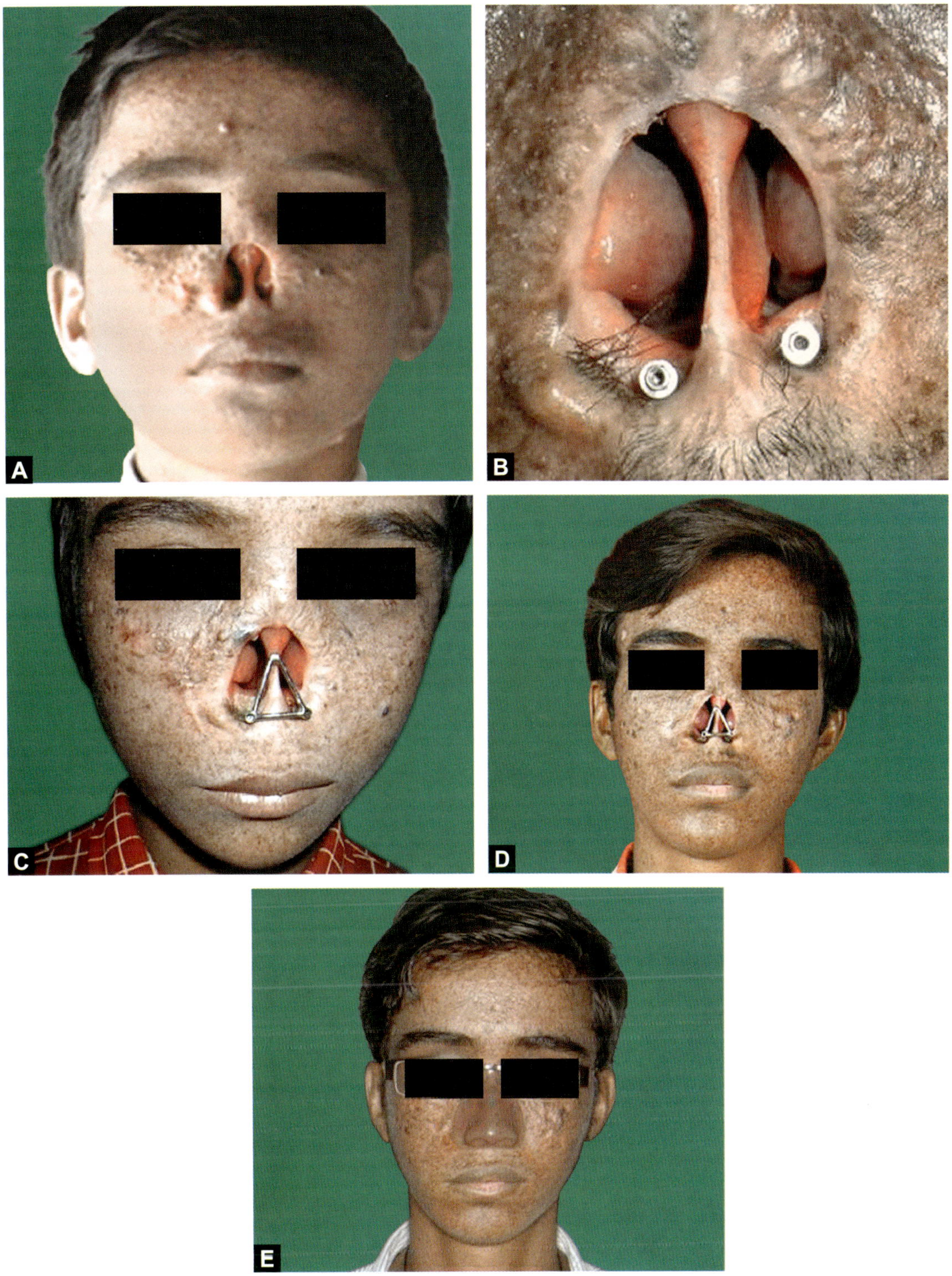

Figs.18A to E: Implant supported nasal prosthesis in xeroderma pigmentosa patient

Extraoral Prosthesis and QoL

Psychosocial perception scale is developed at Tata Memorial Hospital in coordination with of Department of Psychiatry, King Edward Memorial Hospital, Mumbai. The psychosocial perception scale questionnaire was filled by thirty patients (20 male: 10 female) before and after 3 months of use of prosthesis. This questionnaire comprised

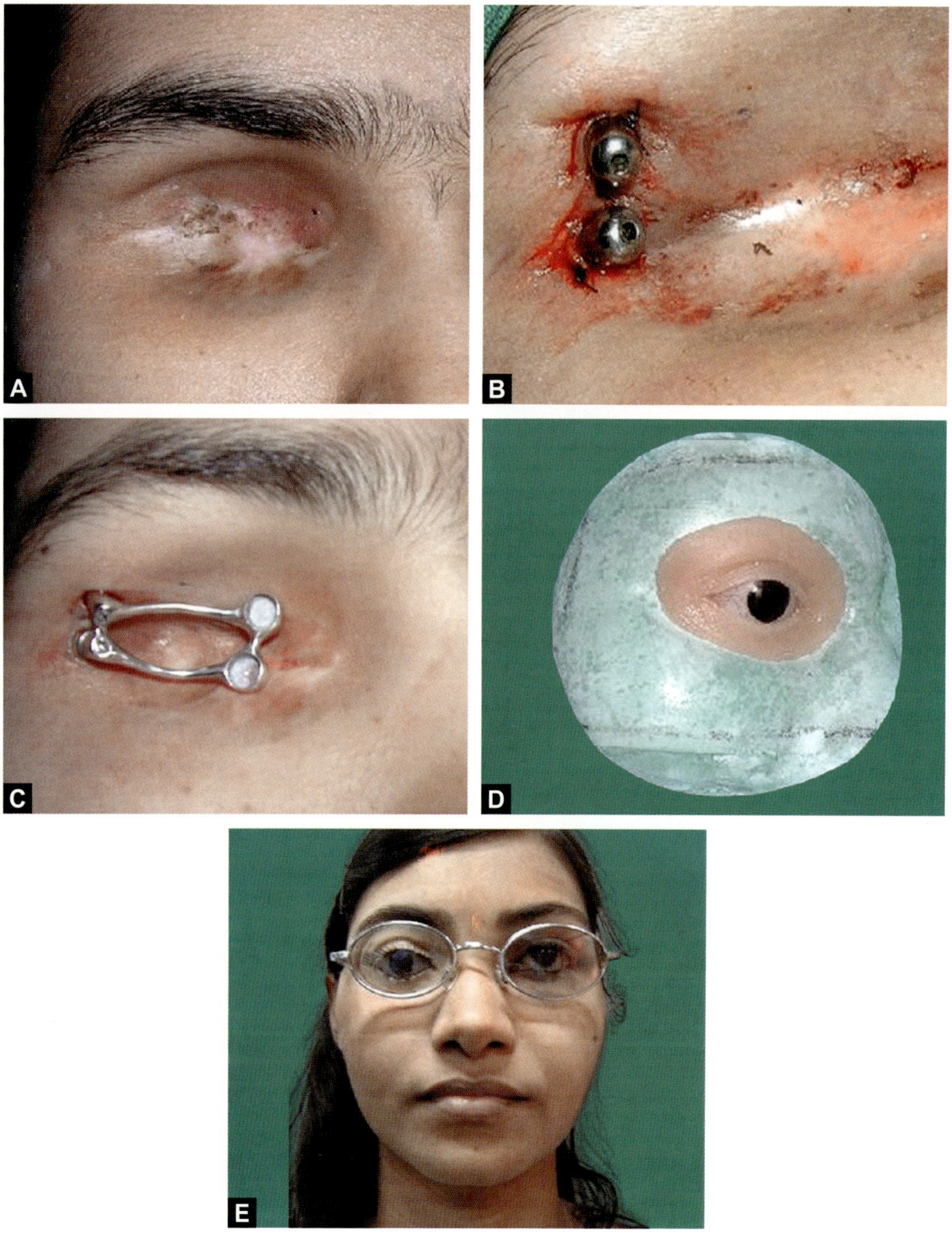

Figs. 19A to E: Implant retained—orbital prosthesis

of 14 items covering appearance, satisfaction, confidence, ability to work, self-contentment, social respect, family spouse friends liking, hope from life, social and daily activities, helpless and worthlessness. All the items showed significant improvement with use of extra oral prosthesis over the period of three months. The results of this study showed improvement in self-reported psycho-social perception with use of extra oral prosthesis.

REFERENCES

1. Dholam KP, Gurav SV. Dental implants in irradiated jaws: a literature review. J Cancer Res Ther. 2012;8 Suppl 1: S85-93.
2. Kumar VV, Jacob PC, Ebenezer S, et al. Implant supported dental rehabilitation following segmental mandibular reconstruction-quality of life outcomes of a prospective randomized trial. J Craniomaxillofac Surg. 2016;44(7):800-10.

3. Kumar VV, Ebenezer S, Kämmerer PW, et al. Implants in free fibula flap supporting dental rehabilitation: Implant and peri-implant related outcomes of a randomized clinical trial. JCraniomaxillofac Surg. 2016;44(11):1849-58.
4. Schepers RH, Slagter AP, Kaanders JH, et al. Effect of postoperative radiotherapy on the functional result of implants placed during ablative surgery for oral cancer. Int J Oral Maxillofac Surg. 2006;35(9):803-8.
5. Dholam KP, Bachher GK, Yadav PS, et al. Assessment of quality of life after implant-retained prosthetically reconstructed maxillae and mandibles postcancer treatments. Implant Dent. 2011;20(1):85-94.
6. Gbara A, Darwich K, Li L, et al. Long-term results of jaw reconstruction with microsurgical fibula grafts and dental implants. J Oral Maxillofac Surg. 2007;65: 1005-09.
7. Wu YQ, Huang W, Zhang ZY, et al. Clinical outcome of dental implants placed in fibula-free flaps for orofacial reconstruction. Chin Med J. 2008;121:1861-65.
8. Kumar VV, Jacob PC, Kuriakose MA. Sub-Periosteal Dissection with Denture-Guided Epithelial Regeneration: A Novel Method for Peri-Implant Soft Tissue Management in Reconstructed Mandibles. J Maxillofac Oral Surg. 2016 Dec;15(4):449-55.
9. Dholam KP, Pusalkar HA, Yadav PS, et al. Implant-retained dental rehabilitation in head and neck cancer patients: an assessment of success and failure. Implant Dent. 2013 Dec;22(6):604-9.
10. Dholam KP, Pusalkar HA, Yadav P, et al. Implant-retained orbital prosthesis. J Indian Prosthodont Soc. 2008;8:55-8.

CHAPTER 17

Composite Tissue Allotransplantation

Subramania Iyer, Mohit Sharma

INTRODUCTION

Composite tissue allotransplant (CTA) or vascularized composite allotransplant (VCA) is a transplant of combination of tissues like skin, muscles, bones, nerve, blood vessels, ligaments and tendons.

Deformities which defy conventional reconstructive and rehabilitative attempts may be benefitted by these transplants.

The replacement of tissues of similar structure and function is best achieved by VCA.

However, the immunosuppression needed for preventing rejection of the transplanted tissue remains the main barrier in wider adoption of this in the reconstructive armamentarium. The interplay between immunological competence and cancer biology makes the adoption of these methods for cancer reconstruction highly debatable.

The discovery of cyclosporine in 1976 gave a boost to organ transplantation as effective immunosuppression was made available. After the first successful hand transplant performed in Lyon, France in1998 (1) over 150 composite tissue transplants have been performed worldwide including more than 100 upper limbs and 35 partial/complete faces. There have been reports of abdominal wall, tongue, trachea, larynx, uterus, penis, bone and joint transplants.

WHY VCA IS CHALLENGING?

VCA have some special features that make it different from solid organ transplant:

- The solid organ transplants are done for life-threatening conditions whereas in VCA the purpose is only to enhance quality of life.
- Solid organs like liver and kidney can be procured from live as well as brain dead donors. VCA can be procured only from deceased donors.
- Donation of these body parts is externally mutilating and hence less accepted by the grieving families.
- Rigorous psycho-social assessment and counseling is essential to make sure the compliance to lifelong immunosuppression especially since this is done for a non-lifesaving procedure.

IMMUNOLOGICAL CONSIDERATIONS

Recognition and rejection of the allogeneic tissue is by the recipient's immune system and initiated by ABO (blood group) antigens and the Human Leucocyte Antigens (HLA). HLAs are cell surface glycoproteins encoded by the Major Histocompatibility Complex located on chromosome 6 and expressed on all nucleated cells. HLA and ABO antigens determine compatibility of transplants. Antigens are presented to the recipient T cells and activate them. T cell response is central to the pathogenesis of transplant rejection. Unlike solid organ transplant, heterogeneous tissues in CTA express different amounts of MHC antigens and hence elicit stronger degree of host immune response. In general, skin and bone marrow are rejected earlier and more aggressively than muscle, cartilage, tendon, nerve or bone.

To prevent rejection induction of immunosuppression is achieved by depletion of T cell population in perioperative and immediate postoperative period.

The common agents used for induction include methyl prednisolone and either ATG or the monoclonal antibodies.

The maintenance of lifelong immunosuppression is achieved using immunosuppressant medications.

The common drugs used include:

- Steroids
- Anti-proliferative drugs which block DNA synthesis and proliferation (Azathioprine, Mycophenolate mofetil, Cyclophosphamide)

- Calcineurin inhibitors which block IL-2 production acting as anti T cell agents (Cyclosporine, Tacrolimus)

Acute episodes of rejection, which occur in almost all cases occasionally are managed with pulse doses of methyl prednisolone.

The common complications of immunosuppression are opportunistic infections and malignancies (lymphoma and skin cancer being the common ones). Other systemic complications include diabetes, hypertension and chronic renal failure.

Most transplant programs incorporate prophylactic antimicrobial therapy against CytoMegalo Virus.

CURRENT APPLICATIONS OF VCA

The areas where VCA has been established its mark are in hands and face. The other areas where it is emerging as an alternative to conventional methods of reconstruction is abdominal wall defects, penis and uterus.

Hand Transplants

The safety and efficacy of hand transplants is well established. So it is being used more frequently across the world.

The ideal candidate for hand transplantation is usually a bilateral amputee, but unilateral amputations have also received transplants which could only be justified if the lost hand is dominant one and its loss is causing profound psychological disturbance and body image alteration in the patient.

Distal transplants do very well with functional recovery. Above elbow transplants have also been successfully carried out. But higher the level of the transplants longer is the re innervation time leading to poorer return of intrinsic muscle function.

The argument against hand transplants is that a good or acceptable functional outcome may be obtained with a myoelectric prosthesis without risk of immunosuppression. But activities of daily living that are highly dependent on sensory recovery and fine movements can not be at present provided by any prosthesis.

Face Transplantation

Burn injuries, high speed trauma, gunshot wounds, animal attacks, and extensive tumor surgery are the primary causes of complex facial deformities.

These defects may involve skin, muscle, and/or bone, as well as different functional and aesthetic units. When all the reconstructive options are exhausted or when will not be able to provide functional rehabilitation face transplants become an option. The transplant could include partial or full face and may include soft tissues only or even the facial bones.

Ethical issues related to both the recipient and the donor are more important in face transplant. The concern for mutilation following face donation is valid and may be a deterrent for it especially in the Indian context. The other major ethical issue is in relation to the morbidity to the recipient if the transplant fails due to primary vascular failure, acute rejection or chronic rejection.

More than 35 partial/full facial transplants have been performed world over. The first face transplant patient had multiple episodes of rejection and recently succumbed to a cancer which probably is unrelated to the transplant. The patients who have had face transplants have gained good aesthesis and functions like nasal breathing, smelling, drinking, eating and intelligible speech. Sensory recovery occurred between 3 to 8 months' post-transplant whereas motor recovery took up to 18 months.

Abdominal Wall Transplantation

Abdominal wall transplantation is generally done in conjunction with small bowel transplantation to accommodate the increased volume of abdominal cavity. This was first reported by Levi et al. in 2003 and later by Cipriani et al in 2007. Recently a remote revascularization technique has been described by Giele et al, in 2014 with the intention of reducing the cold ischemia time to the abdominal wall transplant. The indications for simultaneous abdominal wall transfer would include loss of domain, poor and scarred native abdominal wall due to repeated laparotomies, stoma and wound infections.

Tracheal Transplant

Reconstruction of long segments of trachea is a challenging task. Prefabricating the trachea using cartilages or alloplastic materials or tissue engineered constructs has been attempted with variable results. The first allogenic trachea that was transplanted was in 1979 as reported by Rose et al.

The problems with tracheal transplants is the difficulty in vascularizing the trachea due the absence of a vascular pedicle necessitating heterotopic implantation before transfer to the recipient site. Sternocleidomastoid muscle, omentum and radial forearm site has been used for this remote revascularization. Deleare and group reported the first successful allotransplant of trachea along with immunosuppression in 2010. Even though initially the patient was immunosuppressed they withdrew it after few months when the necrosed membranous trachea was removed and replaced with buccal mucosal graft from the same patient. They further reported 4 more cases with variable immunosuppression with only one failure. The Amrita experience was of one similar case, which was successfully transplanted maintaining its viability for 3 months, but the patient succumbing to a mediastinal bleed due to tumor erosion

Uterine Transplant

Several successful uterine transplants have been carried out for congenital absence of a uterus in presence of functioning ovaries. The advantage of uterine transplant is that they could be procured from matching live donors who have finished their child-bearing requirement and that immunosuppression can be withdrawn after the transplanted uterus has served its purpose of child-bearing in the recipient. The uterus retrieval is along with its vasculature and supporting sacro-uterine and vesico-uterine peritoneal folds and vaginal fornix which are refixed. The uterine transplants done by the Swedish team has resulted in successful pregnancy in many.

ALLOTRANSPLANTS IN CANCER DEFECTS

The limiting factors for widespread use for the VCA in reconstruction are the need for lifelong immunosuppression. The same makes it to be difficult to be used for reconstruction of cancer defects. Cancer immunology and transplant immunology are two faces of the same coin. In cancers, immunomodulation by the cancer cells help them to escape immune surveillance, whereas in transplants the inability to develop immune tolerance leads to rejections. Reported incidence of cancers are in higher rate in immunosuppressed patients who have undergone transplants. At the same time immunosuppression necessitated by the transplants may reactivate the dormant cancer cells in a previously treated cancer survivor. But the rapid strides in immunology research both in cancers and transplants may help in bridging the gap between them and facilitate more wider use of VCA in these.

CONCLUSION

Composite tissue allotransplantation has immense potentials. Functional results after composite tissue allotransplantation, specially the hand and face transplants have been excellent. More organs are being transplanted in a sporadic fashion. Reports of successful penile transplant and that of the scalp and skull bones are examples of ingenious use of this technique to solve problems that cannot be tackled with conventional reconstructive methods.

The reasons for its less widespread use is the issues related with immunosuppression and the technical challenges each surgery throws up.

Current research is heavily concentrated on bringing in an immune tolerance to the transplant without causing harmful effects on the general health of the recipient. Hence more safe and simple methods of immunosuppression may develop in future ushering in a revolutionary change in reconstruction by wider use of VCA principles in the future.

BIBLIOGRAPHY

1. Brenner MJ, Tung TH, Jensen JN, et al. The spectrum of complications of immunosuppression: is the time right for hand transplantation? J Bone Joint Surg Am. 2002;84-A:1861-70.
2. Cendales LC, Kanitakis J, Schneeberger S, et al. The Banff 2007 working classification of skin-containing composite tissue allograft pathology. Am J Transplant. 2008;8(7): 1396-400.
3. Dubernard JM, Owen E, Herzberg G, et al. Human hand allograft: Report on first 6 months. Lancet. 1999;1:1315.
4. Duquesnoy RJ. Is histocompatibility testing needed for composite tissue transplantation? Transplant Proc. 1998;30:2724.
5. Graham B, Adkins P, Tsai TM, et al. Major replantation versus revision amputation and prosthetic fitting in the upper extremity: a late functional outcomes study. J Hand Surg Am. 1998;23(5):783.
6. Jones ND, Morris PJ, Wood KJ. Differential susceptibility of heart, skin and islet allografts to T cell-mediated rejection. J Immunol. 2001;166:2824-30.
7. Joseph E Imbriglia, Robert J Goitz, Jaimie T Shores, et al. Technical aspects of the recipient operation in hand transplantation. Journal of Reconstructive Microsurgery, Thieme Medical Publishers, Aug 2011;28(1):27-34.
8. Levi DM, Tzakis AG, Kato T, et al. Transplantation of the abdominal wall. Lancet 2003;28:2173-76.

9. Murray JE, Merrill JP, Harrison JH. Renal homotransplantation in identical twins. Surg Forum. 1955;6:432.
10. Najarian JS, Simmons RL, eds. Clinical transplantation: Bone and cartilage: Transplantation. Philadelphia: Lea and Febiger; 1972:685-86.
11. Peacock EE Jr. Restoration of finger flexion with homologous composite tissue tendon grafts of the digital flexor mechanism in human beings. Trans Bull. 1960;7:418.
12. Petruzzo P, Dubernard JM. The International Registry on Hand and Composite Tissue Allotransplantation. Clin Transpl. 2011;247-53.
13. Petruzzo P, Lanzetta M, Dubernard JM, et al. The International Registry on Hand and Composite Tissue Transplantation 2010;90(12):1590-94. Unique immunological challenge—long been known that skin is more susceptible to rejection than any other tissue.
14. Shores JT, Brandacher G, Schneeberger S, et al. Composite tissue allotransplantation: hand transplantation and beyond. J Am Acad Orthop Surg. 2010;18(3):127-31.
15. Zamfirescu DG, Owen E, Lascar I, et al. Sentinel skin allograft—a reliable marker for monitoring of composite tissue transplant rejection. Transplant Proc. 2009;41:503–08.

Chapter 18

Future Directions in Reconstruction

Saumya Mathews, Tasneem Belgaumwala, Prabha Yadav

INTRODUCTION

As we complete 5000 free flaps over the past 12 years and look back , we realize that the process of learning has been constant and we have tried to imbibe and implement new technology and refine techniques in our practice.

Looking into the future we hope to continue to do the same, by complementing our skills with the ever-evolving technology. Advancements in functional imaging,application of robotic surgery in microvascular anastomosis and the incorporation of artificial intelligence, nanotechnology and bionics will usher in a new era in field of reconstruction.

Tissue Regeneration in Cancer Reconstruction

Controlled tissue regeneration is the Holy Grail of all wound healing and reconstruction. The fact that there will be no donor site morbidity and no dependence on donors for organ transplant makes this dream so fascinating. The advances in stem cell technology has spurred great interest and promise for regenerative medicine.

Stem cells are defined as a population of cells capable of self-renewal and differentiation subsequently to, functional tissues.

The technology to harvest pluripotent and multipotent stem cells and use them on pre-fabricated scaffolds along with growth factors is currently being investigated. It is postulated that plastic surgeons will be at the forefront of using adipogenic stem cells for tissue generation. Numerous in vivo and in vitro studies are currently underway investigating the role of adipogenic stem cells, fat derived mesenchymal cells, induced pluripotent stem cells and transcription factors. However, the use of stimulated stem cells and viruses which will aid in regeneration of tissue in the setting of malignancy is debatable. The hope is that combining cell-based research and bioengineered models will aid in simultaneously creating multiple cell lines with the potential of growth as well as stopping cell division as required.

Prelamination and Prefabrication

These are methods where time and preconditioning are employed as the bedrock to achieve superior desired results or to actually design and use a flap where it would not be possible conventionally.

Prefabrication is method wherein a blood vessel is selectively implanted to vascularize a particular tissue such as muscle or skin.

Prelamination is a technique wherein different tissues are grafted around the pedicle in order to be transplanted as a composite tissue graft (e.g. tracheal prefabrication on a free radial forearm flap).

Tissue engineers in tandem with plastic surgeons are involved in ongoing research to establish intrinsic circulation into a bioengineered device by incorporating a vascular pedicle or loop into a tissue plane. This process stimulates a proinflammatory reaction causing the release of growth factors and inflammatory mediators into the device. When such a device is embedded in live tissue the body initiates an inflammatory reaction thereby releasing proangiogenic factors that promote neoangiogenesis thereby filling the device with fibroblastic tissue and linking it to the preexisting vasculature.

The application of flap prefabrication into practice requires multi-staged approach, and a high level of expertise and access to safe bioengineered material. Time is a luxury we do not have in oncology as most cases require primary reconstruction followed by immediate adjuvant radiotherapy. In order to shorten the time taken for reconstruction hybrid biomaterials containing cells, growth factors and nonbiological scaffolds are being developed in *in vivo* models. These biomaterials change their mechanical and biochemical properties in response to the environment. Hopefully in the future these techniques may evolve to be important tools in a cancer surgeon's armamentarium.

Robotic Surgery in Plastic Surgery

Robotic surgery has many benefits like:

- 3D imaging
- High magnification
- Removing involuntary hand tremors
- Better ergonomics due to 7 degrees of freedom
- Digital case recording

Improved ergonomics has been used for flap inset in the pharyngeal region and also to facilitate minimal access resection and reconstruction. The use of robots for tele surgery for reconstruction is another possibility for performing major procedures in remote locations. Telepresence and telementoring methods are also to be employed simultaneously to prevent surgical errors and endangering patients. MMI_{TM} a bioengineering company based in Italy has successfully developed robotic micro instruments which can be programmed by the surgeon to perform microanastomoses. The technology is still in nonhuman subject testing phases.

Surgical Simulators

The paradigm of "see one, do one, teach one" will soon be of the past with the advent of surgical trainers based on simulators.

The Mimic Technologies dV-Trainer™, a simulator for the da Vinci system, is a tabletop virtual environment with a two- handed haptic device with force feedback and tracking system. A similar system has been developed for training for flap harvest currently being tested with the latissimus dorsi flap harvest simulator.

Simulators for Surgical Planning

The advent and availability of 3D printing technology has made it possible to create 3D models of the defect to plan reconstruction. This is especially useful in reconstruction of extensive, multidimensional facial defects. The sky is the limit for the development of functional imaging. It may be possible to create a model mimicking skeletal and neurovascular anatomy in real time to aid surgical planning.

Telemedicine

Telemedicine can be used in the preoperative, operative, and postoperative phases of a given plastic surgical procedure.

Software and video conferencing applications can be used for preoperative assessment and counseling. It is especially useful to get an expert consult for a patient residing in a remote location. However, to ensure quality care and patient safety the patient must be examined at least once prior to the procedure to confirm finding and surgical plan.

Telementoring and telepresence can be used during the surgical procedure.

Postoperative follow-up visits can be reduced by means of online follow-up complemented with appropriate documentation and permissions.

Nanotechnology

The development of microbots that can be injected into blood circulation to monitor anastomoses or clear thrombi will be a boon to microvascular surgeons.

Free Flap Monitoring

Devices like implantable or skin adhering Doppler probes, ICG fluorescence devices, mounted portable video recording devices are being used to enable remote monitoring of the free flaps in the postoperative period by the surgeon. The hope is that reduction of skilled man power will translate in the eventual reduction of health care costs.

CONCLUSION

Plastic surgeons have historically been at the forefront of innovation. The future demands multimodality and multispecialty collaboration and co operation for improved patient care. Plastic surgeons along with biomedical engineers, tissue engineers and computer experts will be responsible for creating and shaping a better future in reconstructive surgery.

Chapter 19

A Year in Review: 2016

Prabha Yadav, Dushyant Jaiswal, Vinay K Shankhdhar, Tanmay Mohan Joshi, Neeraj Rao, Namrata Joshi

"Surgery without audit is like playing cricket without keeping the score"

Hugh Devlin

The department of plastic surgery at Tata Memorial Centre (TMC) performs 3 to 4 free tissue transfers every day 4 days a week, and complete more than 600 free flaps in a single year. By continuing this over a period of 12 years we have reached the unique milestone of 5000 free flaps.

	FFOCF	FRAFF	FALT	DIEP	Jejunum	TDAP	Gracillis/ Groin	LD	PAPF/ VRAM	MSAP	SGAP	SC Par-aSC	Total	Success rate
2005	85	84	43	2									214	95%
2006	81	128	38	9	2								258	96%
2007	66	80	64	4									214	92%
2008	77	66	73	8	6								230	91%
2009	109	89	72	13	4								287	95%
2010	123	57	73	16	5								274	93%
2011	146	75	79	29	5								334	95.30%
2012	149	62	124	23	10		2						370	96%
2013	161	90	191	39	7		11		1				500	94%
2014	217	119	201	44	9		12		1				603	96.19%
2015	203	73	228	48	7	10	19		5				593	94.13%
2016	220	56	287	44	7	5	6	1	2	3			631	92.89%
Nov-17	211	43	207	26	11	9	3	10	1	3	2	3	529	93.87%
Total	1848	1022	1680	305	73	24	53	11	10	6	2	3	5037	94.18%

We thus completed the celebratory figure of 5000 flaps in November 2017

Tata Memorial Hospital receives 65000 patients every year. Of the 11000 odd patients with head and neck cancer, 2100 undergo surgery, only 500 receive a free tissue transfer. Similarly, out of the 5000 Breast cancer patient registrations, 1/3 of which are operable, a meager 50 receive a free tissue transfer. 50 more free tissue transfers are done for limbs and trunk. These appear astounding figures for a single institute. We are actually unable to provide microsurgical reconstruction to all patients who get operated at TMC, and deserve one for best outcomes. Providing the same service to the city, state or whole country is an unfulfilled dream.

The purpose of this chapter is to give a bird's eye view into the workload handled by our unit. We have intentionally chosen one year data to highlight the state which we have reached, not the trend over the years.

This " Service evaluation" is essentially data of **'what we do'** and **'how much we do'** cold facts of the reconstructive work we do in year. The **'when to do what'** is covered in Algorithm chapter. The rest of book is about **'how we do it'** and **'why we do it'**.

The Year 2016

Number of major surgeries - 1287 surgeries

1. Free flaps - 631
2. Pedicle flaps-249
3. Other major surgeries -172
4. Minor procedures/surgeries - 235

Free Flaps

Chart of flap-wise distribution

	Jan	Feb	Mar	Apr	May	Jun	Jul	Aug	Sep	Oct	Nov	Dec	Total
FFOCF	17	19	20	16	19	20	18	19	17	16	18	20	220
FRAFF	8	4	7	2	4	7	3	7	3	3	3	5	56
FALT	20	27	25	27	24	26	19	26	24	22	20	27	287
DIEP	3	7	1	4	5	3	2	2	3	5	4	3	44
SGAP	1	–	–	–	–	–	–	–	–	–	–	–	1
TDAP	1	–	–	–	2	–	–	–	1	–	–	1	5
MSAP	–	–	–	–	–	–	–	–	1	1	–	–	2
Free LD	–	–	–	–	–	–	1	–	–	1	–	–	2
PAP	–	–	–	–	–	–	–	–	–	1	–	–	1
GRACILLIS	–	2	1	–	–	–	2	–	–	–	–	–	5
JEJUNUM	–	–	1	1	-	1	1	2	–	1	–	–	7
LAT thigh	–	–	–	–	–	–	–	–	–	–	1	–	1
	50	59	55	50	54	57	46	56	49	50	46	56	631

Charts of **site-wise** distribution of each flap.

FFOCF	Total (220)
Mandible	173
For Maxilla	37
Long Bone Defects	10

Deep inferior epigastric artery Perforator flap	Total (44)
Primary breast reconstruction	36
Secondary breast reconstruction	3
Head neck	5

FRAFF	Total (56)
Buccal mucosa	23
Tongue	23
Maxilla	1
Outer paddle	1
Failed free flap	2
Lip	4
Palate	1
Foot	1

FALT	Total (287)
Buccal mucosa composite resection	64
Buccal mucosa with maxilla and mandibular alveolectomies	53
Tongue	34
Extremity	32
Maxilla	20
Skull base	16
Breast	13
Posterior segmental mandibulectomy	8
Orbital exenteration	8
Failed free flap	8
Parotid	7
PMMC	6
Outer paddle (double free flap)	5
Chest	5
Osteoradionecrosis mandible	4
Scalp	2
Lip	2

Re-explorations for the major flaps

Re-explorations	FFOCF	FALT	FRAFF	DIEP	Jejunum	Total
POD <1	10	18	4	1	-	33
POD 2–5	10	11	4	0	0	25
POD >5	6	6	0	0	–	12
Arterial	6	13	2	0	–	21
Venous	12	21	4	1	0	38
Hematoma	7	7	1	0	–	15
Others	1	–	–	0	–	1
Salvaged	16	21	4	0	0	41
Lost	9	14	4	1	0	28
Re-explorations	26	35	8	1	0	**70**
Re-exploration rate	11.81	12.19	14.28	2.27	0	**11.4**
Salvage rate	61.53	60	50	0	0	**58.57**

	FFOCF	FALT	FRAFF
PMMC	5	2	
FALT	2	11	1
FFOCF	1		
LD		3	
FRAFF		1	
PMMF			2

FALT Morbidities

Neck complications						Donor complications	
Gape of inset	Neck gape	Parotid fistula	Chyle leak	Serous collection	OC fistula	Graft loss	Wound gape
2	1	13	3	13	18	12	9

FFOCF Morbidities

Gape of inset	Neck complications				Donor complications	
	Neck gape	Parotid	Chyle	Seroma	Graft loss	Tendon exposure
9	8	10	6	13	10	1

FRAFF Morbidities

Gape of inset	Neck complications				Donor complications	
	Neck gape	Parotid	Chyle	Seroma	Graft loss	Tendon exposure
2	2	2	1	6	4	2

PRECAUTIONS TO BE TAKEN TO AVOID COMPLICATIONS

Monitoring

Good postoperative monitoring is essential during the first 48 to 72 hours as early explorations are salvageable. Late explorations (after 5 days) are usually due to other causes like orocutaneous fistula or infection and are rarely due to technical problems. Late explorations are difficult to salvage.

Arterial Complications

- Intraoperatively the lie of the vessel should be checked to avoid kinking of the vessel
- Recipient vessel blood flow should be checked
- Recipient vessel should be checked for any inadvertent injury proximally due to cautery
- Avoid milking to confirm patency of the anastomosis
- There is no substitute for meticulous technique

Venous Complications

- Minimal adventectomy to avoid thinning the venous wall especially in patient post chemotherapy/radiotherapy.
- If vessel caliber discrepancy is >1:3, it's better to do an end to side anastomosis
- Check the vessel lie before closure
- Inadvertent vessel injury should be ruled out
- Meticulous technique

Hematoma

- Intra operative blood pressure of the patient should be near the base line pressure and subsequently hemostasis should be achieved
- Hematoma evacuation during exploration should be done with plenty of saline irrigation

Orocutaneous Fistula

Late explorations are usually due to infection or orocutaneous fistulas, hence one should be very careful while doing intraoral inset.

Intra oral inset should have good approximation.

Neck Complications

- Care should be taken during raising of the neck skin flaps
- Valsalva maneuver should be done to rule out chyle leak, which, if detected should be controlled.
- Parotid gland should be underrun to prevent parotid leak

Donor Site Complications

- Tendons should be kept moist during flap harvest to avoid dessication of the paratenon
- If primary closure is under undue tension and skin is blanching excessively on approximation then do not hesitate to put skin graft.
- Hemostasis should be achieved to prevent graft loss
- If the underlying muscle looks nonviable, debridemnt should be done before placing the skin graft.
- Skin graft should be immobilized well.

Chapter 20

Algorithms for Common Defects

Prabha Yadav, Dushyant Jaiswal, Vinay K Shankhdhar, Amrita Rao

Plastic surgery is best described as a problem solving branch. We pride ourselves in offering personalized solutions. This is what makes it surgery such a fascinating and beautiful branch. Though the variable nature of every defect is best served by a customized approach, we are sharing some algorithms we broadly follow.

These algorithms are general guidelines and not absolute commandments. They are protocols which have evolved at Tata Memorial Centre over the years. They are a distillate of experience and wisdom of a lot of bright minds. We have included the algorithms for the most common sites only.

We do believe that many people do a lot of reconstructions differently, which are equally good, if not better. Deviating from these protocols produces better cosmetic and functional results, we as a department will consider the purpose of this book well served.

BUCCAL MUCOSA

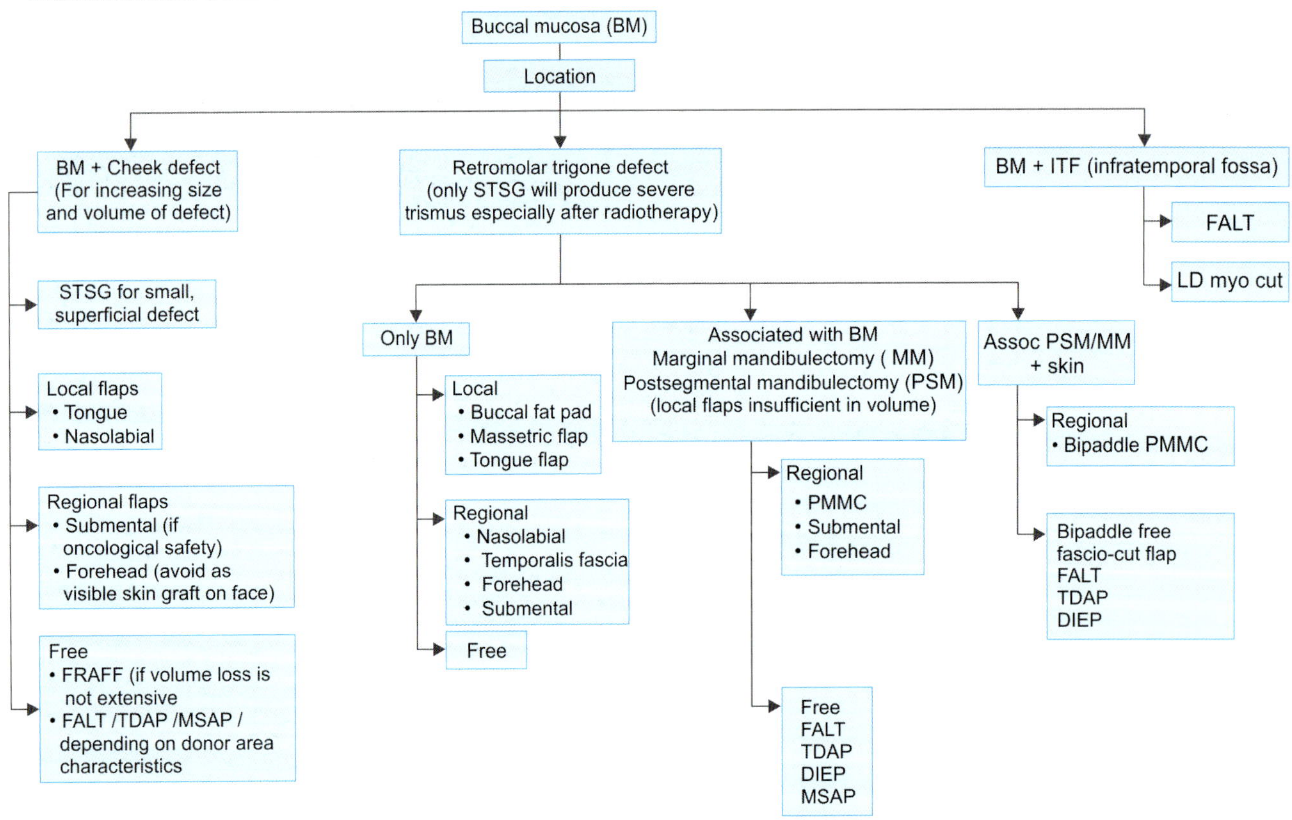

LIP

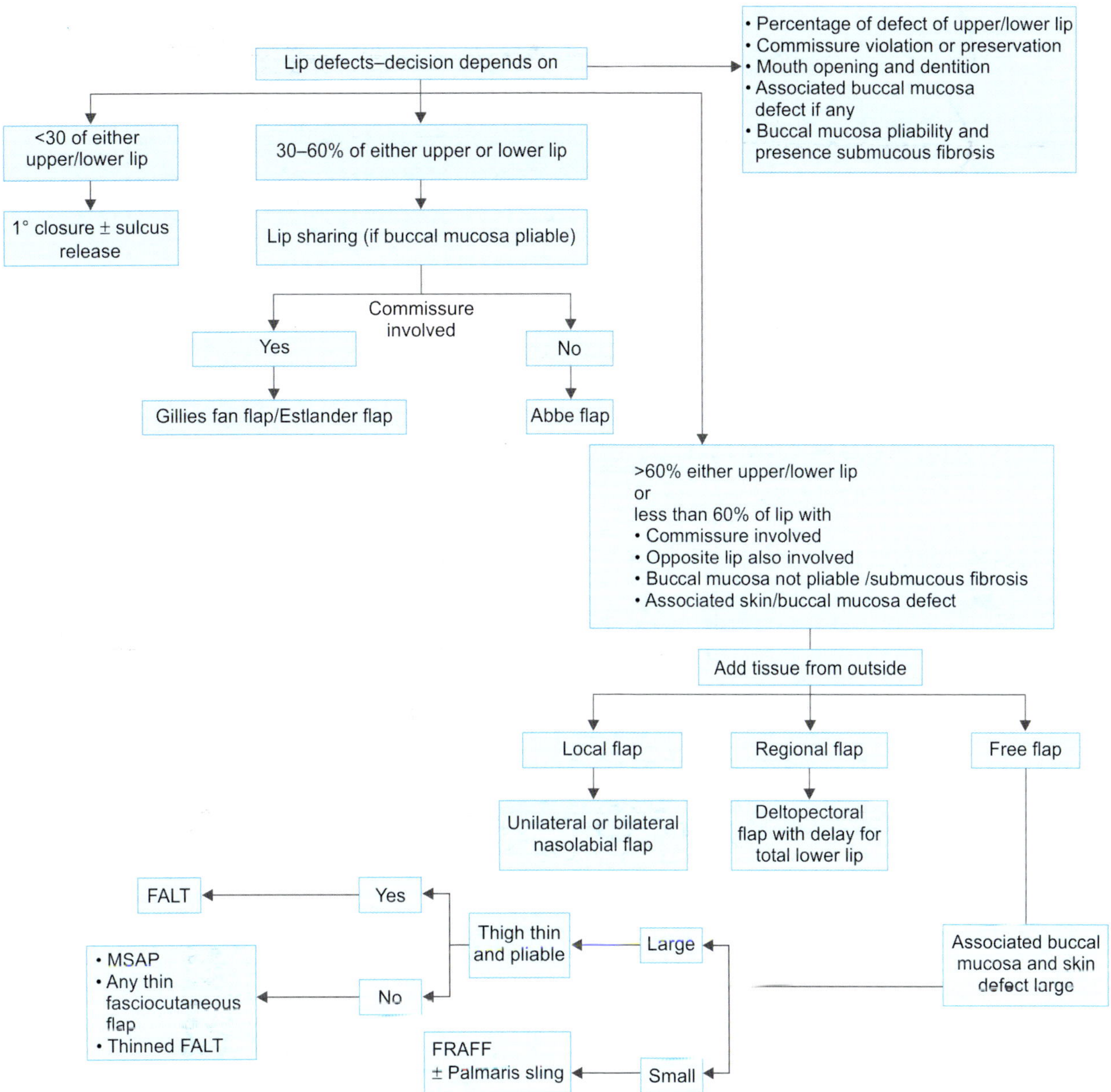
Lip defects–decision depends on
• Percentage of defect of upper/lower lip
• Commissure violation or preservation
• Mouth opening and dentition
• Associated buccal mucosa defect if any
• Buccal mucosa pliability and presence submucous fibrosis
<30 of either upper/lower lip
1° closure ± sulcus release
30–60% of either upper or lower lip
Lip sharing (if buccal mucosa pliable)
Commissure involved
Yes
No
Gillies fan flap/Estlander flap
Abbe flap
>60% either upper/lower lip
or
less than 60% of lip with
• Commissure involved
• Opposite lip also involved
• Buccal mucosa not pliable /submucous fibrosis
• Associated skin/buccal mucosa defect
Add tissue from outside
Local flap
Regional flap
Free flap
Unilateral or bilateral nasolabial flap
Deltopectoral flap with delay for total lower lip
Associated buccal mucosa and skin defect large
Large
Small
Thigh thin and pliable
Yes
No
FALT
• MSAP
• Any thin fasciocutaneous flap
• Thinned FALT
FRAFF
± Palmaris sling

MANDIBLE

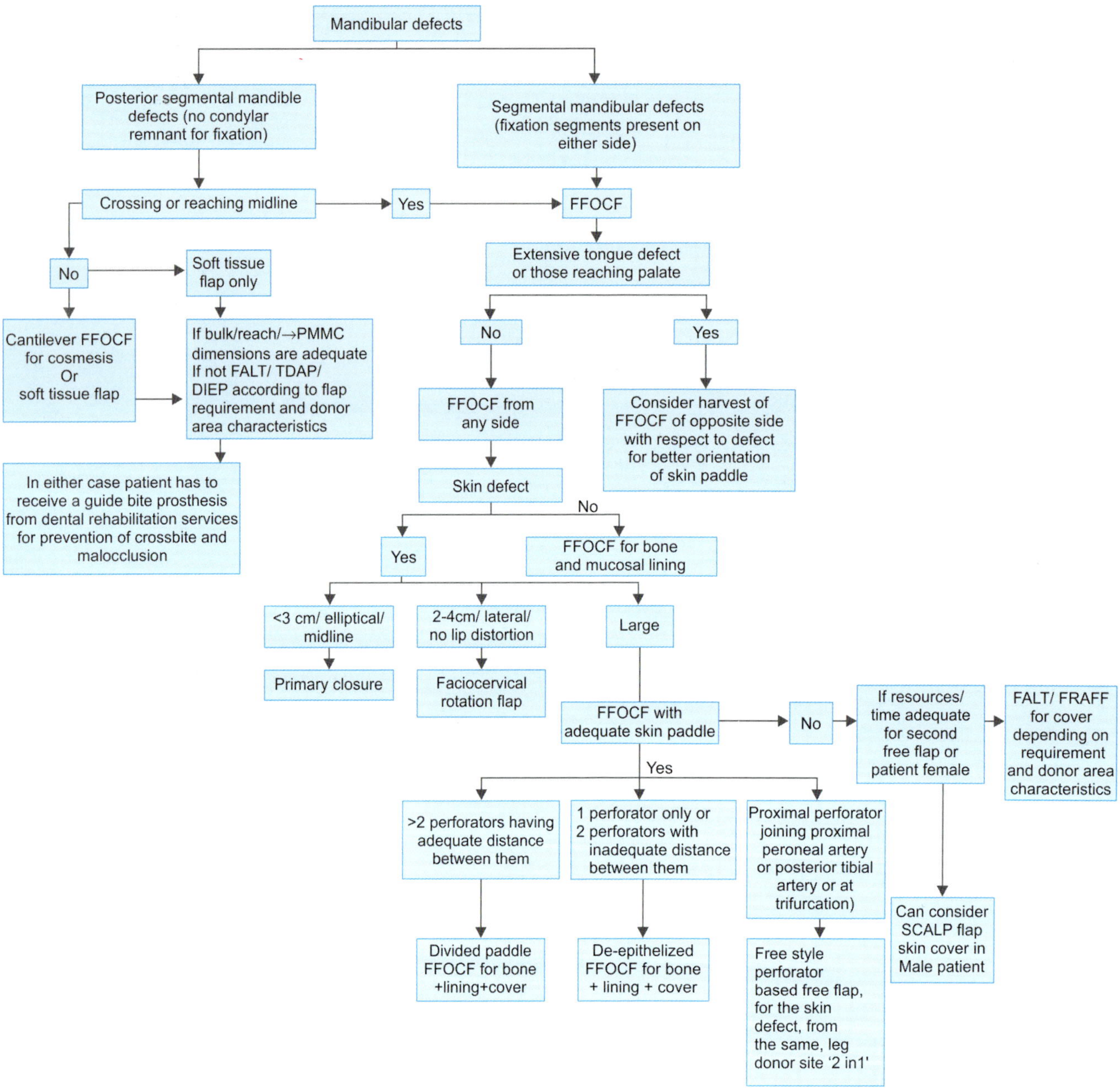
Mandibular defects
Posterior segmental mandible defects (no condylar remnant for fixation)
Segmental mandibular defects (fixation segments present on either side)
Crossing or reaching midline
Yes
FFOCF
No
Soft tissue flap only
Cantilever FFOCF for cosmesis Or soft tissue flap
If bulk/reach/→PMMC dimensions are adequate If not FALT/ TDAP/ DIEP according to flap requirement and donor area characteristics
In either case patient has to receive a guide bite prosthesis from dental rehabilitation services for prevention of crossbite and malocclusion
Extensive tongue defect or those reaching palate
No
Yes
FFOCF from any side
Consider harvest of FFOCF of opposite side with respect to defect for better orientation of skin paddle
Skin defect
No
Yes
FFOCF for bone and mucosal lining
<3 cm/ elliptical/ midline
2-4cm/ lateral/ no lip distortion
Large
Primary closure
Faciocervical rotation flap
FFOCF with adequate skin paddle
No
If resources/ time adequate for second free flap or patient female
FALT/ FRAFF for cover depending on requirement and donor area characteristics
Yes
>2 perforators having adequate distance between them
1 perforator only or 2 perforators with inadequate distance between them
Proximal perforator joining proximal peroneal artery or posterior tibial artery or at trifurcation)
Can consider SCALP flap skin cover in Male patient
Divided paddle FFOCF for bone +lining+cover
De-epithelized FFOCF for bone + lining + cover
Free style perforator based free flap, for the skin defect, from the same, leg donor site '2 in1'

MAXILLA

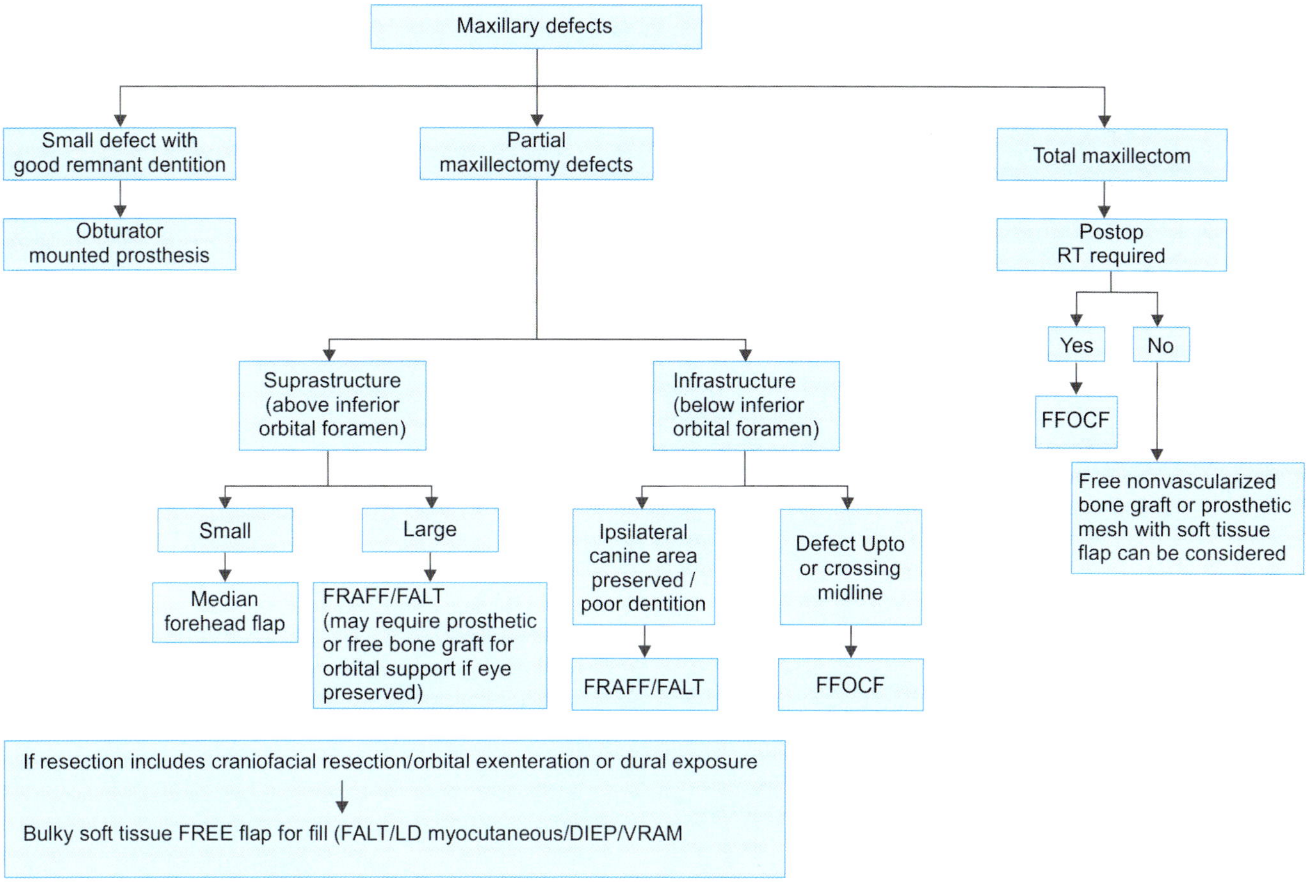
Maxillary defects
Small defect with good remnant dentition
Obturator mounted prosthesis
Partial maxillectomy defects
Suprastructure (above inferior orbital foramen)
Small
Median forehead flap
Large
FRAFF/FALT (may require prosthetic or free bone graft for orbital support if eye preserved)
Infrastructure (below inferior orbital foramen)
Ipsilateral canine area preserved / poor dentition
FRAFF/FALT
Defect Upto or crossing midline
FFOCF
Total maxillectom
Postop RT required
Yes
FFOCF
No
Free nonvascularized bone graft or prosthetic mesh with soft tissue flap can be considered
If resection includes craniofacial resection/orbital exenteration or dural exposure
Bulky soft tissue FREE flap for fill (FALT/LD myocutaneous/DIEP/VRAM

PHARYNX

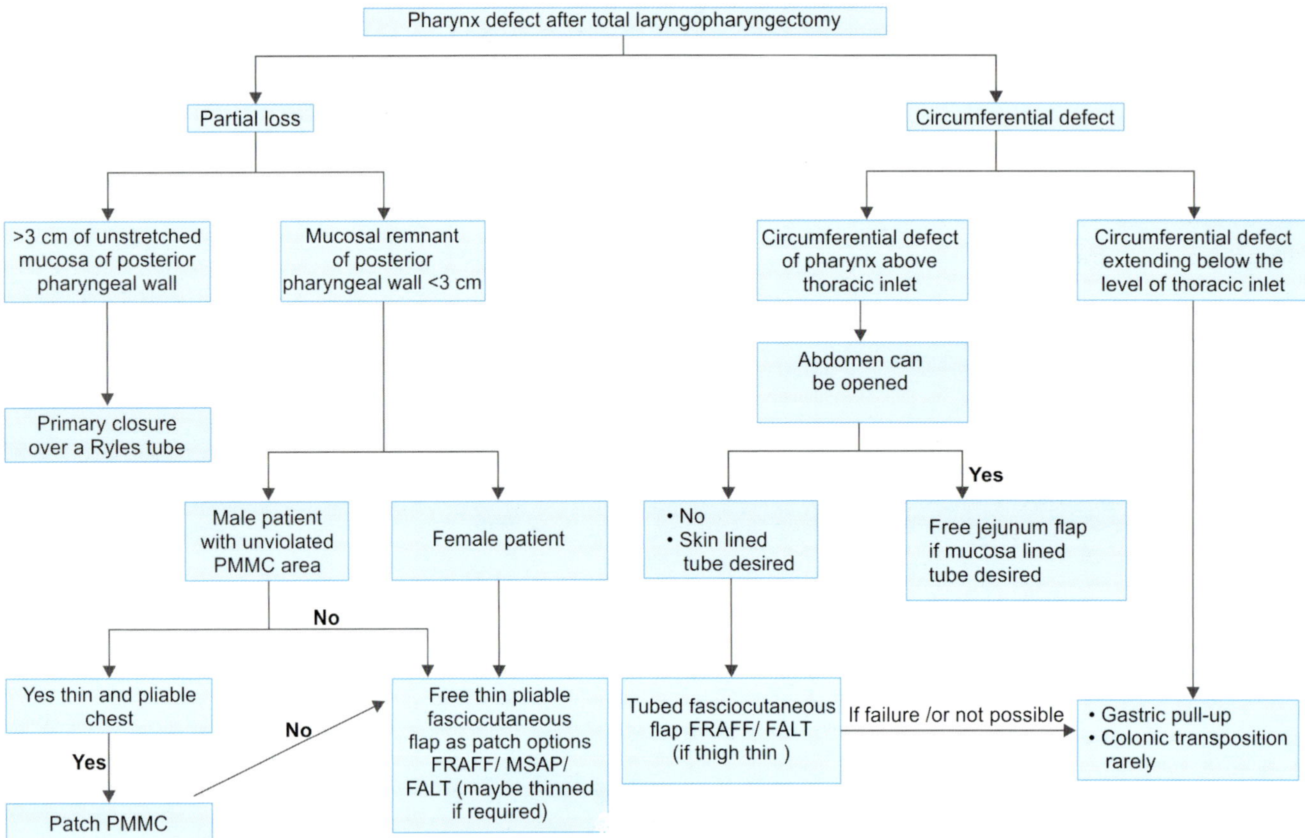

* As per a study done of TMH by head 2 neck DMG no buttressing with PMMF required even in post radiation during primary surgery this may be done to patch a leak if it accours

TONGUE

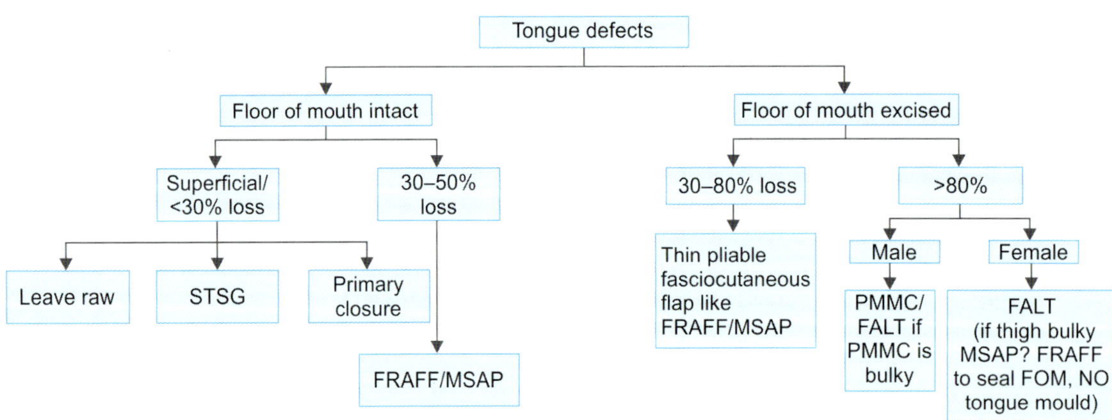

Note
If resection includes segmental mandibulectomy ⟶ FFOCF
If resection includes PSM/Supraglottic laryngectomy ⟶ Soft tissue flap (pedicled or FREE)

REEXPLORATION

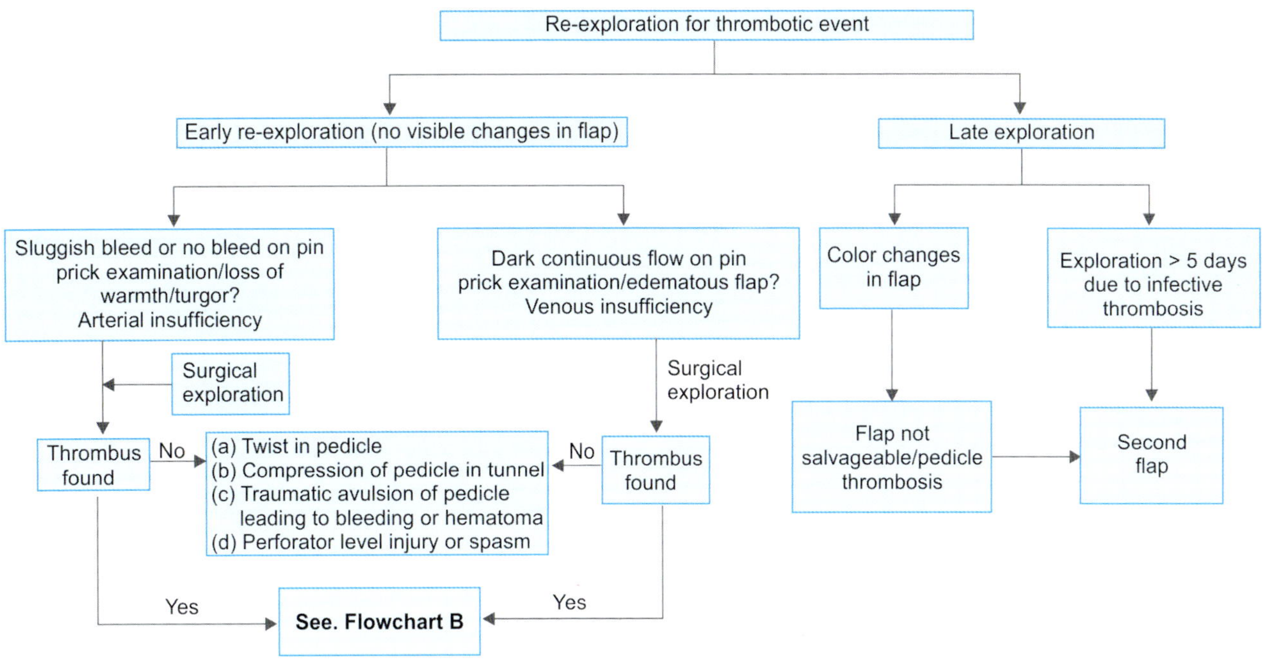

A

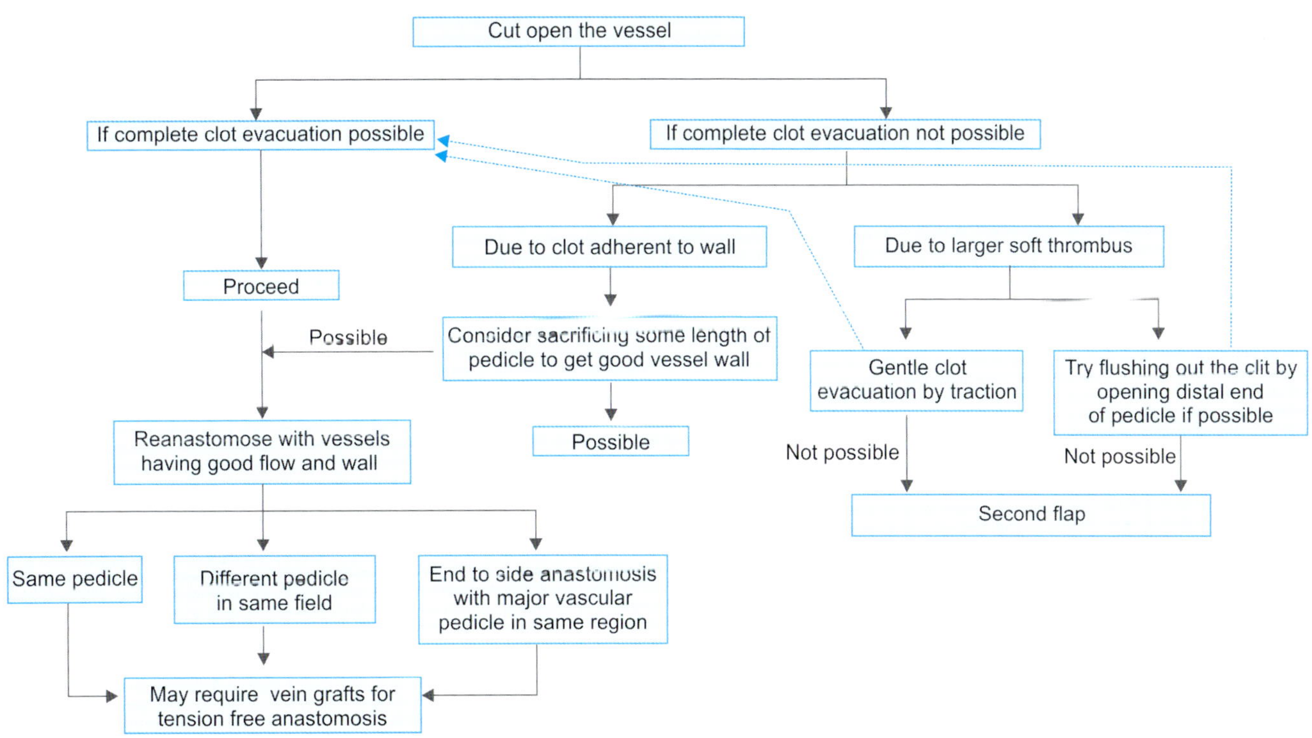

B

SECOND FLAP

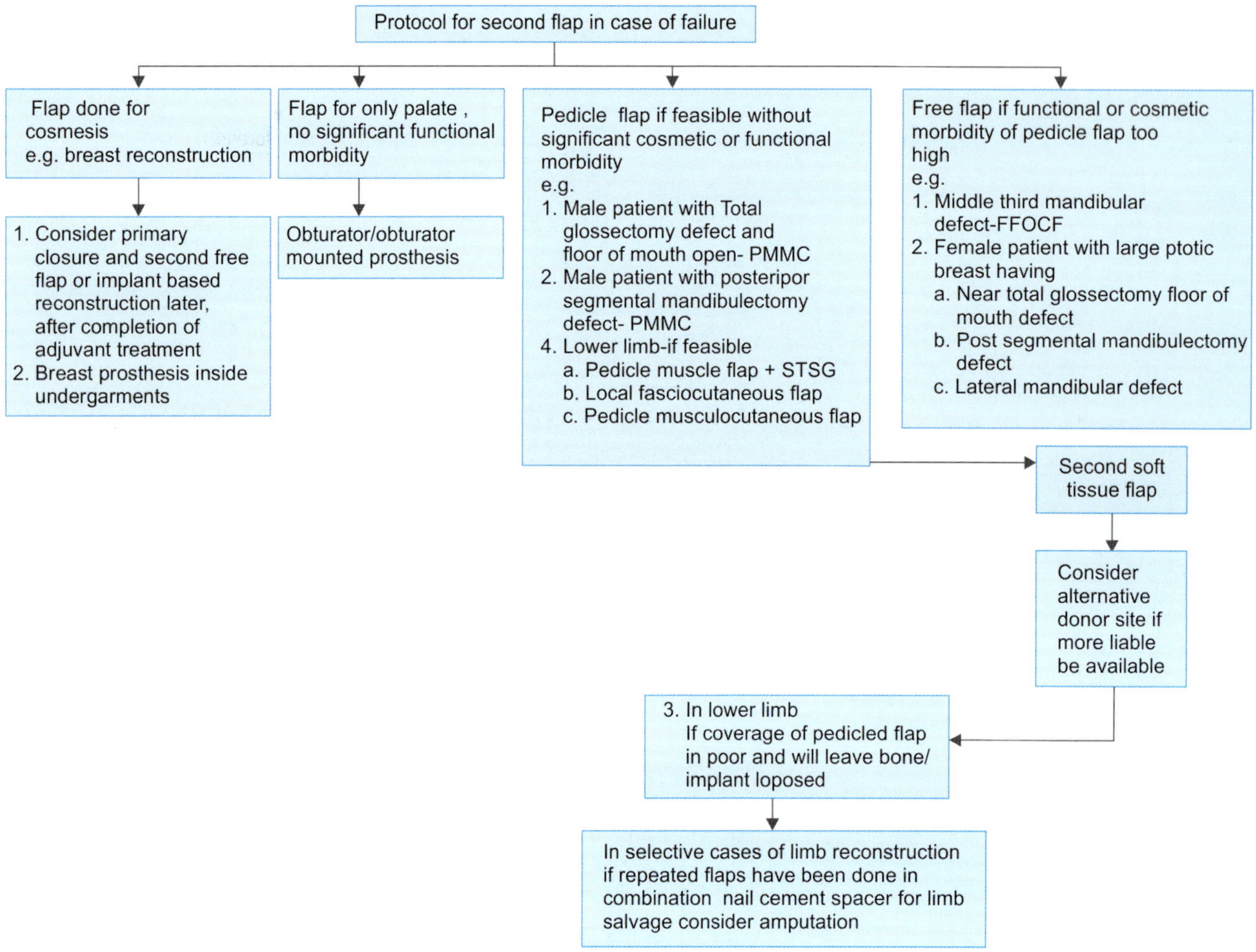
Protocol for second flap in case of failure
Flap done for cosmesis e.g. breast reconstruction
1. Consider primary closure and second free flap or implant based reconstruction later, after completion of adjuvant treatment
2. Breast prosthesis inside undergarments
Flap for only palate , no significant functional morbidity
Obturator/obturator mounted prosthesis
Pedicle flap if feasible without significant cosmetic or functional morbidity
e.g.
1. Male patient with Total glossectomy defect and floor of mouth open- PMMC
2. Male patient with posteripor segmental mandibulectomy defect- PMMC
4. Lower limb-if feasible
a. Pedicle muscle flap + STSG
b. Local fasciocutaneous flap
c. Pedicle musculocutaneous flap
Free flap if functional or cosmetic morbidity of pedicle flap too high
e.g.
1. Middle third mandibular defect-FFOCF
2. Female patient with large ptotic breast having
a. Near total glossectomy floor of mouth defect
b. Post segmental mandibulectomy defect
c. Lateral mandibular defect
Second soft tissue flap
Consider alternative donor site if more liable be available
3. In lower limb
If coverage of pedicled flap in poor and will leave bone/ implant loposed
In selective cases of limb reconstruction if repeated flaps have been done in combination nail cement spacer for limb salvage consider amputation

BREAST

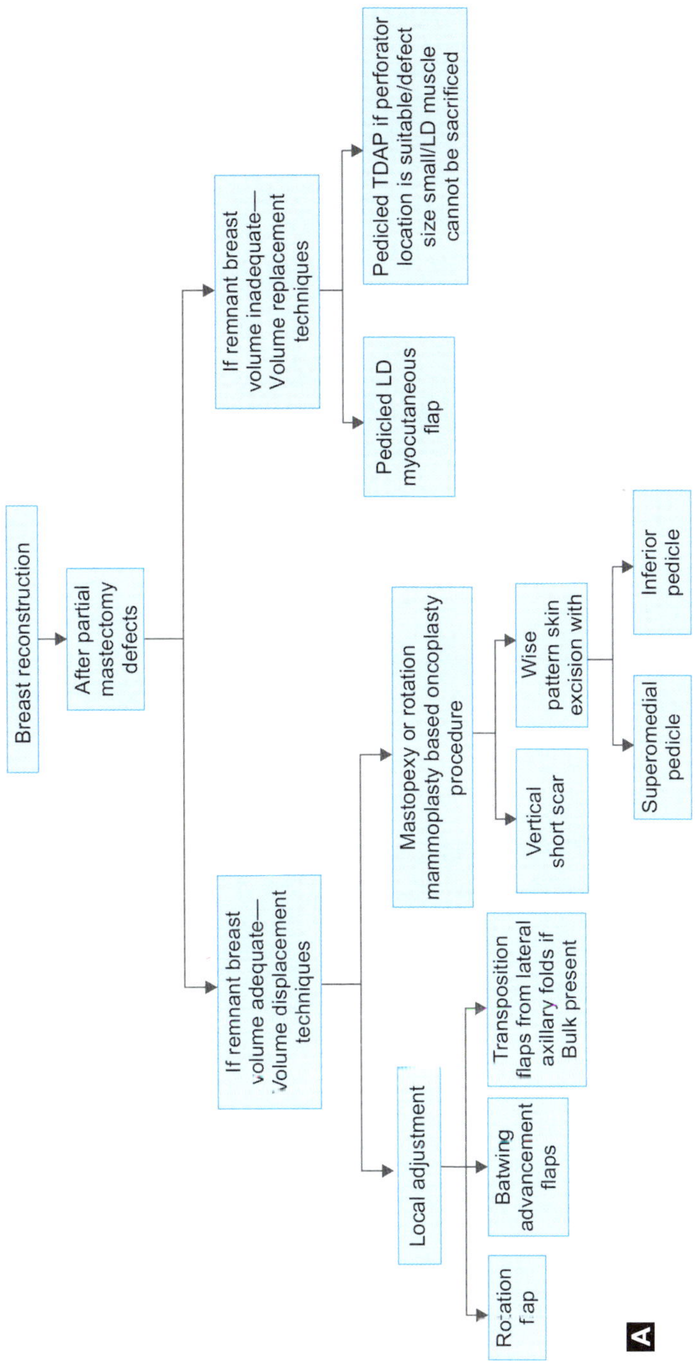
Breast reconstruction
After partial mastectomy defects
If remnant breast volume inadequate—Volume replacement techniques
Pedicled LD myocutaneous flap
Pedicled TDAP if perforator location is suitable/defect size small/LD muscle cannot be sacrificed
If remnant breast volume adequate—Volume displacement techniques
Local adjustment
Rotation flap
Batwing advancement flaps
Transposition flaps from lateral axillary folds if Bulk present
Mastopexy or rotation mammoplasty based oncoplasty procedure
Vertical short scar
Wise pattern skin excision with
Superomedial pedicle
Inferior pedicle
A

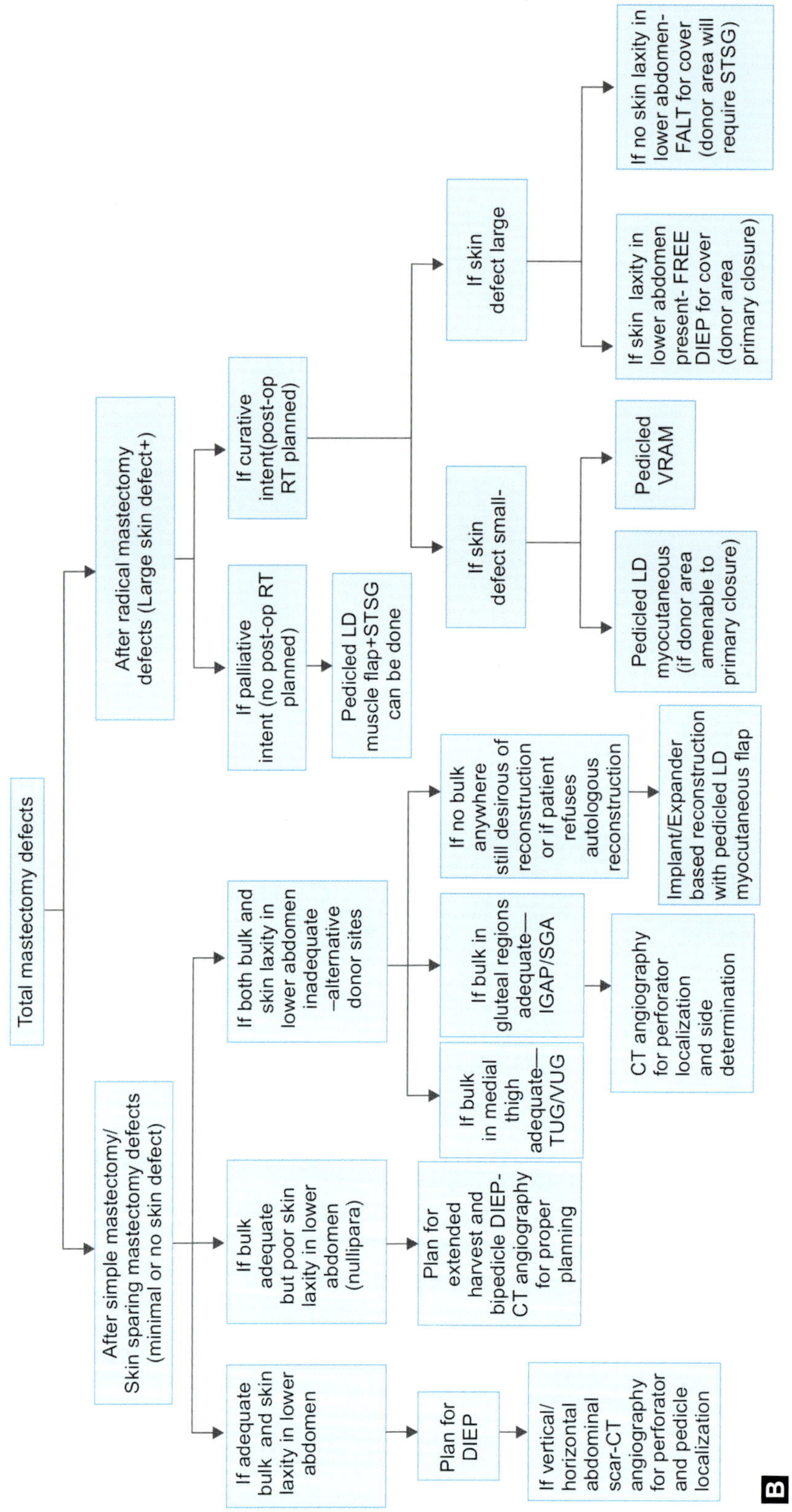
Total mastectomy defects
After simple mastectomy/ Skin sparing mastectomy defects (minimal or no skin defect)
After radical mastectomy defects (Large skin defect+)
If adequate bulk and skin laxity in lower abdomen
Plan for DIEP
If vertical/ horizontal abdominal scar-CT angiography for perforator and pedicle localization
If bulk adequate but poor skin laxity in lower abdomen (nullipara)
Plan for extended harvest and bipedicle DIEP-CT angiography for proper planning
If both bulk and skin laxity in lower abdomen inadequate -alternative donor sites
If bulk in medial thigh adequate—TUG/VUG
If bulk in gluteal regions adequate—IGAP/SGA
CT angiography for perforator localization and side determination
If no bulk anywhere still desirous of reconstruction or if patient refuses autologous reconstruction
Implant/Expander based reconstruction with pedicled LD myocutaneous flap
If palliative intent (no post-op RT planned)
Pedicled LD muscle flap+STSG can be done
If curative intent(post-op RT planned)
If skin defect small-
Pedicled LD myocutaneous (if donor area amenable to primary closure)
Pedicled VRAM
If skin defect large
If skin laxity in lower abdomen present- FREE DIEP for cover (donor area primary closure)
If no skin laxity in lower abdomen- FALT for cover (donor area will require STSG)
B

Index

Page numbers followed by f refer to figure.

A

B

C

D

E

F

M

N

O

P

R

U

V

X